Statistical Models for
Longitudinal Studies of Health

Monographs in Epidemiology and Biostatistics
Edited by Jennifer L. Kelsey, Michael G. Marmot, Paul D. Stolley, Martin P. Vessey

MONOGRAPHS IN EPIDEMIOLOGY AND BIOSTATISTICS   VOLUME 16

Statistical Models for Longitudinal Studies of Health

Edited by

James H. Dwyer, PH.D.
Manning Feinleib, M.D., DR. P.H.
Peter Lippert, M.D.
Hans Hoffmeister, PH.D.

New York   Oxford
OXFORD UNIVERSITY PRESS
1992

Oxford University Press

Oxford   New York · Toronto
Delhi   Bombay   Calcutta   Madras   Karachi
Petaling Jaya   Singapore   Hong Kong   Tokyo
Nairobi   Dar es Salaam   Cape Town
Melbourne   Auckland

and associated companies in
Berlin   Ibadan

Published by Oxford University Press, Inc.,
200 Madison Avenue, New York, New York 10016

Oxford is a registered trademark of Oxford University Press

Library of Congress Cataloging-in-Publication Data
Statistical models for longitudinal studies of health
edited by
James H. Dwyer ... [et al.].
p.   cm.—(Monographs in epidemiology and biostatistics; v. 16)
Consists mostly of papers from the Workshop on the Analysis
of Longitudinal Data, held in Berlin in June of 1987, sponsored
by the Institute for Epidemiology in Berlin and others.
Includes bibliographical references and index.
ISBN 0-19-505473-3
1. Epidemiology—Longitudinal studies—Statistical methods—Congresses.
I. Dwyer, James H., 1946–xxxx.   II. Institute
for Epidemiology (Berlin, Germany).   III. Workshop on the Analysis
of Longitudinal Data (1987: Berlin, Germany).   IV. Series.
[DNLM: 1. Epidemiology—congresses.   2. Health—congresses.
3. Longitudinal Studies—congresses.   4. Models, Statistical—congresses.
W1 MO567LT v. 16 / W 900.1 S797 1987]   RA652.2.M3S73   1991
614.4′2′072—dc20   DNLM/DLC   90-14332

9 8 7 6 5 4 3 2 1

Printed in the United States of America
on acid-free paper

Preface

The fundamental goal of epidemiology and related fields is the promotion of health and the prevention of disease.

Epidemiology and many related fields involved in the study of human health are thus concerned with change in health status (change from healthy to diseased, change from alive to dead, change from low risk to high risk) and change in those factors that may influence health status. Relative to cross-sectional studies, then, the attraction of longitudinal studies is the opportunity they afford to actually observe change in both determinants and outcomes within individuals—rather than infer it from differences among individuals. However, this attractiveness is to some extent counterbalanced by myriad problems that confront the researcher who chooses to conduct longitudinal studies.

One category of such problems is statistical analysis. Many of these problems were recognized by the researchers who carried out the Berlin–Bremen Study, an investigation of cardiovascular risk factors in the German cities of Berlin and Bremen. This longitudinal study of adolescents was sponsored by the Institute for Epidemiology in Berlin, the German Ministry for Research and Technology, and the Ministry of Health for the state of Bremen, and was directed by Drs. Peter Lippert and Norbert Semmer. Coincidentally, the National Center for Health Statistics in the United States was planning longitudinal studies and was eager to consolidate current knowledge about the interpretation of these data. This international consortium thus sponsored the Workshop on the Analysis of Longitudinal Data, which was held in Berlin in June 1987. The goal was to bring together a group of accomplished statisticians from different fields that conduct longitudinal studies in order to review the state-of-the-art in this area. We aimed to achieve some common understanding (and some consensus) concerning the fundamental statistical issues that confront longitudinal researchers in epidemiology and the social sciences. Jargon specific to disciplines often masks important commonalities across approaches, and this leads to unnecessary delays while techniques are reinvented.

Virtually all the participants in the workshop have indicated that they were introduced to important new ideas from the exchange between disciplines, and it is our hope that this volume will achieve that goal for a much wider audience. Most of the chapters included in this volume are derived from papers presented at the workshop.

Finally, many persons have contributed to the production of this volume, and we would like to thank a few of them here: Diane Rehfeld, Martha Petrov, Vasiliki Leventakou, three anonymous reviewers, and the patient guidance of Jeffrey House.

Alhambra, Calif.	J.H.D.
Hyattsville, Md.	M.F.
Hamburg	P.L.
Berlin	H.H.
October 1990	

Contents

Part II Models for Categorical Data

Part III Special Problems in the Modeling
of Longitudinal Observations

Part IV Future Directions

Contributors

Gerhard Arminger
Professor of Statistics
Department of Economics
Bergische Universität Wuppertal
Wuppertal, Germany

Peter M. Bentler
Professor of Psychology
University of California
Los Angeles, California

Norman E. Breslow
Professor and Chairman
Department of Biostatistics
School of Public Health and
  Community Medicine
University of Washington
Seattle, Washington

William Clarke
Associate Professor of Biostatistics
Department of Preventive Medicine
University of Iowa
College of Medicine
Iowa City, Iowa

David G. Clayton
Senior Lecturer
Medical Statistics
Cambridge University
Cambridge, England

Lester Curtin
Chief
Statistical Methods Staff
National Center for Health Statistics
Hyattsville, Maryland

James H. Dwyer
Associate Professor
Institute for Prevention Research
Department of Preventive Medicine
University of Southern California
School of Medicine
Alhambra, California

Manning Feinleib
Director
National Center for Health Statistics
Hyattsville, Maryland

Hans Hoffmeister
Professor
Institute for Epidemiology
Federal Health Office
Berlin, Germany

John M. Kaldor
Biostatistician
National Centre in HIV
  Epidemiology and Clinical
  Research
Faculty of Medicine
University of New South Wales
Sydney, Australia

Gary G. Koch
Professor
Department of Statistics
University of North Carolina
School of Public Health
Chapel Hill, North Carolina

Ulrich L. Küsters
Assistant Professor of Statistics
Department of Economics
Bergische Universität Wuppertal
Wuppertal, Germany

James D. Leeper
Associate Professor
University of Alabama
College of Community Health
  Sciences
Tuscaloosa, Alabama

Kung-Yee Liang
Associate Professor
Department of Biostatistics
Johns Hopkins University
School of Hygiene and Public Health
Baltimore, Maryland

Peter Lippert
Vice Minister of Health
Hamburg Ministry of Health
Hamburg, Germany

Lawrence Moulton
Assistant Professor
Department of Biostatistics
University of Michigan
School of Public Health
Ann Arbor, Michigan

Alvaro Muñoz
Associate Professor
Department of Epidemiology
Johns Hopkins University
School of Hygiene and Public Health
Baltimore, Maryland

Michael D. Newcomb
Associate Professor
Program in Counseling
Department of Education
University of Southern California
Los Angeles, California

Joan L. Pinsky
Health Statistician
National Heart, Lung and Blood
  Institute
Bethesda, Maryland

Bernard Rosner
Associate Professor
Preventive Medicine
Harvard Medical School
Boston, Massachusetts

Julio M. Singer
Associate Professor
Departamento de Estatistica
Universidade de São Paulo
São Paulo, Brazil

Maura E. Stokes
Manager
Statistical Testing and Application
SAS Institute, Inc.
Cary, North Carolina

Duncan C. Thomas
Associate Professor
Department of Preventive Medicine
University of Southern California
Los Angeles, California

James Ware
Professor of Psychiatry
Department of Biostatistics
Harvard Medical School
Boston, Massachusetts

Christine Waternaux
Professor of Psychiatry and Lecturer
Department of Biostatistics
Harvard Medical School
Boston, Massachusetts

Robert Woolson
Professor
Department of Preventive Medicine
University of Iowa
College of Medicine
Iowa City, Iowa

Scott Zeger
Associate Professor
Department of Biostatistics
Johns Hopkins University
School of Hygiene and Public Health
Baltimore, Maryland

Statistical Models for
Longitudinal Studies of Health

1

Introduction to Statistical Models for Longitudinal Observation

JAMES DWYER AND MANNING FEINLEIB

Longitudinal studies are both attractive and problematic. Compared with cross-sectional data, the attractiveness of longitudinal data derives from the richer set of analytic questions that can be addressed. Longitudinal studies also circumvent some potential sources of bias due to selection, heterogeneity, directionality, and confounding. The problems that are peculiar to longitudinal data are of three types: statistical, logistical, and theoretical. The major statistical problem is that repeated observations on the same individual are not independent of one another. The logistical problem is that some persons are usually lost to follow-up which raises a source of bias (attrition) specific to longitudinal observation. The theoretical problem is one of selecting an appropriate model from the large number of alternative models that can be assumed when analyzing and interpreting change through time. These alternative models can yield different substantive conclusions, and care must be exercised in selecting which model or class of models is most appropriate. The chapters that make up this volume present a range of statistical models that can be applied to longitudinal data.

The main purpose of this introduction is to provide a typology of alternative statistical models that can be applied to data from longitudinal studies. This should be generally useful and also helpful for understanding the more specialized discussions in the subsequent chapters. Emphasis is placed on how different types of models address potential sources of bias and on the implicit assumptions that each estimable discrete-time model makes about the continuous-time process that generates the observed data. The central section is preceded by brief discussions of nomenclature, reasons for conducting longitudinal studies, and special problems that arise in them. This chapter builds on previous reviews from mathematics (Karlin & Taylor, 1981) and biostatistics (*Biometrics*, 1988, Vol. 44, No. 4; Cook & Ware, 1983; Goldstein, 1979; Grizzle & Allen, 1969; Jöreskog, 1970a; Koch, Amara, Stokes, & Gillings, 1980; Ware, 1985; Wu & Kusek, 1988) as well as from such other fields as psychology

(Nesselroade & Baltes, 1979; Jöreskog, 1970b), economics (Heckman, 1981; Hsaio, 1986), and sociology (Duncan & Kalton, 1987; Plewis, 1985).

TYPES OF LONGITUDINAL STUDIES

The definining characteristic of a longitudinal study *design* is that a sample of persons, or other units, is observed prospectively through time (is "tracked"). Longitudinal *data*, on the other hand, may be collected retrospectively (Duncan & Kalton, 1987). For example, a study of coronary heart disease (CHD) employing a longitudinal design would define a sample at baseline and follow the individuals to observe risk factors and morbidity through time. However, longitudinal CHD data could be obtained retrospectively by reviewing health records or by asking persons to recall past events. Retrospective data are likely to involve recall errors and to suffer from selection bias. Health records in countries with national record systems that cover most of the population, however, may yield retrospective data that are of comparable quality with prospectively collected data when variables are measured with time-invariant procedures.

Prospective longitudinal studies have been referred to in the biomedical literature as *cohort studies* or *follow-up studies* to distinguish them from retrospective *case-control studies*. Survey statisticians have tended to use the term *panel* to delineate prospective longitudinal studies. Because "cohort" is also used to refer to birth cohorts (persons born in a particular calendar year), it is probably less confusing to use "panel" to refer to the sample of persons followed in a longitudinal study. Thus a longitudinal study can follow a panel from a single birth cohort (persons born in New York in 1945) or from multiple birth cohorts (persons born in New York in 1945, 1950, and 1955). More often, however, the panel is determined by region of residence (or school attended, place of work, or some other characteristic) and year of birth at baseline observation. This type of panel is representative of a *dynamic population* that includes leavers and stayers from numerous geographically defined birth cohorts. A dynamic population of children in a school district might consist of those children in the first grade in 1970, those in the second grade in 1971, and so on. This dynamic population is distinct from a panel of children identified in the first grade in 1970 who are subsequently followed—wherever they may move— and to which no new entrants are allowed.

In the context of survey research, Duncan and Kalton (1987) have proposed the distinction among four types of longitudinal study measurement designs: panel survey, repeated survey, rotating panel survey, and split panel survey. The *repeated survey* (or repeated cross-sectional survey) involves repeated sampling and observation from a consistently defined population (e.g., geographic region and age range). Different persons are sampled at each time point as a population moves through time. The repeated survey is a series of independent cross-sectional surveys. Repeated surveys may be refined to follow a dynamic population defined by birth cohort and current geographic location. An example would be surveys of 20-year-olds living in California in 1970, 25-year-olds living there in 1975, and so on.

The *rotating panel* involves replacing some members of the panel with new persons at specified time intervals. This strategy may be necessary when effects of repeated measurement are expected or measurement places considerable burden on the respondent. Finally, the *split panel* is a combination of a panel and a repeated survey. This strategy allows measurement of the change both in a dynamic population and in individuals. Advantages of alternative designs are discussed further in Chapter 2.

Longitudinal studies can also be classified as observational or experimental. Experimental studies involve a manipulated intervention, such as the clinical trial. Experiments may be randomized (e.g., random assignment to treatment or control conditions) or nonrandomized. Nonrandomized studies are sometimes called *quasi-experiments* (Cochran & Rubin, 1973; Cook & Campbell, 1979). Longitudinal observations are useful in randomized experiments because they allow verification that randomization has produced equivalent groups at baseline and because the course of response to treatment (actual change) can be tracked. However, longitudinal observation is even more important in nonrandomized studies, since a series of pretreatment observations can be used to determine the trajectory of the two treatment groups prior to the intervention. Assurance that the two treatment groups not only are at the same level at baseline but also have been following the same time path reduces the plausibility of pretreatment nonequivalence as an alternative explanation of posttreatment differences. If initial trajectories do differ between groups, this difference can be incorporated into the estimate of intervention effect (Dwyer, 1984).

Our primary concern in this volume is with observational (i.e., nonexperimental) panel surveys. It is in observational studies and nonrandomized clinical trials that the form of the statistical model is of particular importance.

REASONS FOR CONDUCTING LONGITUDINAL STUDIES

Study of Age- and Time-Related Variables

The most obvious reason for conducting longitudinal studies in the biomedical sciences is the investigation of change over time and its determinants. An important example of change over time is growth. Cross-sectional surveys relating body height or weight to time-related variables such as age, bone age, or stages of sexual maturation are subject to several biases in the shape of the resulting growth curves. One is that persons may be heterogeneous with regard to the shape of the curve: there may be subgroups of children with distinctly different growth curves. A second is that there may be differences in growth curves between birth cohorts. These could arise from differences in nutrition, health care, and so on. Longitudinal observation of several birth cohorts, on the other hand, allows measurement of individual differences in growth patterns (and their relation to other variables) as well as of cohort differences (Goldstein, 1979).

The impact of aging on level of functioning provides another example. Cross-sectional studies may suggest that various mental and physiologic functions deteriorate with age. However, longitudinal studies may find heterogeneity: that there is a subset of persons who do not suffer declines of certain functions as they age. The cross-sectional findings may have been due to increased morbidity of cohorts of more advanced age. In the absence of longitudinal observation, attribution of age trends to aging *per se* is more dubious.

Many variables are defined in terms of change with time. Labile hypertension could, for example, be defined in terms of both the level and the variance of blood pressure over time. Similarly, the variability of individual body weight within adults over time has been identified as a possible risk factor for CHD. Clearly, the study of such variables provides strong motivation for the collection of longitudinal data.

The shift in emphasis in epidemiology from infectious to chronic diseases, such as heart disease and cancer, focuses research attention on progressive disease processes that can occur over much of the life span. Many of the factors increasing the risk of these diseases cannot be characterized as an event bounded by a few days or months. Rather, many are environmental or psychosocial patterns that contribute to the progression of the disease over years or decades.

Temporal Sequence

An important prerequisite for interpretation of an association as due to a causal effect is that change in the hypothesized cause precedes (in time) change in the effect. Information about the temporal sequence of events in longitudinal observational studies can be very useful in this regard. For example, the clinical finding of elevated serum cholesterol level in patients with CHD could be explained by a biologic model in which the disease gives rise to the elevated cholesterol level. However, a longitudinal study in which the elevation is found to be *predictive* of subsequent development of CHD reduces the plausibility of the "reverse causation" explanation.

When attempting to sort out such "directionality" questions it is useful to distinguish among several research situations based on characteristics of the hypothesized cause-and-effect variables at baseline:

1. No variation across individuals in the dependent variable at baseline (e.g., effect of smoking on risk of CHD, starting with youthful population free of disease; effect of beliefs about smoking on risk of becoming a smoker, starting with nonsmoking children; effect of dietary fiber on risk of colon cancer, starting with youthful population free of disease)
2. No variation in the causal variable at baseline (e.g., effect of smoking on high-density lipoprotein cholesterol, starting with children who are nonsmokers at baseline)
3. Variation in *neither* variable at baseline (follow children until some become smokers and cardiovascular morbidity occurs)
4. Variation in *both* variables at baseline (relative body weight and blood pressure)

Longitudinal observation is particularly useful in sorting out temporal sequence in the first three of these circumstances. However, the fourth presents some difficulties. When both the hypothesized *cause* and the hypothesized *effect* variables vary across persons at baseline, the two variables may equilibrate such that identification of a temporal sequence of changes in annual or biannual observations is difficult.

It is important to bear in mind that clues about causal directionality gleaned from longitudinal studies do not resolve problems of confounding or spuriousness. That is, an unknown or unmeasured variable could be causing both the elevated serum cholesterol and the development of CHD. Also it is possible that manifestations of the hypothesized response actually preceded the hypothesized cause, even when longitudinal observation suggests the opposite. This could arise when early manifestations of the hypothesized response (e.g., disease) are not detectable. Thus the presumption of no variance in disease in a "disease-free" population is always subject to error. An example is the finding that level of serum cholesterol is predictive of subsequent increased risk for neoplastic disease. It is quite plausible that asymptomatic malignancies could alter cholesterol metabolism for many years prior to diagnosis.

Filtering of Unmeasured Confounders

One of the most powerful advantages of longitudinal observation is that change scores remove the effects of confounders that do not change over time. For example, suppose that a positive cross-sectional association is observed between level of serum calcium and blood pressure. Among the numerous plausible explanations of this finding are those involving genetic and social-class factors that confound the observed relationship. However, now suppose that six-month change in serum calcium level is found to be associated with change in blood pressure. This finding would exclude time-invariant factors with time-invariant effects as a plausible source of confounding—even though such factors were not measured. There are, of course, a host of (unmeasured) *time-varying factors* that remain as plausible confounders. The conclusion that a factor has been filtered by change scores relies on the assumption, rather than the observation, of the temporal dynamics of the unmeasured variable.

The filtering of unmeasured time-invariant confounders can lead to a striking contrast between cross-sectional associations and longitudinal associations between change scores. For example, reported level of dietary calories from saturated fats tends to show little correlation with serum cholesterol level in cross-sectional surveys of humans. However, change scores in these two variables generally yield positive associations. This result may be due to the filtering of confounders that bias the cross-sectional correlations.

Heterogeneity

Models estimated with cross-sectional data must include the assumption that the model is invariant across unmeasured individual differences in persons. For example, suppose that the random variables y and x are presumed to relate linearly:

$$y_i = \alpha + \beta x_i + \zeta_i$$

where i indicates the ith member of a population, α and β are constant parameters, and ζ is a random disturbance. To estimate α and β, additional assumptions are necessary. One is that α and β are identical across all persons in the population; another is that $E(\zeta_i) = \mu_\zeta$ is identical for all i. For some pairs of variables y and x these assumptions may be plausible. For many variables, however, we might expect some heterogeneity in α (or μ_ζ), β, or $\sigma_{\zeta\zeta} = E[(\zeta_i - \mu_\zeta)^2]$ across persons; it may also be plausible that some of these parameters change over time.

Now suppose that y and x are observed at several points in time ($t = 1$, $2, \ldots, T$). Heterogeneity across persons can then be incorporated by specifying the model as

$$y_{it} = \alpha_i + \beta_i x_{it} + \zeta_{it}$$

where α_i and β_i vary across persons. The individual parameters β_i may then serve as variables in a "second stage" equation model. Similarly, heterogeneity across time can be incorporated:

$$y_{it} = \alpha_t + \beta_t x_{it} + \zeta_{it}$$

where α_t, β_t, and var(ζ_{it}) may change with time. Finally, the specification

$$y_{it} = \alpha + \beta x_{it} + \eta_i + \zeta_{it}^*$$

where $\zeta_{it} = \eta_i + \zeta_{it}^*$ allows $E(\zeta_{it})$ to vary across persons. This specification is of particular prominence in the analysis of longitudinal data (it is known as either the *random-* or the *fixed-* effects model, depending on how η_i is defined). It is also a special case of how longitudinal data can be used to "filter" unmeasured variables (η_i) from the observed variables.

It is important to distinguish between heterogeneity and *state dependence*. For example, suppose that the prevalence of flu infection is 15 percent in repeated cross-sectional surveys. This may arise because all persons are at 15 percent risk of flu (homogeneity), or because some subset of susceptible persons are at even greater risk (heterogeneity). The presence or absence of heterogeneity in susceptibility can then be addressed with longitudinal observation by assessing the dependence of current flu status on past flu status. A finding of such dependence suggests heterogeneity of susceptibility. However, "true" state dependence may also be operating: Homogeneity of susceptibility applies initially, but the incidence of infection alters subsequent susceptibility.

Longitudinal data can also be used to study the determinants of state dependence, if it is found. Suppose that positive flu status at t_1 ($f_1 = 1$) is related to the risk of flu at t_2 (f_2). Then if π_2 (probability $f_2 = 1$) is positively related to f_1, is this because flu infection increases susceptibility to subsequent flu infection, or is it because the characteristics of the person or the environment that make the person susceptible are stable over time (or both)? These two possibilities may be referred to as *true state dependence and spurious state dependence*, respectively. True state dependence can be differentiated from spurious state dependence with longitudinal data in a manner analogous to that discussed for the random-effects model (but with a model adapted to categorical variables).

Estimation of Dynamic Models

Longitudinal data also provide the opportunity to estimate equation systems that model the rate of adjustment of change in an effect variable to change in a causal variable. For example, imagine an experiment in which a person with a steady body weight increases calorie intake by a constant amount without increasing the level of physical activity. Daily measurement of body weight after the increase in calorie intake begins would reveal an adjustment curve that eventually levels off at a new equilibrium body weight.

Dynamic models fit to longitudinal data can yield similar information, except that the shape of the adjustment curve must be constrained by assumption. These continuous-time dynamic models provide a link between the discrete-time observations of panel studies and the continuous-time models in which researchers theorize about the processes underlying their data. These models necessarily involve more assumptions and are therefore more speculative; however, they have the virtue of shedding light on the temporal sequence of changes in variables.

Selection Bias

Often persons above or below a certain threshold of the dependent variable are not included in a sample. This exclusion produces selection bias in estimated regression slopes. For example, suppose that persons with systolic blood pressure (SBP) above a certain level are less likely to be included in a community sample because of increased mortality and morbidity. If the goal of the study is to estimate the relationship between SBP and relative body weight (RW), regression of SBP on RW for members of such a sample will yield an attenuated estimate: RW will be associated with the residual in the regression model, and the usual ordinary least squares assumption of independence yields a biased estimate. However, longitudinal data provide the opportunity to estimate this association (between RW and the residual) and to obtain an unbiased estimate of the SBP–RW relation.

Modeling Group Nonequivalencies in Quasi-experiments

Often units cannot be assigned to experimental conditions according to a randomization scheme. A longitudinal measurement design may then be used to assess baseline (pretreatment) differences between intervention and control groups. If baseline nonequivalence is found, a statistical model is used to adjust the estimate of intervention effect for baseline differences.

Most such designs involve a single baseline measure. In this circumstance it is necessary to make a strong assumption about the fate of a baseline group nonequivalence in the outcome variable y in the absence of an intervention effect. Two common assumptions are that the baseline difference will remain over time (unconditional model) and that the difference will regress over time (conditional model). These two models (cf. Dwyer et al., 1989) may be specified as

$$y_{i1} = \beta_0 + \beta_1 y_{i0} + \beta_2 x_i + \zeta_i$$

where x is a dichotomous dummy variable indicating experimental condition (treatment or control); the constraints that $E(\zeta) = \sigma_{x\zeta} = \sigma_{y_0\zeta} = 0$ specify the conditional version of the model; and the constraints $\beta_1 = 1$, $E(\zeta) = \sigma_{x\zeta} = 0$ specify the unconditional version. The unconditional model may also be specified as a multiple equation regression; this is especially useful when more than two waves of observation are being analyzed.

The unconditional model is a "change score" $(y_{i2} - y_{i1})$ model; the conditional model is the classic analysis of covariance model (Cochran & Cox, 1957). Each provides the same point estimate of the intervention effect if study groups are equivalent on y at baseline. They differ in their definition of β_2 only when $\sigma_{y_0x} \neq 0$:

$$\beta_2 = (\mu_{y_1|x=1} - \mu_{y_1|x=0}) - \beta_1(\mu_{y_0|x=1} - \mu_{y_0|x=0})$$

where $\beta_1 = 1$ in the unconditional case and β_1 is the within-group regression of y_1 on y_0 in the conditional case. The conditional model is appropriate when units of analysis were randomized to conditions and baseline nonequivalence is entirely due to sampling variation; the unconditional model is appropriate when variables omitted from the model operate as η in the following model:

$$y_{i0} = \alpha_0 + \alpha_1 x_i + \eta_i + \zeta_{i0}$$

$$y_{i1} = \gamma_0 + \gamma_1 x_i + \eta_i + \zeta_{i1}$$

where ζ is uncorrelated with x and η, but η may be correlated with x. Note that the confounders represented by η are time invariant and thus are filtered by difference scores in y $(y_{i1} - y_{i0})$.

The major limitation of these models is that they only assess baseline nonequivalence in level of the dependent (and other covariate) variable. What is also of interest in quasi-experiments is the time trajectory of the dependent variable within each group. The obvious approach to determining the time course that group differences would have taken in the absence of an intervention is to take several pretreatment measures so that the trajectory, as well as the level, can be determined. Taking account of the trajectory in the estimation of the treatment effect can then be accomplished with the following model (cf. Dwyer, 1984):

$$y_{i,-1} = \alpha_0 + \eta_i + \zeta_{i,-1}$$

$$y_{i0} = \beta_0 + \beta_1 y_{i,-1} + \lambda\eta_i + \zeta_{i0}$$

$$y_{i1} = \gamma_0 + \beta_1 y_{i0} + \beta_2 x_i + \lambda\eta_i + \zeta_{i1}$$

$$\vdots$$

where measurements $y_{i,-1}$ and y_{i0} precede the intervention; η has zero mean and is free to correlate with x; α, β, and λ are fixed parameters to be estimated; the ζ have zero mean, $E(\zeta_{it}x_i) = E(\zeta_{it}\eta_i) = 0$ for $t \geqslant 0$, and $E(\zeta_{it}y_{i,t-1}) = 0$. This more flexible model uses the pretreatment pattern of change in y to project the expected difference between groups into the future. The model can be identified with two pretreatment observation points, but the necessary constraints are less restrictive if additional points are available.

SPECIAL PROBLEMS IN ANALYSIS OF LONGITUDINAL DATA

Estimation of Variances

Suppose that the random variable y is defined across a population of persons with variance σ_{yy} and mean μ. Then a sample of N observations of y from this population yields the data set $\{y_i\}_{i=1,...,N}$. If we are then interested in estimating σ_{yy} with sample data, we might begin with computing the sample variance $S_{yy} = (1/N)\sum_{i=1}^{N}(y_i - \sum y_i/N)^2$. A major concern is then the relationship between sample values of S_{yy} and the population parameter σ_{yy}. This is investigated taking the expectation across samples of size N where, for simplicity but without loss of generality, we assume that $\mu = 0$:

$$
\begin{aligned}
E[S_{yy}] &= \left(\frac{1}{N}\right) E\left[\sum_{i=1}^{N}\left(y_i - \frac{\sum y_i}{N}\right)^2\right] \\
&= \left(\frac{1}{N}\right) E\left[\left\{y_1 - \frac{(y_1 + y_2 + \cdots)}{N}\right\}^2 + \left\{y_2 - \frac{(y_1 + y_2 + \cdots)}{N}\right\}^2 + \cdots\right] \\
&= \left(\frac{1}{N}\right) E\left[y_1^2 + \frac{(y_1^2 + y_1y_2 + \cdots + y_2y_1 + y_2^2 + \cdots)}{N^2}\right. \\
&\qquad \left. - 2\frac{(y_1^2 + y_1y_2 + y_1y_3 + \cdots)}{N} + \cdots\right]
\end{aligned}
$$

Clearly, the expectation of the sample variance is a complex function of squares and products of elements of the sample. However, there are two assumptions (which can be rendered plausible by proper sampling designs) that greatly simplify this expression. The first is that each member of the sample is equally likely to be selected. It is then the case that $E[y_i^2] = \sigma_{yy}$ for every i, and

$$
\begin{aligned}
E[S_{yy}] &= \frac{1}{N}\left(1 - \frac{1}{N}\right)[E(y_1^2) + E(y_2^2) + \cdots + E(y_N^2)] \\
&\quad + \frac{1}{N}\left[\sum_i\sum_j\left(-\frac{2}{N}\right)E(y_iy_j)\right] \\
&= \left(1 - \frac{1}{N}\right)\sigma_{yy} + \frac{1}{N}\sum_i\sum_j\left(-\frac{2}{N}\right)\sigma_{ij}
\end{aligned}
$$

where $i \neq j$ and σ_{ij} is the covariance of the ith and jth observations. Further simplification is then achieved by the additional assumption that $\sigma_{ij} = 0$ when $i \neq j$; this assumption is appropriate when sampling occurs such that every sampled unit is independent of every other unit (random sampling).

And this is precisely why longitudinal observation creates some difficulty. When a set of observations is derived from repeated measurement of a random sample of individuals, observations are not independent and σ_{ij} is often not zero when i and j refer to observations from the same individual. Thus estimates of the population variance, and subsequent standard errors of means and regression coefficients that contain that estimate, will be biased if it is assumed that $\sigma_{ij} = 0$ for all $i \neq j$. The extent of the bias depends, of course, on the magnitude and direction of the covariances. When the covariances are positive, the estimated variance will be biased upwards. Thus a major statistical goal when analyzing longitudinal data is to obtain estimates of σ_{ij} and incorporate them into analyses. Failure to do so can result in substantial losses of statistical power.

Two solutions to this problem are available. The first is to model the dependence among related observations. This is the subject of much of the fourth section of this chapter. The second is to compute "robust" variance estimates (cf. Royall, 1986; White, 1982).

Estimation of Standard Errors in Regression Models

Suppose that the association between two random variables y and x is described by the model

$$y_i = \alpha + \beta x_i + \zeta_i \tag{1a}$$

where $E(\zeta_i) = 0$, $E(\zeta_i^2) = \sigma$ for all i, and $\sigma_{x\zeta} = 0$. Now suppose that the variables y and x are observed at T equally spaced points in time for a panel of N persons. In addition, suppose that ζ is autocorrelated (i.e., $\sigma_{\zeta_{it}\zeta_{i,t+\tau}} \neq 0$ for $\tau \neq 0$). If we ignore the dependence among the multiple observations of the same persons we might estimate the model

$$y_{it} = a + bx_{it} + \varepsilon_{it}$$

by ordinary least squares. While it can be shown that $E(\hat{b}) = \beta$ and $E(\hat{a}) = \alpha$ if the model in (1a) holds, failure to take account of the autocorrelation in ζ can reduce the precision of the estimate. Thus a more powerful estimate is obtained if the model in (1a) is assumed and the covariances among ζ_{it} and $\zeta_{it'}$ are specified in the model as the matrix Ψ. Generalized least-squares and maximum likelihood estimators of Ψ and the regression parameters are then available under the assumption of multivariate normality (see "Estimation Summary").

When the sample size is large, the loss of precision from assuming that Ψ is diagonal will be small. Furthermore, robust estimates of the true standard errors can be computed without explicit modeling of the covariance among residuals (Royall, 1986; White, 1982). However, if Ψ is nondiagonal because of excluded determinants of y that are correlated with x, then the mean response portion of the model in (1a) is misspecified. The estimated regression coefficient is then biased whether Ψ is incorrectly assumed diagonal or if it is estimated. This topic will be discussed in more detail in the section concerning fixed- and random-effects models.

When sample size is small and autocorrelation is large, loss of precision due to the assumption that Ψ is diagonal may be substantial. This can arise in observation of aggregates such as communities or countries, where sample size is necessarily restricted to only a few dozen units of analysis. Repeated observation can yield substantial statistical power if the autocorrelations are strong, and if this autocorrelation structure is incorporated into the model. In simple cases (balanced designs and multivariate normal variables) this may be achieved with multivariate regression or analysis of covariance models.

In instances where categorical outcomes are of interest, ignoring the serial dependence among the disturbances produces bias in estimators even when the presumption of independence of disturbances and x_{it} holds. Thus it is of greater importance to estimate the nondiagonal elements of Ψ or to model the serial dependence (Zeger, Liang, & Albert, 1988). Alternative approaches to such modeling are addressed in Chapters 8, 9, and 15.

Compounded Measurement Error

Assuming independent random (nonsampling) measurement error in two variables, taking the mean of the variables measured on the same sample yields a variable with reduced measurement error. This arises because uncorrelated errors tend to cancel each other when summed. However, the situation is contrary with difference scores. This is developed as follows.

Suppose that y is observed at $t = 1$ and $t = 2$ and that y is related to the true (unobserved) score (η) as follows for the ith member of a population:

$$y_{i1} = \eta_{i1} + \varepsilon_{i1} \qquad y_{i2} = \eta_{i2} + \varepsilon_{i2}$$

where ε_{i1} and ε_{i2} are random variables (measurement errors) uncorrelated with one another [$\text{cov}(\varepsilon_{i2}, \varepsilon_{i1}) = 0$], uncorrelated with the true scores, and with expectations of zero. If the covariance of η with itself over time is $\sigma(\eta_2, \eta_1) = \rho$, the mean and variance ($\sigma_{\eta\eta}$) of η are constant over time, and $\sigma(\varepsilon_1, \varepsilon_1) = \sigma(\varepsilon_2, \varepsilon_2) = \sigma_{\varepsilon\varepsilon}$, then the proportion of the variance in y_1 or y_2 due to measurement error is $\sigma_{\varepsilon\varepsilon}/(\sigma_{\eta\eta} + \sigma_{\varepsilon\varepsilon})$. In contrast, the variance of the mean $(y_1 + y_2)/2$ attributable to measurement error is derived from

$$\text{var}\left[\frac{(y_1 + y_2)}{2}\right] = \text{var}\left[\frac{(\eta_1 + \eta_2 + \varepsilon_1 + \varepsilon_2)}{2}\right] = \frac{(\sigma_{\eta\eta} + \sigma_{\eta\eta} + 2\rho + \sigma_{\varepsilon\varepsilon} + \sigma_{\varepsilon\varepsilon})}{4}$$

From this we see that $\sigma_{\varepsilon\varepsilon}/(\sigma_{\eta\eta} + \rho + \sigma_{\varepsilon\varepsilon})$ is the proportion of variance in the mean that is due to measurement error. Clearly, if $\rho > 0$, then $\sigma_{\varepsilon\varepsilon}/(\sigma_{\eta\eta} + \sigma_{\varepsilon\varepsilon}) > \sigma_{\varepsilon\varepsilon}/(\sigma_{\eta\eta} + \rho + \sigma_{\varepsilon\varepsilon})$, and the mean has reduced measurement error. However, consider the variance of the difference score $(y_2 - y_1)$:

$$\text{var}(y_2 - y_1) = \text{var}(\eta_2 - \eta_1 + \varepsilon_2 - \varepsilon_1) = \sigma_{\eta\eta} + \sigma_{\eta\eta} - 2\rho + \sigma_{\varepsilon\varepsilon} + \sigma_{\varepsilon\varepsilon}$$

which reveals that the proportion of error variance in the difference score is

$\sigma_{\varepsilon\varepsilon}/(\sigma_{\eta\eta} - \rho + \sigma_{\varepsilon\varepsilon})$, which will exceed that of either score or their mean when $\rho > 0$. In addition to these relative measurement error variances being larger for difference scores, the absolute measurement error variances show the same pattern. Error variance in y_1, $(y_2 - y_1)/2$, and $(y_2 - y_1)$ is $\sigma_{\varepsilon\varepsilon}$, $\sigma_{\varepsilon\varepsilon}/2$, and $2\sigma_{\varepsilon\varepsilon}$, respectively.

Thus when difference scores are of interest, power can be reduced in longitudinal studies relative to cross-sectional studies. Furthermore, when estimation of parameters is biased by random measurement error (Stefanski, 1985), that bias will be greater in analyses of longitudinal data involving change scores than in cross-sectional analyses. For example, when a predictor variable in a linear regression model is measured with error, the estimated regression coefficients are biased. Thus it is important in longitudinal studies to incorporate a measurement submodel into the statistical model. The submodel can use information from multiple measurements or from external sources to correct for bias in estimates due to measurement error (see Chapter 12).

The foregoing discussion has assumed that errors of measurement at $t = 2$ were uncorrelated with those at $t = 1$. If this is not the case ($\sigma_{\varepsilon_2\varepsilon_1} \neq 0$), and $\sigma_{\varepsilon_2\varepsilon_1} > 0$, measurement errors will tend to be filtered in difference scores whereas they will compound in means. Many measurements in medicine may involve consistent measurement errors. For example, artifacts in imaging techniques, such as thallium scintigraphy of myocardial perfusion, may persist because of fixed constitutional differences between patients. Artifacts due to adipose tissue, for example, will be present on repeated scans. However, change between repeated scans will be independent of these consistent sources of error.

A problematic implication of substantial measurement error in change scores is that associations between change and initial level are biased in the negative direction. This can be seen in the following expression for the covariance of y_1 and $(y_2 - y_1)$:

$$\sigma[y_1, (y_2 - y_1)] = \sigma[(\eta_1 + \varepsilon_1), (\eta_2 + \varepsilon_2 - \eta_1 - \varepsilon_1)]$$
$$= [\sigma(\eta_2, \eta_1) - \sigma(\eta_1, \eta_1)] - \sigma(\varepsilon_1, \varepsilon_1)$$
$$= \sigma[\eta_1, (\eta_2 - \eta_1)] - \sigma(\varepsilon_1, \varepsilon_1)$$

Thus the covariance of interest, $\sigma[\eta_1, (\eta_2 - \eta_1)]$, is estimated with a negative bias when $\hat{\sigma}[y_1, (y_2 - y_1)]$ is the estimator. This arises because the amount of change in y, $(y_2 - y_1)$, is not independent of ε_1—even though ε_1 is uncorrelated with y_1 and y_2:

$$\sigma[\varepsilon_1, (y_2 - y_1)] = -\sigma(\varepsilon_1, \varepsilon_1)$$

and this is precisely the bias in $\sigma[y_1, (y_2 - y_1)]$.

Empirical Example

To demonstrate the extent of bias in the relationship between initial level and subsequent change when a variable is measured with error, consider a measurement model fit to measurements of systolic blood pressure. The data for this demonstration come from 576 men aged 32 through 38 at baseline in the

Framingham Heart Study (Dawber, 1980). These data will be used repeatedly in subsequent examples and are taken from the third and fourth biannual examinations. (The first two examinations are often excluded to avoid artifacts due to elevated readings in these initial screenings.) The observed means and standard deviations of SBP at each examination are given in Table 1-1.

Suppose the following measurement model for these observations:

$$\text{SBP}a_{i1} = \eta_{i1} + \varepsilon_{i1} \qquad \text{SBP}b_{i1} = \lambda\eta_{i1} + \delta_{i1}$$

$$\text{SBP}a_{i2} = \eta_{i2} + \varepsilon_{i2} \qquad \text{SBP}b_{i2} = \lambda\eta_{i2} + \delta_{i2}$$

where η_{i1} is the expected SBP on replicated measurement (unobserved true score) at $t = 1$ for the ith member of the population; η_{i2} is expected SBP at $t = 2$; SBPa is the recorded SBP of a first examiner and SBPb is that measured by a second examiner; the measurement errors ε and δ are presumed uncorrelated with the true scores, uncorrelated with one another, and to have zero expectation; λ is a parameter reflecting the relative slope of SBPb on η relative to SBPa on η.

Maximum likelihood estimates of the parameters of this model can be obtained if the observed variables are assumed multivariate normal. The fit of the model with the data is acceptable ($\chi^2 = 1.48$, df $= 2$).

The goal now is to compare the covariance of the observed initial level and change (e.g., for SBPa) with the initial level and change in η:

$$\hat{\sigma}[\text{SBP}a_{i1}, (\text{SBP}a_{i2} - \text{SBP}a_{i1})] = -64.9 \ (8.3)$$

$$\hat{\sigma}[\eta_1, (\eta_2 - \eta_1)] = -17.5 \ (7.0)$$

These covariances correspond to regression slopes of $-.28$ and $-.09$ for observed and true scores, respectively. The dramatic two-thirds reduction in the negative association that results from adjustment for measurement error is apparent. The remaining negative association may be real, or it may also be

Table 1–1. Data from Framingham Heart Study examinations 3–6 (576 men aged 32–38 at baseline)

	1	2	3	4	5	6	7	8
1 SBP$_3$[a]	1.00							
2 SBP$_4$	.66	1.00						
3 SBP$_5$	.62	.68	1.00					
4 SBP$_6$	.61	.63	.67	1.00				
5 RW$_3$	.33	.26	.23	.24	1.00			
6 RW$_4$	.31	.29	.23	.26	.95	1.00		
7 RW$_5$	.30	.29	.30	.27	.92	.95	1.00	
8 RW$_6$	.27	.25	.23	.27	.90	.93	.95	1.00
Mean	126.2	127.9	128.5	130.3	120.3	121.0	121.1	121.5
SD	15.3	16.7	17.6	17.3	16.0	16.1	16.5	16.4

[a]SBP$_3$, systolic blood pressure at examination 3, etc. RW$_3$, relative weight at examination 3, etc. SBP is first examiner, relative weight is Metropolitan.

explained by measurement errors not common to repeated measurements on the same day.

An alternative approach to estimation of the association between initial level and subsequent slope is necessary when multiple indicators of a variable are not available. One such alternative involves the estimation of the slope of y over time for each case and relating this slope to its own intercept (rather than to the initial observation). This model requires more than two observation time points to achieve identification of parameters. The model may be specified in a manner analogous to that for a measurement model. For the case of four examinations ($t = 0, 1, 2, 3$) we have

$$y_{i0} = \alpha_0 + \eta_{i0} + \varepsilon_{i0}$$

$$y_{i1} = \alpha_1 + \eta_{i0} + \eta_{i1} + \varepsilon_{i1}$$

$$y_{i2} = \alpha_2 + \eta_{i0} + 2\eta_{i1} + \varepsilon_{i2}$$

$$y_{i3} = \alpha_3 + \eta_{i0} + 3\eta_{i1} + \varepsilon_{i3}$$

where the α_t are constants; η_{i0} is the individual intercept for y regressed on time and η_{i1} is the slope; $E(\eta_{i0}) = E(\eta_{i1}) = 0$; the ε_{it} are deviations of y about the line $(\alpha_t + \eta_{i0} + t\eta_{i1})$; $E(\varepsilon_{it}) = 0$; autocorrelation of ε_{it} with $\varepsilon_{i,t-1}$ may be estimated. The parameter of interest is then the covariance of η_{i0} and η_{i1} (or the slope of η_{i1} regressed on $\eta_{i0} = \beta = \sigma_{\eta_1\eta_0}/\sigma_{\eta_0\eta_0}$). Note that the terms ε_{it} include both measurement error and sampling error. Computation of individual values of η_0 and η_1 will necessarily incorporate these errors and result in bias. Maximum likelihood estimation of the parameters of the equation model avoids this bias (Blomqvist, 1977). For the data from the third to sixth examinations in Framingham, where y is SBP (first examiner only), initial level and slope are unrelated:

$$\hat{\rho}_{\eta_1\eta_0} = .009 \qquad \hat{\beta}_{\eta_1\eta_0} = .002 \; (.023)$$

where it has been assumed that $E(\varepsilon_{it}\varepsilon_{i,t-1}) = 0$. Both the multiple indicator and multiple examination approaches to estimating the relation between change and initial level, therefore, indicate no relationship in these blood pressure data.

To this point the discussion has focused on the implications of nonsampling measurement error on the estimation of models involving continuous variables. In this case, random error in the dependent variable reduces precision but does not introduce bias in the estimation of slopes or intercepts (unless standardized coefficients are of interest). Random error in a predictor variable, however, does produce bias in estimates of slopes and intercepts. In the case of a single predictor, random error in the predictor attenuates the slope estimator toward zero. This can be seen by comparing β in the model

$$\eta_i = \alpha + \beta\xi_i + \zeta_i \; (\sigma_{\xi\zeta} = 0)$$

with b in the model

$$y_i = a + bx_i + \varepsilon_i \; (\sigma_{x\varepsilon} = 0)$$

where y is a flawed measure of η and x is a flawed measure of ξ ($y_i = \eta_i + \delta_{yi}$;

$x_i = \xi_i + \delta_{xi})$. By the method of moments we find that

$$b = \frac{\sigma_{yx}}{\sigma_{xx}} = \frac{\sigma_{\eta\xi}}{\sigma_{\xi\xi} + \sigma_{\delta_x\delta_x}} = \beta\left(\frac{\sigma_{\xi\xi}}{\sigma_{\xi\xi} + \sigma_{\delta_x\delta_x}}\right)$$

Note that the error in y does not introduce bias into b, whereas error in x biases b downward. In the case of multiple predictors, random measurement error among the predictors can produce upward or downward bias.

In contrast to the instance of a continuous dependent variable, models involving a categorical dependent variable are more problematic. Random error in the dependent variable (i.e., classification error) produces bias in logistic or probit regression slopes. Thus the use of multiple measures to correct for bias due to such error takes on special importance in the categorical context. This issue, and a proposed solution, are described in Chapters 12 and 15.

Regression to the Mean

The preceding discussion of measurement error leads us to another potential source of confusion in the interpretation of longitudinal data: the phenomenon often referred to as regression to the mean, or the regression artifact. In the blood pressure data just given, for example, we find that ordinary least squares (OLS) regression of SBPa$_{i2}$ on SBPa$_{i1}$ yields the following:

$$y_{i2} = 37.0 + .72y_{i1} + \hat{\zeta}_{i2}$$

where the slope .72 corresponds to a correlation of .66. The extent of regression is then $(1 - .72)$ in the natural metric and $(1 - .66)$ in a standardized metric. Regression is the extent to which the conditional expected value of y_{i2} given y_{i1}, $E(y_{i2} | y_{i1})$, is closer to $E(y_{i1})$ than y_{i1}. This amount of regression $(1 - .72 = .28)$ is identical to the slope of change $(y_{i2} - y_{i1})$ regressed on initial level (y_{i1}) calculated above for these two measures of SBP $(-.28)$. Thus adjustment for measurement error in this instance reduces the extent of regression over the two-year lag from $-.28$ to $-.09$ mm Hg millimeter of mercury at the initial measurement.

These observations make clear that random measurement error can be a source of exaggerated regression to the mean between observations. It may be useful to fit longitudinal observations of a variable to alternative models that explain regression patterns. For example, when only measurement error is responsible for change and cross-sectional variance is constant, there will be no additional regression from the first to the third and subsequent observation occasions. A simple linear model that corresponds to this circumstance may be specified as follows:

$$y_{it} = \alpha_t + \lambda_t\alpha_i + \varepsilon_{it} \tag{1b}$$

where α_t is a set of fixed constants corresponding to the expected value of y at each wave $(t = 0, \ldots, T-1)$; $\lambda_0 = 1$, λ_t is a fixed parameter for $t > 0$ (this allows the variance of y to change over time); α_i is a random variable that does not change over time but varies over individuals; ε_{it} is random measurement error with zero expectation for all i and t, $\sigma_{\varepsilon_{it}}$ is identical for all i within t, and ε_{it} is uncorrelated with α_i at each t. In this case, then, suppose that regressing y_{i1} on y_{i0} yields the regression coefficient β [$=\sigma_{y_{i1}y_{i0}}/\sigma_{y_{i0}y_{i0}} = \lambda_1\sigma_{\alpha\alpha}/(\sigma_{\alpha\alpha} + \sigma_{\varepsilon\varepsilon})$]. It then follows that when y_{i2} is regressed on y_{i0}, $(\lambda_2/\lambda_1)\beta$ is the expected regression coefficient. If $\lambda_{t+1} \geqslant \lambda_t$ (as is the case with many biologic measurements), the lagged autoregression coefficient will remain constant, or even increase, as the lag increases. When this pattern is found, serial measurements can simply be averaged to estimate α_i, or a measurement model as specified above can be constrained such that $\eta_{it} = \eta_i$.

However, generally β does not remain constant or increase as the lag between observations increases. Rather β often decreases as the lag increases—even after adjustments are made for measurement error. This pattern may arise because time-varying factors, rather than time-invariant factors (i.e., α_i), are determining y through time. In the extreme case, this type of process leads to complete regression to the mean: $\beta_{y_ty_0} \to 0$ as the lag between measures increases ($t \to \infty$). To the extent that other time-varying determinants of y are uncorrelated with y_{i0}, they produce a reordering of persons rank ordered on y. This reordering is equivalent to regression to the mean. A simple linear model of such a process is the following:

$$\eta_{it} = a_t + a_3\eta_{i,t-1} + \zeta_{it} \qquad (2a)$$

where y has been replaced by η from a measurement model involving multiple observations of y_{it} ($y_{it} = \eta_{it} + \varepsilon_{it}$); a_t is a series of constants; a_3 is a parameter; ζ_{it} is a random disturbance with zero expectation and constant variance at each t. Identification of the model can be achieved by assuming that $\sigma[\zeta_{it}, \eta_{i,t-\tau}] = 0$ for some values of $\tau \geqslant 1$. Alternatively, identification can be achieved by specifying difference equations such as

$$\eta_{it} - \eta_{i,t-1} = (a_t - a_{t-1}) + a_3(\eta_{i,t-1} - \eta_{i,t-2}) + \zeta_{it} - \zeta_{i,t-1}$$

where it is assumed that $(\zeta_{it} - \zeta_{i,t-1})$ is uncorrelated with $\eta_{i,t-2}$. This assumption is plausible if (2a) is misspecified because of excluded variables that are filtered by differencing.

A mathematical advantage of this type of model is that it is the discrete time form of a continuous time model:

$$\frac{d\eta_i(t)}{dt} = \alpha_1 + \alpha_3\eta_i(t) + \frac{d\zeta_i(t)}{dt} \qquad (2b)$$

where $\eta(t)$ is a continuous variable in continuous time, and $d\zeta_i(t)/dt$ is a stochastic process whose integral is random at a discrete point in time. Such "dynamic" models are attractive in many biologic contexts because they describe systems that can come to equilibrium (with "negative feedback", $\alpha_3 < 0$), oscillate, or become catastrophic. This model is analogous to the autoregressive equations used in the analysis of time series (Box & Jenkins, 1970).

An alternative to the autoregressive model in equation (2a) is one in which it is assumed that there is no feedback of η on itself. Rather, η is determined by ξ and ζ, where ξ does involve feedback:

$$\eta_{it} = \alpha_t + \xi_{it} + \zeta_{it} \tag{3a}$$

$$\xi_{it} = \beta_0 + \beta_1 \xi_{i,t-1} + \omega_{it} \tag{3b}$$

where α_t is a set of intercepts; ζ_{it} is a random disturbance with zero autocorrelation over the observation lag; ω_{it} is a random disturbance uncorrelated with $\xi_{i,t-1}$. Identification is achieved by assuming that ξ_{it} is uncorrelated with ζ_{it}, for all t and t'. The factors ξ and ζ represent time-varying factors that determine change in η over time; and to the extent that ξ is stable over time, it provides stability as well. Cox (1981) referred to (2) as an "observation-driven" model (since response at t is dependent on observed response at $t-1$) and to (3) as a "parameter-driven" model (since response at t is dependent on unobserved ξ).

Many biologic variables evidence a pattern of serial covariance that is intermediate between the two extremes represented by models in equations (1) and (2). The intermediate situation is one where the decay of autocovariance increases with time but does not drop toward zero. Such data may be consistent with a model that combines equations (1) and (2), or one that combines (1) and (3). We first combine (1) and (2) to specify a dynamic model:

$$\eta_{it} = a_t + \lambda_t a_i + a_3 \eta_{i,t-1} + \zeta_{it} \tag{4a}$$

or

$$\frac{d\eta_i(t)}{dt} = \alpha_1 + \gamma \alpha_i + \alpha_3 \eta_i(t) + \frac{d\zeta_i(t)}{dt} \tag{4b}$$

where $\lambda_0 = 1$ and $\lambda_t = \lambda$ for $t > 0$. Identification is achieved by constraining ζ_{it} to be uncorrelated with $\eta_{i,t-\tau}$. In biologic applications the a_i are often referred to as *stochastic environmental* effects, while ζ represents *demographic* effects (Karlin & Taylor, 1981).

An extension of (1) that has been used extensively for the analysis of growth curves involves polynomial functions of time. Equation model (1) allows for the intercept in a linear equation to vary across individuals. The growth curve extension to variable polynomial coefficients may be specified as follows:

$$\eta_{it} = \alpha + \alpha_i + \beta_i t + \gamma_i t^2 + \cdots + \zeta_{it} \tag{5}$$

where the variable coefficients $\alpha_i, \beta_i, \ldots$ are random variables describing the time path of η for each case; ζ_{it} is assumed random with zero mean, constant variance within t, and zero correlation with the variable coefficients. A further variant of this model is obtained by assuming that ζ is first-order autoregressive ($\zeta_{it} = \rho \zeta_{i,t-1} + \delta_{it}$; $\sigma[\zeta_{i,t-1}, \delta_{it}] = 0$). Equation model (5) is used most often as a component of a two-stage model in which relations between exogenous variables and the variable coefficients are estimated (Rao, 1965).

Empirical Examples

Each of the foregoing models explains change, stability, and regression to the mean for a single longitudinally observed variable in terms of different processes. The utility of these models derives either from the ability to adapt the model to known characteristics of a variable or from fitting observations of poorly understood variables to alternative models. The latter strategy may be fruitful in that certain of the alternatives can be rejected because of poor fit. Those that "fit" may then provide clues concerning the process generating the variable. However, it is likely that these simplified models are misspecified due to the strong assumptions necessary to achieve identification. Thus interpretation of fit should be cautious.

The alternative models were fitted to the blood pressure data described previously (from examinations 3 through 8 of the Framingham Heart Study, two readings per visit). Maximum likelihood procedures were used for estimation and assessment of fit, assuming multivariate normality.

The measurement model for the six waves of SBP measurements (twelve measures in all) was specified as

$$\text{SBP}a_{it} = \eta_{it} + \varepsilon_{ita} \qquad \text{SBP}b_{it} = \eta_{it} + \varepsilon_{itb}$$

$$\eta_{it} = \alpha_t + \zeta_{it}$$

where $E(\zeta_{it}) = 0$ for each t, and the variance–covariance matrix of ζ (Ψ) was unconstrained; the ε are assumed random, uncorrelated with one another, uncorrelated with η, and $E(\varepsilon_{it}) = 0$ for each t. While the variances of the observed variables increased from 208 to 318 over the ten years of observation, the estimated variance in η increased from 173 to 278. The model yielded a goodness-of-fit χ^2 of 207.9 with 51 degrees of freedom. Since it is well known that sequential measurements of SBP decline within one examination period, the means of SBPa and SBPb were allowed to differ. These additional six parameters reduced the degrees of freedom to 45, and the χ^2 declined to 125.6 This χ^2 provides a baseline against which to compare the fit of the various structures imposed on the data; the difference between this χ^2 and one for a model with additional constraints is distributed as a χ^2 with degrees of freedom equal to the number of additional constraints.

The model in equation (1) was then specified as

$$\eta_{it} = \alpha_t + \lambda_t \alpha_i + \zeta_{it}$$

where the matrix Ψ is constrained to be diagonal. The χ^2 increased to 258.5 with an increase to 54 degrees of freedom ($\Delta\chi^2 = 258.5 - 125.6 = 132.9$, Δdf $= 54 - 45 = 9$). Estimates of α_t increased steadily from 124.7 ($t = 0$) to 130.6 ($t = 5$) mm Hg over the ten-year period. The time-invariant factor explaining stability over time had variance $\hat{\sigma}_{\alpha\alpha} = 118.7$ (SE $= 10.2$), which accounted for 69 percent of the variance of η_{io} (173) and 51 percent of the variance in SBPa_{io} (233). $\hat{\lambda}_t$ increased from 1 ($t = 0$) to 1.30 ($t = 2$) and then remained stable. Clearly this model depicting stability in blood pressure as due to time-invariant factors (e.g., genotype), and change as due to factors with zero autocorrelation over a two-year period, is inconsistent with these data.

Next we fit the model in (4) to the data. This is equivalent to adding feedback to the previous model:

$$\eta_{it} = a_t + \lambda_t a_i + a_3 \eta_{i,t-1} + \zeta_{it}$$

where the coefficient a_3, or $(a_3 - 1)$, reflects the feedback in the system. The fit for this model $(\chi^2 = 167.5, \text{df} = 53)$ is an improvement over the model without feedback $(\Delta\chi^2 = 258.5 - 167.5 = 91, \Delta\text{df} = 54 - 53 = 1)$, but the constraints implied by (4) do yield a significant deterioration in fit relative to the measurement model $(\Delta\chi^2 = 167.5 - 125.6 = 41.9, \Delta\text{df} = 53 - 45 = 8)$. Some of the parameter estimates for this combination model are as follows (some standard errors are in parentheses):

$$\hat{\lambda}_t = 0.80(.07), 0.88, 0.81, 0.83, 0.86 \qquad t = 1, \ldots, 5$$

$$\hat{\sigma}_{\alpha\alpha} = 117.8(11) \qquad \hat{a}_3 = .33(.04)$$

Notice that $\hat{\sigma}_{\alpha\alpha}$ is virtually unchanged from the previous model. Also note that $\hat{a}_3 = .33$ implies considerable regression in SBP; however, this regression is now to α_i for each case rather than a group mean.

While there is substantial evidence of negative feedback mechanisms for blood pressure, a researcher might hypothesize that the two-year lag between examinations is too lengthy for such mechanisms to be detected. An alternative to (4) is then to assume that the autoregressive structure applies to an unmeasured factor, as in (3). An alternative combined model may then be specified as

$$\eta_{it} = \alpha_t + \lambda_t \alpha_i + \xi_{it} + \zeta_{it}$$

$$\xi_{it} = \gamma \xi_{i,t-1} + \omega_{it}$$

where $\lambda_t = \lambda$ for $t > 0$; α_i, ξ, and ζ are uncorrelated; ω_{it} is uncorrelated with $\xi_{i,t-\tau}$ $(\tau = 1, \ldots)$; all random variables have zero expectation and constant variance (this latter constraint is one approach to identification of the model). The fit of the model $(\chi^2 = 163.6, \text{df} = 60)$ was comparable to the model with feedback in η, although they are not hierarchically related. Model estimates are as follows:

$$\hat{\sigma}_{\alpha\alpha} = 121.4 \ (17.8) \quad \hat{\sigma}_{\zeta\zeta} = 32.8 \ (3.8) \quad \hat{\sigma}_{\psi\psi} = 33.2 \ (5.3)$$

$$\hat{\gamma} = .82 \ (.06) \qquad \hat{\lambda} = 1.1 \ (0.1)$$

where λ could have been constrained to 1 (since its standard error includes 1). These parameter estimates imply that the estimated variance of ξ increased from 49.2 $(t = 1)$ to 90.6 $(t = 5)$. The model then decomposes the observed variance of SBPa_{i5} (311) into the following components:

$$\hat{\lambda}^2 \hat{\sigma}_{\alpha\alpha} + \hat{\sigma}_{\xi\xi} + \hat{\sigma}_{\zeta\zeta} + \hat{\sigma}_{\varepsilon\varepsilon} = 147 + 91 + 33 + 34$$

where all but $\sigma_{\varepsilon\varepsilon}$ can also be considered the partitioning of the variance of η_{i5}

(245). These results suggest that 11 percent of the variance in measured SBP ($\sigma_{\varepsilon\varepsilon}/\sigma_{yy}$) is due to "between-examiner" variability, short-term change in SBP, and "within-examiner" errors of measurement. Of the "true" variance in η (271), 54 percent is attributable to factors that are invariant over time (α_i), 34 percent is attributable to first-order autoregressive factors (ξ), and the remaining 12 percent is attributable to "occasion" factors (ζ) with no stability over the two years between examinations. The variability associated with the autoregressive factors may offer the best opportunity for intervention; some of the invariant component, however, may be due to fixed environmental or behavioral variables that are amenable to change.

Substantive interpretation of such models is highly speculative, since all the determinants of variance are unmeasured. However, such modeling can give clues to the role of time-variant and -invariant factors in explaining regression patterns in an observed variable. These clues can then be used to build models involving other measured variables. Varieties of these models are discussed under "Statistical Models for Longitudinal Data" in this chapter.

Categorical Outcomes

Models of processes analogous to regression in categorical variables are also available. For the case of ordered categories, there are two main types: those with, and those without, an absorbing barrier. The presence or absence of certain types of morbidity, such as flu symptoms, is an example of an ordered category without an absorbing barrier. An individual may alternate back and forth between two or more categories during a lifetime. Vital status, on the other hand, includes the essential absorbing barrier: the mortality transition. Processes involving absorbing barriers are not subject to regression effects at the individual level; however, hazard rates of interacting groups may evidence stability and regression over time. These rates may then be modeled with equations for continuous variables.

Processes involving transitions between ordered categories without absorbing barriers may also evidence patterns of stability and change over time for individuals. A general model of such processes may be specified as follows:

$$y_{it}^* = \gamma_0 + \beta_1 y_{i,t-1} + \beta_2 y_{i,t-2} + \cdots + \phi(y_{i,t-1} + y_{i,t-1} y_{i,t-2} + \cdots) + \alpha_i + \zeta_{it}$$

$$y_{it} = 0 \quad \text{if } y_{it}^* < 0$$

$$\phantom{y_{it}} = 1 \quad \text{if } y_{it}^* \geq 0 \qquad\qquad (y^* \text{ standard logistic or normal})$$

where the observed categorical variable y_{it} measures the state of the ith person at time t ($y = 0, 1, \ldots$); y^* is a logistically or normally distributed *unmeasured* variable; $\beta_{t-\tau}$ reflects the dependence of state at time t on earlier states; ϕ reflects dependence of the current state on the length of time in the current state; α_i is a random variable reflecting time-invariant factors; and ζ is a random disturbance. Identification of various forms of this model involves constraints on the parameters, covariances, and means. The unmeasured variable y^* can be treated as a mathematical device or as a "latent" variable.

Missing Data

A discussion of several approaches to missing data in longitudinal studies is provided in Chapter 11. Missing data are not, of course, peculiar to longitudinal studies, but they are generally a more severe problem in these studies than in other models. To presume that data are missing completely at random (MCAR) in longitudinal studies is often implausible. This is demonstrated in Chapter 10 for the Framingham Study.

The most frequently applied approaches to MCAR data are (1) deletion of cases with incomplete data (listwise deletion), (2) use of all available data to estimate means and covariances (pairwise deletion), and (3) iterative imputation of missing data (the Expectation Maximization algorithm; Beale & Little, 1975). The EM approach is an extension of pairwise deletion in which the means ($\hat{\mu}_0$) and covariances ($\hat{\Sigma}_0$) based on all available data are used to impute values for missing data by linear regression. The resulting complete data matrix is then used to estimate new means $\hat{\mu}_1$ and covariances $\hat{\Sigma}_1$, which are used to impute new values for the missing observations. This iterative algorithm continues until the covariance estimates converge (if they converge). Under the condition of multivariate normality, the EM algorithm yields estimates with a smaller mean squared error than the simpler methods. In general, the extent of this advantage increases as the extent of missing data increases. However, a larger advantage of the EM over pairwise deletion is seen for some patterns of nonrandom missing data, where the EM yields unbiased estimates while the other two methods yield biased estimates (Little & Rubin, 1987).

The three alternative approaches to adjustment of covariance matrices for the estimation of regression coefficients from incomplete continuous data have recently been evaluated in a simulation study reported by Azen, Guilder, and Hill (1989). Their particular focus was on nonnormally distributed data and patterns of missing data involving dependence of missing status on other variables or on censoring (in which the probability of a missing value of a variable is dependent on its own level). They also restricted their simulation to the cross-sectional instance where the dependent variable was complete. They concluded that the EM algorithm also performs well with log-normal or mixed-normal variables and with dependent or censored patterns of missing data. It is important to remember, however, that missing status can produce bias because such status is dependent on unmeasured or poorly measured variables; the EM algorithm is of no assistance in this case.

Considerable recent work has focused on the application of missing-value methods to estimation of longitudinal models (Hui, 1984; Laird & Ware, 1982), as outlined in Chapters 4 and 11.

In longitudinal experiments, a problematic type of missing data is that which arises from a systematic process in which the probability that observation of the ith person is missing on the tth occasion (π_{it}) interacts with the experimental condition (x) and the outcome variable (y). In general, suppose that the structural model is

$$y_{it} = \beta_0 + \beta_1 x_{1it} + \beta_2 x_{2it} + \cdots + \alpha_i + \zeta_{it} \qquad \begin{aligned} i &= 1, \ldots, N \\ t &= 0, \ldots, T-1 \end{aligned}$$

where the disturbance ζ_{it} is normally distributed and uncorrelated across time or persons; the random effect α_i varies between persons but is constant over time; x_1 is a dummy variable indicating experimental group ($x_{1i1} = 0$ for all i, $x_{1it} = 1$ when $t > 1$ and ith case in the intervention/0 otherwise); $x_2, \ldots$ are time-varying or time-invariant determinants of y. For simplicity, assume that $T = 2$. Suppose that $d_i = 1$ if y_{i2} is observed at $t = 2$, and $d_i = 0$ if y_{i2} is not observed, and that $d_i = 1$ if the latent variable

$$d_i^* = \gamma y_{i2} + \theta_1 x_{1i2} + \theta_2 x_{2i2} + \cdots + \underline{\delta} w_i + \varepsilon_i^* \geqslant 0$$

where $\underline{w}_i$ is a time invariant variable (or vector of variables) that does not affect y but does affect the probability of attrition, θ and $\underline{\delta}$ are coefficients, and ε_i^* is normally distributed. Estimation of β_1 utilizing only complete observations ($d_i = 1$) will lead to a biased estimate if γ and θ_1 are nonzero. To correct for this bias, the two defining equations just given can be combined into a joint model, and maximum likelihood procedures can be used to obtain an estimate of program effect. If the specified model is correct, then unbiased estimates are obtained. The success of this approach depends on measurement of factors $\underline{w}$ that are associated with attrition but are not determinants of drug use. This approach was applied to the Gary income maintenance experiment (Hausman & Wise, 1979); it could be applied to clinical trials and population experiments with nonrandom attrition.

STATISTICAL MODELS FOR LONGITUDINAL DATA

The following summary is organized around several distinguishing characteristics of statistical models:

1. Continuous versus categorical dependent variables
2. Random versus fixed individual effects
3. Static, growth curve, and dynamic models
4. Constant and variable coefficients
5. Continuous and discrete time models
6. Unidirectional and reciprocal systems

An additional distinction that would be necessary in a more rigorous treatment is that between deterministic and stochastic processes.

Before discussing various types of models it is useful to distinguish three components of a statistical model: measurement, structure, and density. An example of a model with all three components specified is the following, which is presumed to hold for each member of some population:

$$\underline{Y} = \underline{\tau} + \underline{\Lambda}\underline{\eta} + \underline{\varepsilon} \qquad \text{(measurement)} \qquad (6a)$$

$$\underline{\theta} = E(\underline{\varepsilon}\underline{\varepsilon}')$$

$$\underline{\eta} = \underline{\alpha} + \underline{\eta}\underline{B} + \underline{\zeta} \qquad \text{(structure)} \qquad (6b)$$

$$\underline{\Psi} = E(\underline{\zeta}\underline{\zeta}')$$

where E indicates expectation over members of a large population; $\underline{Y}$ is a $p \times 1$ vector of observed random variables; $\underline{\tau}$ is a $p \times 1$ vector of unknown intercepts; $\underline{\Lambda}$ is a $p \times q$ matrix of unknown coefficients relating q latent variables $\underline{\eta}$ to the observed variables; $\underline{\varepsilon}$ is a $p \times 1$ vector of unobserved measurement errors with $p \times p$ covariance matrix $\underline{\theta}$; $\underline{\alpha}$ is a $q \times 1$ vector of unknown intercepts for the structural portion of the model; $\underline{B}$ is a $q \times q$ matrix of unknown coefficients describing relations among latent variables and disturbances; $\underline{\zeta}$ is a $q \times 1$ matrix of unobserved disturbances with $q \times q$ covariance matrix $\underline{\Psi}$; the *density* portion of the model is specified by the assumption that the observed variables $\underline{Y}$ are multivariate normal in distribution.

For the parameters of such a model to be *identified*, it is necessary to place constraints on the elements of the various matrices and to assume that replicate observations are independent of one another. The various models discussed in the following sections may be specified as special cases of this general model. Logit (or probit) models for categorical variables may be similarly specified by replacing $\underline{Y}$ with $\underline{Y}^*$, where $y_j = 1$ if $y_j^* \geqslant 0$, $y_j = 0$ otherwise, and y_j^* is logistically (or normally) distributed with mean of zero and variance of $\pi^2/3$ (or 1). Extension to the case of more than two ordered categories is achieved via the proportional odds (original logit) or ordinal probit models.

The preceding specification assumes that all elements in $\underline{Y}$ are random variables. An alternative approach (for models with a clear distinction between dependent and predictor variables) is to assume that the dependent variables are random while the predictor variables are mathematical. Values of mathematical variables are observable constants rather than observed manifestations of random variables. However, the aspect of the model that is of primary substantive interest to researchers is the mean and covariance structure portion of the model.

The above model specification follows Jöreskog (1970a) and derives from the tradition of fitting linear models to Gaussian data with maximum likelihood. An alternative approach to model specification (see Chapter 8) is that of generalized linear models (GLMs) estimated by quasi-likelihood (cf. McCullagh & Nelder, 1983). Suppose, for example, that a single response random variables y_i is related to a fixed explanatory variable x_i. Then the GLM specification is

$$h[E(y_i)] = \alpha + \beta x_i \qquad \mathrm{var}(y_i) = g[E(y_i)]\phi$$

where E denotes expectation, h is a "link" function, g is a "variance" function, and ϕ is a "scale" or "shape" parameter. When y is Gaussian, h is the identity function, and g is $\mathrm{var}[E(y_i)]$, we have the usual linear regression model with $\phi = 1/r^2$ (where r is the correlation between y and x). When y is dichotomous (0 or 1), h is the logit transformation and $g[E(y_i)] = E(y_i)[1 - E(y_i)]$, the logistic regression model is obtained with $\phi = 1$.

Continuous versus Categorical Variables

A continuous variable is defined on a contiguous subset of real numbers, and it may change with continuous time. Blood pressure, for example, is a continuous variable with a continuous time path $y(t)$. Categorical variables, on the other hand, may be mapped onto a finite set of integers, and transitions between levels may occur in continuous or discrete time. Categorical variables may or may not be ordered and may or may not include an absorbing boundary. Diagnostic categories are examples of categorical variables; vital status is an example of a categorical variable with an absorbing boundary (mortality).

A simple model for continuous longitudinal data is the usual linear regression equation:

$$y_{it} = \alpha + \beta x_{it} + \zeta_{it} \tag{7}$$

where y and x are continuous variables observed at times t ($=0,\ldots,T-1$). Given appropriate constraints, the parameters α and β may be estimated.

A simple model for a dichotomous categorical outcome is the probit (or logistic):

$$\eta_{it} = \alpha + \beta x_{it} + \zeta_{it} \tag{8}$$

$$\text{prob}(y_{it} = 1) = \text{prob}(\eta_{it} \geq 0) = \int_{-\infty}^{\alpha+\beta x} N(z; 1, 0)\,dz \tag{9}$$

where "prob" indicates probability; y_{it} is the observed outcome (0 or 1) for the ith case on the tth occasion; η_{it} is a latent variable that may be interpreted as a mathematical convenience or as an unobserved continuous variable; ζ_{it} is uncorrelated with x_{it} and is conditionally distributed as the unit normal $[N(z; \sigma = 1, \mu = 0)]$; the covariance of ζ_{it} and $\zeta_{i't'}$ is zero if $i \neq i'$, is equal to $\psi_{tt'}$ (i.e., the elements of $\boldsymbol{\Psi}$) if $i = i'$. The logistic version of the model is specified by replacing $N(z; 1, 0)$ with the logistic distribution $G(z; \sigma^2 = \pi^2/3, \mu = 0)$. A more flexible version of this model allows the variance of ζ to change with time. Estimation of such probit models can be obtained with LISREL (Jöreskog & Sorbom, 1988) or LISCOMP (Muthèn, 1987).

The model specified in equations (8) and (9) is linear in the probit or logit of the probability of an event. For example, (8) can be rewritten for two predictor variables as

$$\log\left[\frac{\text{prob}(y_{it} = 1)}{1 - \text{prob}(y_{it} = 1)}\right] = \alpha + \beta_1 x_{1it} + \beta_2 x_{2it}$$

or

$$\frac{\text{prob}(y_{it} = 1)}{1 - \text{prob}(y_{it} = 1)} = e^{\alpha} e^{\beta_1 x_{1it}} e^{\beta_2 x_{2it}}$$

where, for events with low probability, the relationship of x_1 or x_2 with the probability of the event is presumed logarithmic, and the form of the multivariate model is multiplicative for the odds of an event. There may, of course, be circumstances in which such an assumption is inappropriate. A simple alternative is a linear relation between the probability and predictors; the multivariate model is additive in this instance, rather than multiplicative. Thomas (1981) has proposed an empirical approach to the choice of model by including a parameter in a composite model that selects the form of the model that is least interactive. However, when one of the two models is preferred on theoretical grounds, the presence or absence of interaction becomes the empirical issue.

A more specialized model for longitudinally observed categorical outcomes is one suited to mortality studies. The proportional hazards model (Cox, 1972) stems from a continuous-time differential equation with negative feedback. The model is appropriate when the dichotomous outcome involves a transition to an absorbing category (one from which there is no return). This model will be discussed further in the section of this chapter concerned with continuous-time models.

Random versus Fixed Individual Effects

Suppose that we observe the continuous random variables $y(t)$ and $x(t)$ at T discrete points in time ($t = 0, \ldots, T - 1$) among a sample of persons from a population. We may then suppose that y_{it} is generated by the following static process:

$$y_{it} = \alpha_i + \beta x_{it} + \zeta_{it} \tag{10}$$

where α_i is an "individual effect" and ζ_{it} is a random disturbance. This is a modification of (7), in which the terms α_i are variable intercepts; they allow the intercept to differ for each member of a population, whereas the slope is constrained to be the same for all members. These individual effects may be treated as manifestations of a random variable (random effects) or as fixed constants (fixed effects). In the case of the *random*-effects model we have the specification

$$E(\alpha_i) = \alpha \qquad E[(\alpha_i - \alpha)^2] = \sigma_{\alpha\alpha}$$

$$E[(\alpha_i - \alpha)(\alpha_{i'} - \alpha)] = 0 \qquad \text{if } i \neq i'$$

$$E(\zeta_{it}) = 0 \qquad E(\zeta_{it}, \zeta_{i't'}) = 0 \quad \text{if } i \neq i' \text{ or } t \neq t'$$

$$= \sigma_{\zeta\zeta} \quad \text{if } i = i'$$

$$E(\alpha_i \zeta_{it}) = E(x_{it} \zeta_{it}) = 0$$

where the variance of y_{it} conditional on x, $\sigma_{yy|x}$, is ($\sigma_{\alpha\alpha} + \sigma_{\zeta\zeta}$). An important additional constraint in the classic random-effects model (Wishart, 1938) is that $E[(\alpha_i - \alpha)x_{it}]$ is zero at each t.

The *fixed*-effects version of the model in (10) is specified as follows:

$$E(\alpha_i) = \alpha_i \qquad \text{(i.e., } \alpha_i \text{ is a fixed constant)}$$

$$E(\zeta_{it}) = 0, \qquad E(\zeta_{it}, \zeta_{i't'}) = \begin{cases} 0 & \text{if } i \neq i' \text{ or } t \neq t' \\ \sigma_{\zeta\zeta} & \text{if } i = i' \end{cases}$$

$$E(x_{it} \zeta_{it}) = E(\zeta_{it} | \alpha_i) = 0$$

where the variance of y_{it} conditional on x_{it} *and* α_i is $\sigma_{\zeta\zeta}$. Note that, in contrast to the random-effects model, there is no constraint on the dependence of x_{it} on α_i. In practice, β can be estimated by OLS in either of two ways: A dummy variable can be included for each individual or y_{it} and x_{it} can be transformed as deviations about their time series means ($y_{it} - \bar{y}_i$ and $x_{it} - \bar{x}_i$) before estimates are computed.

The choice between the random- and fixed-effects models should depend on how the individual effects are assumed to operate. It turns out, however, that the important difference between the two models is the assumption concerning the dependence between α_i and x_{it} (Mundlak, 1978). The random-effects model, estimated with a generalized least squares (GLS) estimator, assumes that these two random variables are uncorrelated. The fixed-effects model, estimated with an OLS estimator, allows an association. This association can be seen if we rewrite (10) as

$$y_{it} = \sum_{j=1}^{N} \alpha_i D_j + \beta x_{it} + \zeta_{it}$$

where the dummy variable $D_j = 1$ if $j = i$, and $D_j = 0$ when $j \neq i$. This dummy variable form of the model, estimated by OLS, makes it clear that the association between D_j and x_{it} is unconstrained. Furthermore, the random-effects model can be respecified such that $E[(\alpha_i - \alpha)x_{it}]$ $(\sigma_{\alpha x})$ is a free parameter, and then the GLS estimator of β in the random-effects model is equivalent to the OLS estimator of β in the fixed-effects model. Since it is reasonable to specify individual effects as random variables in most epidemiologic panel studies (because the particular individuals included in a sample are not of interest), this "modified" random-effects model will probably be more useful than the fixed-effects model.

The fact that the random-effects and modified random-effects models yield different estimators of β indicates that β is construed differently in the two models. The slope in the modified random-effects (or fixed-effects) model, β_m, is most easily understood. It is the expected value of the individual slope obtained from a time series regression of y_t on x_t for the ith member of a large population. Any differences between persons in level of y or x averaged over time are thus ignored. This kind of information, of course, is a major reason for conducting longitudinal studies: Individual differences in starting points due to unmeasured factors are removed. In contrast, the slope β_r from the random-effects model represents a mixture of cross-sectional *and* longitudinal information. And the mix is determined by the magnitude of "within-occasion" variance in x (interindividual variance) relative to "between-occasion" variance in x (intraindividual variance).

When there is considerable stability over time in x—as is the case with most variables of interest to epidemiologists—β_r tends to reflect primarily the cross-sectional association between y and x. What is of particular interest in longitudinal studies, however, is the difference between interindividual and intraindividual relations between y and x. In general, we expect the intraindividual covariances to be less confounded by selection bias and background variables than the interindividual covariances.

The case of only two occasions of measurement is instructive about the distinction between random-effects and modified random-effects models. If we include time effects in the modified random-effects version of (10)

$$y_{it} = \alpha_t + \alpha_i + \beta_m x_{it} + \zeta_{it} \tag{11}$$

(the α_t are constants, $E[\alpha_i] = 0$), then the ML estimator $\hat{\beta}_m$ is identical to the OLS estimator of b in the model

$$y_{i1} - y_{i0} = b_0 + b(x_{i1} - x_{i0}) + \varepsilon_i \tag{12}$$

where ε_i is uncorrelated with $(x_{i1} - x_{i0})$ and $T = 2$ (only two occasions of measurement). In fact, the estimators $\hat{\beta}_m$, the fixed-effects estimator of (11), and $\hat{b}$ are all identical in this instance. This can be seen by applying the method of moments to (12) to obtain

$$b = \frac{\sigma_{y_1 x_1} + \sigma_{y_0 x_0} - \sigma_{y_1 x_0} - \sigma_{y_0 x_1}}{\sigma_{x_1 x_1} + \sigma_{x_0 x_0} - 2\sigma_{x_1 x_0}} \tag{13a}$$

The OLS estimator $\hat{b}$ is then obtained by replacing moments with sample estimates. The parameter β_m is defined from (11) as follows:

$$\beta_m = \frac{\sigma_{y_0 x_0} - \sigma_{\alpha_i x_0}}{\sigma_{x_0 x_0}}$$

$$= \frac{\sigma_{y_1 x_1} - \sigma_{\alpha_i x_1}}{\sigma_{x_1 x_1}}$$

$$= \frac{\sigma_{y_0 x_1} - \sigma_{\alpha_i x_1}}{\sigma_{x_0 x_1}}$$

$$= \frac{\sigma_{y_1 x_0} - \sigma_{\alpha_i x_0}}{\sigma_{x_0 x_1}}$$

Solving these four equations for $\sigma_{\alpha_i x_0}$, $\sigma_{\alpha_i x_1}$, and β_m (and replacing population moments with sample estimates) yields the same estimator of slope found in (13a). Furthermore, estimation of $\sigma_{\alpha_i x_0}$ and $\sigma_{\alpha_i x_1}$ allows a test of the random-versus modified random-effects models; if the null hypothesis that $\sigma_{\alpha_i x_0} = \sigma_{\alpha_i x_1} = \cdots = \sigma_{\alpha_i x_t} = \cdots = 0$ can be rejected, then the random-effects model can be rejected in favor of the modified model.

An important general point here is that researchers are often confused when substantive differences in model specification (i.e., which parameters are fixed to specific values and which are estimated) become confounded with estimation techniques or variable definitions that are of primarily mathematical interest. In the case of models for longitudinal data, this has been the case. The constraint that individual effects in y are uncorrelated with x has been confounded with generalized least squares estimation and random effects; allowing this covariance to be a free parameter has been confounded with OLS or ML and fixed effects.

Individual effects may also be incorporated into models for categorical variables. For example, suppose that the model in (8) and (9) is rewritten as

$$\eta_{it} = \alpha_i + \beta x_{it} + \zeta_{it}$$

$$\text{prob}(y_{it} = 1) = \text{prob}(\eta_{it} \geq 0) = \int_{-\infty}^{\alpha+\beta x} N(z; 0, 1)\, dz$$

where α_i is a modified random effect and N is the normal density (or logistic density) with zero mean and unit variance (zero mean and variance $\pi^2/3$). The estimate of β is then derived from the relationship between change in risk and change in x. In the ordinal probit form, software is readily available for the computation of weighted least squares estimates for large samples (Jöreskog & Sorbom, 1988).

An alternative approach to specification of models with individual specific parameters is in terms of GLMs (Zeger, Liang, & Albert, 1988). For example, a random-response y_{it} observed at T points in time may be related to the fixed covariate x_{it} by the model

$$h[E(y_{it} \mid a_i, b_i)] = \alpha + a_i + (\beta + b_i)x_i$$

$$\text{var}(y_{it} \mid a_i, b_i) = g[E(y_i \mid a_i, b_i)]\phi$$

where α and β are fixed effects; a_i and b_i are random effects from a mixture distribution. This very general model allows heterogeneity in both level (a_i) and slope (b_i) regression parameters for continuous or categorical y. However, estimation techniques for categorical y_i are in the developmental stage. Such models are variously described by different authors as "individual specific" or "subject-specific," or as including "random coefficients" or "random effects."

Empirical Examples

The blood pressure and relative weight data from the Framingham study can be used to clarify further the distinction between the random- and modified random-effects models. We use data from the third through the fifth examinations for men aged 32 through 38 years at baseline ($N = 576$). Multivariate normal ML estimates of the three cross-sectional regression coefficients are as follows:

$$y_{it} = \alpha_t + \beta_t x_{it} + \zeta_{it} \tag{13b}$$

$$y_{i0} = 88.2(4.6) + .316(.038)x_{i0} \qquad \hat{\rho} = .330 \tag{13c}$$

$$y_{i1} = 91.8(5.1) + .299(.042)x_{i1} \qquad \hat{\rho} = .288 \tag{13d}$$

$$y_{i2} = 89.6(5.2) + .321(.043)x_{i2} \qquad \hat{\rho} = .301 \tag{13e}$$

where estimated standard errors are given in parentheses; y_{it} = systolic blood pressure (SBP, first measurement) at the tth examination, x_{it} = metropolitan relative weight (RW); the only identifying constraint is the within-equation specification that $\sigma_{\zeta_{it}x_{it}} = 0$ (while $\sigma_{\zeta_{it}x_{it'}}$ is unconstrained when $t \neq t'$); ρ is the product-moment correlation between y_{it} and x_{it}. The mean of SBP increased from 126.2 to 127.9 to 128.5 mm Hg, and the standard deviation of SBP increased from 15.3 to 16.7 to 17.6 over the three examinations. The mean and standard deviation of RW also showed slight increases: 120.3 (16.0 SD), 121.0 (16.1), 121.1 (16.5) percent of ideal weight.

Constraining the three slopes (β_t) in (13b) to be equal across examinations yields a goodness of fit χ^2 of 0.45 with 2 degrees of freedom ($p = .80$) for the model

$$y_{it} = \alpha_t + \beta x_{it} + \zeta_{it} \tag{14}$$

where $\hat{\alpha}_t = 88.5$ (4.2), 90.0 (4.2), 90.6 (4.2); $\hat{\beta} = .313$ (.034) for $t = 0, 1, 2$; $\sigma_{\zeta_{it}\zeta_{i't'}}$ is unconstrained if $i = i'$ and zero if $i \neq i'$ (that replications are independent is assumed throughout the following); $\sigma_{x_{it}\zeta_{it'}}$ is zero for $t = t'$ and unconstrained for $t \neq t'$. The small χ^2 value indicates that the hypothesis of constant slope over the three examinations cannot be rejected. The smaller standard error for the constrained model reflects the increased precision achieved from pooling the three cross-sectional sets of data. The model in (14) makes use of the longitudinal observations to increase precision, but uses only the cross-sectional information to define β: β in (14) is a weighted average of the β_t in (13b).

The "random-effects" alternative to (13b) is specified by

$$y_{it} = \alpha_t + \alpha_i + \beta x_{it} + \zeta_{it} \tag{15}$$

where α_t are fixed constants; $\sigma_{\zeta_{it}\zeta_{it'}}$ is unconstrained when $t = t'$ and zero when $t \neq t'$ (Ψ is diagonal); $\sigma_{x_{it}\zeta_{it'}}$ is zero for all t and t'; α_i is a random variable with $E(\alpha_i) = E(\alpha_i x_{it}) = E(\alpha_i \zeta_{it}) = 0$ and $E(\alpha_i^2) = \sigma_{\alpha\alpha}$ for all t. Assumption of the model in (15) yields the estimate $\hat{\beta} = .366$ (.032), which is 17 percent larger in magnitude than the cross-sectional estimate in (14); the estimate of $\sigma_{\alpha\alpha}$ is 156.0 (11.1). The increase in slope arises because the random-effects estimator is a weighted average of cross-sectional and longitudinal slopes; as we shall see subsequently, the longitudinal slopes are larger than the cross-sectional slopes in this data set. However, the goodness-of-fit chi-square for the model in (15) is considerably larger than its degrees of freedom: $\chi^2 = 45.33$ (df $= 10$, $p < .001$).

This lack of fit suggests that the constraint of no correlation between α_i and x_{it} may be inconsistent with the data. Relaxing this constraint uses 3 degrees of freedom (for estimates of the three covariances) and reduces the χ^2 to 23.88 (df $= 7$). The resulting "modified" random-effects estimates are

$$\hat{\alpha}_t = 49.8 \ (8.6), \ 51.0 \ (8.7), \ 51.5 \ (8.7)$$

$$\hat{\beta} = .635 \ (.071)$$

$$\hat{\sigma}_{\alpha\alpha} = 184.0 \ (17.5)$$

$$\hat{\sigma}_{\alpha_i x_{it}} = -85.6 \ (20.6), \ -86.5 \ (20.8), \ -81.6 \ (21.1)$$

where estimation again assumes multivariate normality of all observed and unobserved variables. The fit of the modified model is improved further by constraining $\sigma_{\alpha_i x_{it}}$ to be equal for all t, and allowing the effect of α_i to vary over time:

$$y_{it} = \alpha_t + \lambda_t \alpha_i + \beta x_{it} + \zeta_{it} \tag{16}$$

where $\lambda_0 = 1$. The χ^2 reduces to 10.65 (df = 7, p = .16), and the estimate of β is 0.620 (.067).

It is clear from these results that the longitudinal slope is much larger than the cross-sectional slope: the estimate from (16) is 1.98 times the cross-sectional estimate in (13). The slopes in equations (13) and (14) indicate that SBP increases with RW across persons of different RW. These are interindividual covariances of interindividual differences, indicating that a 1-unit increase in RW is associated with a 0.33-unit increase in SBP. However, this cross-sectional association may be a biased estimator of the expected *intra*individual change in SBP after *intra*individual change in RW, as we found in these data from Framingham. There are numerous possible sources of such bias. Many of these sources can be summarized in terms of *misspecifications* of the assumed linear model. For example, relevant variables may have been omitted from the model specified in (13) or (14), or the specification that the residuals are uncorrelated with x may be inappropriate because of selection bias (e.g., persons with high SBP are less likely to be included in the observations).

The random-effects (equation [15]) and modified random-effects (equation [16]) models utilize the measures of intraindividual change in longitudinal data to avoid some of the sources of mispecification in the cross-sectional model (equation [14]). The random-effects model controls for time-invariant omitted determinants of y that are uncorrelated with x; the modified random-effects model (or fixed-effects model) allows these omitted variables to be correlated with x. The modified random-effects model also allows for association between disturbances and x due to selection bias. For example, if persons with high blood pressure are less likely to participate, the cross-sectional slope of SBP on RW will be attenuated. This situation can be constructed as equivalent to one in which a determinant of SBP has been omitted from the model.

As mentioned previously, the modified random-effects model (or fixed-effects model) yields similar estimates of slope to a "change score" regression model. The change score model can be derived from (16) (assuming that $\lambda_t = 1$ for all t) by subtraction:

$$y_{it} - y_{i,t-1} = \alpha_t - \alpha_{t-1} + \beta(x_{it} - x_{i,t-1}) + \zeta_{it} - \zeta_{i,t-1} \qquad (17)$$

where $(x_{it} - x_{i,t-1})$ is assumed to be uncorrelated with $(\zeta_{it} - \zeta_{i,t-1})$. Notice that the individual effects (α_i in [16]) have been filtered by the differencing. The ML estimate of β obtained from (17) is 0.600 (.079), which is very similar in magnitude to the modified random-effects estimate from (16): .620 (.067). Notice, however, that the estimated standard error is larger in the difference equation (.079/.067 = 1.18), suggesting greater power for the modified random-effects model.

In addition to the three alternative error structures just described (random effects, fixed effects, modified random effects), there is the specification described previously under "Regression to the Mean." In this case a dynamic (or autoregressive) structure is assumed for the disturbances. Such a model can be considered a generalization of the random-effects or modified random-effects model where, for example,

$$\zeta_{it} = \gamma\zeta_{i,t-1} + v_{it}$$

with $E(v_{it})$ and $E(v_{it}\zeta_{i,t-1})$ equal to zero. In the next section we consider models in which such a dynamic process is incorporated into the observed variable portion of the model.

Static, Growth Curve, and Dynamic Models

Static models relate a dependent variable (say y) to a predictor variable (say x) such that change (or expected change) in y with respect to x (dy/dx) is the focus. Models concerned with change in y with respect to time (dy/dt), where $y(t)$ is an explicit polynomial function of time, are here termed *growth curve models*. A model becomes *dynamic* (or autoregressive) when change in y through time is the focus, and y_{it} is a function of $y_{i,t-\tau}$ for $\tau \geq 1$ (in discrete time), or dy_i/dt is a function of $y_i(t)$ (in continuous time). The derivative dy/dt is, in this instance, not necessarily an explicit function of time, but rather a function of y and other variables. Dynamic models have the advantage that they can come to equilibrium through "negative feedback." Static models do not take account of change through time, while growth curve models explode or collapse in the long run. Dynamic models have the additional advantage that they can include reciprocal relations between variables; the direction of influence must be specified for static and growth curve models—even though the directionality may be in question, or may be reciprocal.

An example of a static model is the modified random effects version of (10) with time effects (see [16]):

$$y_{it} = \alpha_t + \lambda_t\alpha_i + \beta x_{it} + \zeta_{it}$$

where α_i is free to covary with x_{it}. The focus here is the slope β, which is $\partial y/\partial x$; $\partial\zeta/\partial x$ is presumed zero. Static models can be expanded to include multiple predictors, powers of predictors, and interactions among predictors.

Growth curve models are special cases of static models in which the predictor variable is time. They may be derived from continuous time differentials:

$$\frac{dy_i}{dt} = \alpha_1 + \alpha_2 t + \alpha_3 t^2 + \cdots + \frac{d\zeta_i}{dt} \tag{18}$$

where the coefficients are presumed constant across persons; $d\zeta_i/dt$ is the derivative of an approximation to continuous time white noise (e.g., a Wiener process). The metric t is chronologic time. The integrated form of (18) in continuous time is

$$y_i(t) = \alpha_i + \alpha_1 t + \left(\frac{\alpha_2}{2}\right) t^2 + \left(\frac{\alpha_3}{3}\right) t^3 + \cdots + \zeta_i(t) \tag{19}$$

where $\zeta_i(t)$ is a Wiener process (cf. Karlin & Taylor, 1981). The model in (19) can then be adapted to the discrete time circumstance of most longitudinal studies to obtain

$$y_{it} = \alpha_{0i} + \alpha_1 t + \left(\frac{\alpha_2}{2}\right) t^2 + \left(\frac{\alpha_3}{3}\right) t^3 + \cdots + \zeta_{it} \tag{20}$$

where α_i may be a random or modified random (or fixed) effect and ζ_{it} is uncorrelated with α_i and t^p ($p = 1, 2, 3, \ldots$). If individuals in a population differ on some exogenous variable x, then (20) can be extended (Grizzle & Allen, 1969):

$$y_{it} = \alpha_{0i} + \alpha_1 x_i t + \left(\frac{\alpha_2}{2}\right) x_i t^2 + \left(\frac{\alpha_3}{3}\right) x_i t^3 + \cdots + \zeta_{it}$$

where a different growth curve is obtained for each value of x.

When the metric t is replaced by chronologic (or bone) age, there is generally some within-occasion variance in age (interindividual variance). However, if subsequent observations are equally spaced in time, then change in age is identical for all members of the sample. An integrated model in this instance may be written

$$y_{i0} = \alpha_{0i} + \alpha_1 A_{i0} + \left(\frac{\alpha_2}{2}\right) A_{i0}^2 + \cdots + \zeta_{i0}$$

$$y_{i1} = \alpha_{0i} + \alpha_1 (A_{i0} + 1) + \left(\frac{\alpha_2}{2}\right) (A_{i0} + 1)^2 + \cdots + \zeta_{i1}$$

$$\vdots$$

$$y_{it} = \alpha_{0i} + \alpha_1 (A_{i0} + t) + \left(\frac{\alpha_2}{2}\right) (A_{i0} + t)^2 + \cdots + \zeta_{it}$$

$$\vdots$$

where α_{0i} is a modified random effect; $\boldsymbol{\Psi}$ is diagonal; $E(\zeta_{it} A_i^p) = 0$ for all $t > 0$, but is unconstrained for $t = 0$. This specification allows for starting at different ages and for individual differences in the height of the curve; but the shape of the curve (specified by the slopes) is identical for all cases.

When an hypothesis concerning the growth process generates a specific mathematical form of the model, a stronger model results. In this instance the parameters of the model may have biologically meaningful interpretations. This is in contrast to the generic polynomial model. A simple example of a strong model is Robertson's logistic growth curve

$$\frac{dy}{dt} = \alpha_1 y(t) + \alpha_2 y^2(t) = -\alpha_2 y(t) \left[-\left(\frac{\alpha_1}{\alpha_2}\right) - y(t) \right] \tag{21}$$

where $-\alpha_1/\alpha_2$ might be the mature height of an organism. The mature height is the equilibrium value of $y(t)$, where dy/dt is zero. This can be seen by setting (21) equal to zero and solving for $y(t)$:

$$\alpha_1 y + \alpha_2 y^2 = 0 \Rightarrow y(\alpha_1 + \alpha_2 y) = 0$$

which is satisfied by the values $y(t) = 0$ and $y(t) = -\alpha_1/\alpha_2$. The rationale behind (21) is that the height (or other size parameter) "feeds back" to the rate of growth such that the rate of growth, dy/dt, increases until height approaches mature height; then the rate of growth declines until height reaches the equilibrium. The rate of growth increases until $(\alpha_1 + 2\alpha_2 y)$ is zero, where $y(t) = -\alpha_1/2\alpha_2$ (the inflection point obtained from differentiating (21) to obtain the second derivative, $d^2 y/dt^2$, and setting it equal to zero).

Integrating (21) gives

$$y(t) = -\frac{\alpha_1}{\alpha_2}\left(\frac{e^{\alpha_0 + \alpha_1 t}}{1 + e^{\alpha_0 + \alpha_1 t}}\right)$$

which makes it clear that α_1 specifies the rapidity with which $y(t)$ approaches the equilibrium, while the ratio $-(\alpha_1/\alpha_2)$ specifies an equilibrium level of $y(t)$ as $t \to \infty$ (when $\alpha_1 > 0$ and $\alpha_2 < 0$).

The logistic growth curve does not make very strong assumptions about the growth process, but it at least imposes some biologic meaning to the parameters of the model. Other strong models for follow-up data and exposure histories are discussed in Chapter 14.

Since the logistic growth model involves feedback, it serves as an introduction to dynamic models. The dynamic model most analogous to (21) is a continuous-time dynamic model; these models will be discussed in the section of this chapter on continuous-time models and in Chapter 3. The following discussion focuses on discrete-time dynamic models.

Dynamic Models

An example of a discrete-time *dynamic model* for continuous variables is the following:

$$y_{it} = \alpha_i + \beta_1 y_{i,t-1} + \beta_2 x_{it} + \zeta_{it} \tag{22}$$

where $E(\zeta_{it}) = 0$; $E(\zeta_{it}\zeta_{i't'}) = 0$ (if $i \neq i'$) or ψ_{tt} (if $i = i'$ and $t = t'$); ζ_{it} is uncorrelated with x_{it} and $y_{i,t-1}$; the coefficients are constant over individuals and time; x and y are random variables; α_i is a random effect. This model is dynamic in the sense that change in y through time (from y_{t-1} to y_t) is explained by the model. This can be seen by rewriting (22) as

$$y_{it} - y_{i,t-1} = \alpha_i + (\beta_1 - 1)y_{i,t-1} + \beta_2 x_{it} + \zeta_{it}$$

where $(\beta_1 - 1)$ will generally be negative. Dynamic models are sometimes referred to as *conditional* (static and growth-curve models are termed *unconditional*) since the regression of change in y on x is conditioned on the earlier value of y.

While dynamic models have several advantages over static models, the dynamic model in (22) is specified in discrete time, and the parameters of the model are specific to the observation lag in a particular study. Furthermore, the model is necessarily a rough approximation since it depicts change as occurring only at the time of examination. In the section concerning continuous-time models we will construct a dynamic model that is the integrated form of a continuous-time differential. In that instance the coefficients of the differential equation model have a more realistic temporal interpretation.

Empirical Example

To this point we have ignored nonsampling measurement error in the dependent variable because it does not bias estimates in static models. However, dynamic models involve lagged values of the dependent variable as predictors, and measurement error can in this instance introduce bias into estimates of coefficients. Thus we return to the Framingham systolic blood pressure and relative weight data described previously. In this instance, however, we will utilize data from two measurements of SBP (SBPa and SBPb) at each of six examinations (3 through 8).

We begin with the model in equation (22), except that it will be extended to include a model for x (RW) as well as y (SBP) and a measurement error model for y. The measurement portion of the model is specified as it was previously:

$$y_{1it} = \tau_{1t} + \eta_{it} + \varepsilon_{1it} \qquad y_{2it} = \tau_{2t} + \eta_{it} + \varepsilon_{2it} \tag{23}$$

where y_{1it} is the first measure of SBP for the ith person at the tth examination and y_{2it} is the second measurement; τ_{jt} are constant intercepts; η_{it} is the expected SBP (without measurement error); ε_{jit} is the measurement error; $E(\eta_{it}) = E(\varepsilon_{jit}) = E(\eta_{it}\varepsilon_{jit}) = 0$, and $E(\varepsilon_{jit}\varepsilon_{j'i't'}) = \theta_{tt}$ (if $j = j'$ and $i = i'$ and $t = t'$) or 0 (otherwise). Relative weight is presumed to have been measured without error. The structural portion of the model is then specified as follows:

$$\eta_{it} = \alpha_t + \lambda_t\alpha_i + \alpha_1 x_{it} + \alpha_2 \eta_{i,t-1} + \zeta_{\eta it} \tag{24a}$$

$$x_{it} = \beta_t + \gamma_t\beta_i + \beta_2 x_{i,t-1} + \zeta_{xit} \tag{24b}$$

where $\alpha_t, \alpha_1, \alpha_2, \lambda_t, \beta_t, \beta_2,$ and γ_t are unknown coefficients to be estimated; α_1 and β_i are random individual effects with variances $\sigma_{\alpha\alpha}$ and $\sigma_{\beta\beta}$; λ and γ vary over time, but are fixed to 1 at $t = 0$; the random disturbances ζ have zero expectation; and

$$E(\zeta_{\eta it}\zeta_{\eta i't'}) = E(\zeta_{xit}\zeta_{xi't'}) = E(\zeta_{\eta it}\zeta_{xi't'}) = 0$$

(unless $i = i'$ and $t = t'$);

$$E(\zeta_{\eta it}\eta_{i,t-1-m}) = E(\zeta_{\eta it}x_{i,t-1-m}) = E(\zeta_{xit}x_{i,t-1-m}) = E(\zeta_{\eta it}x_{i,t-1-m}) = 0$$

for $t = 1, \ldots, T-1$ and $m = 0, \ldots, t$. Finally, it is assumed that all observed variables have a multivariate normal distribution.

Maximum likelihood estimates of the coefficients in (24) (with standard errors) are as follows:

$$\hat{\alpha}_1 = .040 \; (.018) \qquad \hat{\alpha}_2 = .378 \; (.038)$$

$$\hat{\beta}_2 = .539 \; (.026)$$

$$\hat{\sigma}_{\alpha\alpha} = 59.8 \; (10.9) \qquad \hat{\sigma}_{\beta\beta} = 53.4 \; (7.0)$$

suggesting a small positive effect of RW on change in SBP. However, if the random-effects constraints that $E(\alpha_i x_{it}) = E(\beta_i \eta_{it}) = 0$ are relaxed, yielding a dynamic analog to the "modified" random-effects model above, then $\hat{\alpha}_1$ increases to .146 (.027). These constraints are relaxed by incorporating $E(\alpha_i x_{i0})$ and $E(\beta_i \eta_{i0})$ as parameters in the model. If the random effects are removed from the model entirely, the resulting estimate of α_1 is close to zero: $-.003$ (.012). Thus incorporation of the random effects, and then allowing them to be correlated with the predictor variable, progressively increases the magnitude of the estimated effect of relative weight on blood pressure.

Variable Coefficients

We previously considered random and fixed effects as variable intercepts in a static linear model. The notion of variable intercepts can be extended to include variable slopes as well. For example, the model

$$y_{it} = \alpha_i + \beta_i x_{it} + \zeta_{it} \tag{25a}$$

where $E(\zeta_{it}) = 0$ and $E(\zeta_{it} x_{i't'}) = 0$ if $i = i'$ or $t = t'$ (but is otherwise unconstrained), allows a line with different intercept and slope to be fitted to data from each person in a population. The variables α_i and β_i may be treated as either random variables or fixed constants. When variability in β_i exceeds that expected by sampling error, the relationship between y and x is said to be subject to heterogeneity. When the covariance of α_i and β_i is unconstrained, $E(\beta_i)$ is the slope in the corresponding modified random effects model.

The model in (25a) may be extended to the case in which α_i and β_i are treated as stochastic variables (Rao, 1965). For example, the equation

$$\hat{\beta}_i = \gamma_0 + \gamma_1 Z_i + v_i \tag{25b}$$

$$\hat{\beta}_i = \beta_i + \varepsilon_i \qquad v_i = v_i^* + \varepsilon_i$$

where $\hat{\beta}_i$ is a sample estimate of β_i, Z is a measured variable that is invariant with time, and $E(v_i^*) = E(\varepsilon_i) = E(v_i^* Z_i) = E(\varepsilon_i Z_i) = E(\varepsilon_i \beta_i) = 0$.

A special case of a combined model consisting of (25a) and (25b) is where x is equal to time or age. If powers of t are included in (25a), we have a polynomial stochastic growth curve model. Such a model enables a researcher to assess the relationship between background factors and the shape of the growth curve, or to relate characteristics of growth curves on alternate dimensions.

Estimation of variable coefficient models when the predictor variable in (25a) is time of measurement (or age) can be handled with programs for estimating covariance structures (e.g., Jöreskog & Sorbom, 1988). However, when relations among time-varying variables are used, specialized software is necessary.

Empirical Example

As an illustration of the application of the variable coefficient models we again return to the blood pressure (y) and relative weight (x) data from Framingham. In this instance we use data from examinations 3 through 6.

Lauer, Clarke, and Beaglehole (1984) have analyzed blood pressure and relative weight data from children. The longitudinally observed variables were regressed on age to estimate the slope (trend) and intercept (level). The following model is similar. However, estimated slopes and intercepts for individuals are not actually computed; rather, ML estimates of covariances between the variable coefficients are obtained. The model is specified as follows:

$$y_{it} = \alpha_i + (t - \bar{t})\beta_i + \varepsilon_{it} \qquad\qquad x_{it} = \gamma_i + (t - \bar{t})\lambda_i + \delta_{it}$$

$$\alpha_i = \omega_1 + \omega_2\gamma_i + \omega_3\lambda_i + \zeta_{1i}$$

$$\beta_i = \omega_4 + \omega_5\gamma_i + \omega_6\lambda_i + \zeta_{2i}$$

where α_i and β_i are intercepts and slopes for blood pressure regressed on time; γ_i and λ_i are intercepts and slopes for relative weight regressed on time; the deviations from linearity, ε and δ, are presumed uncorrelated with one another and with the variable coefficients and have an expectation of zero; the coefficients ω are to be estimated; $E(\zeta_1) = E(\zeta_2) = 0$, $E(\zeta_1\zeta_2)$ is unconstrained, and the ζ are uncorrelated with the variable coefficients.

Maximum likelihood estimates of the model parameters from the Framingham data (assuming multivariate normality and letting $\bar{t} = 0$, $t = 0, 1, 2, 3$) are as follows:

$$\hat{\omega}_1 = 89.05 \ (4.59) \qquad \hat{\omega}_2 = .31 \ (.04) \ [.38] \qquad \hat{\omega}_3 = -.55 \ (.37) \ [-.08]$$

$$\hat{\omega}_4 = 2.34 \ (1.51) \qquad \hat{\omega}_5 = -.01 \ (.01) \ [-.07] \qquad \hat{\omega}_6 = .64 \ (.12) \ [.53]$$

where standard errors are given in parentheses and standardized values are given in brackets. The magnitudes of these coefficients suggest their origins. The coefficient ω_2 is an aggregate of cross-sectional slopes; the intercept of SBP at four examinations is being regressed on the intercept of four measures of RW. The coefficient ω_6 relates the time trend in SBP to the time trend in RW; the resulting coefficient is similar to that found for the regression of change on change or the modified random-effects model (see "Random versus Fixed Individual Effects").

Alternative specifications of the model could involve selecting a different value for $\bar{t}$ (e.g., a midpoint), or including α_i as a predictor of β_i. In the case of these particular data, however, such changes alter the estimated regression coefficients only slightly. The reason is that α_i and β_i are virtually uncorrelated ($\hat{\rho} = -.01$).

What is of particular interest here is the lack of relationship between level of RW and trend in SBP ($\hat{\omega}_5$ is actually negative). If it is hypothesized that the association between RW and SBP is due to a causal effect of RW on SBP, then this finding might appear counter to the hypothesis. However, in systems that equilibrate over time periods that are shorter than the observation lag in a longitudinal study, time trend in the dependent variable will tend not to be associated with the level of the causal variable. The reason for this is that adjustment of the dependent variable to change in the independent variable produces a higher equilibrium level for the dependent variable rather than a steeper slope over a period longer than the adjustment phase. This issue is addressed in Chapter 3 and briefly in the next section.

Continuous- versus Discrete-Time Models

As mentioned previously, discrete-time dynamic models are limited by the unrealistic assumption that change occurs at discrete points in time. Linear equations specified in terms of variables observed at examination times are discrete-time models. Interpretation of the coefficients of such models is limited by two factors. First, the process presumed to operate by the researcher is continuous with time, usually involving gradual adjustment of a dependent variable to a new equilibrium level after a change in a causal variable. Second, the coefficients of discrete-time models are tied to the length of time between observations; this characteristic hampers comparison of findings between studies of different design.

The logistic (or probit) regression model applied to mortality data is an example of a discrete-time model for categorical outcomes (see Chapter 7). In contrast, the hazard model is a continuous-time model. As with most continuous-time models, it is cast in terms of a differential equation:

$$\frac{dy}{dt} = -h(t)y(t) \qquad h(t) = \lim_{\Delta t \to 0} \left\{ \frac{y(t) - y(t + \Delta t)}{\Delta t y(t)} \right\}$$

where $h(t)$ is referred to as the hazard rate and $y(t)$ is the number of persons surviving to time t. This simple dynamic model specifies that the level of $y(t)$ feeds back to determine the rate at which $y(t)$ declines. The hazard rate is then -1 times the slope of the survival curve divided by its height: the instantaneous rate of change in the probability of failure per unit time, given survival to t. The rationale for this formulation is that the "hazard" inherent in the rate of decline in the survival curve $(-dy/dt)$ increases as the height of the curve $[y(t)]$ decreases.

The integrated form of the hazard model depends on the form of $y(t)$. If $y(t) = Ne^{-\beta t}$, then $h(t)$ is constant and equal to β, since $dy/dt = -\beta N e^{-\beta t} = -\beta y(t)$. In this instance the probability of mortality between time t_1 and t_2 $(t_2 > t_1)$, conditional on survival to t_1, is then $[y(t_1) - y(t_2)]/y(t_1)$ or $[1 - e^{-\beta(t_2 - t_1)}]$, which is zero when $t_1 = t_2$ and approaches one as $(t_2 - t_1)$ increases.

The advantage of the continuous-time hazard formulation is that differences between groups in $h(t)$ are independent of the length of follow-up used to estimate $h(t)$ for each group. This is clear in the case where $h(t)$ is presumed constant over time in each group. In Cox's "proportional" formulation of the hazard model, the form of $y(t)$ is not specified. It is assumed, however, that the shape of $y(t)$ for the groups being compared (say $y_0(t)$ and $y_1(t)$) is such that $h_1(t)/h_0(t)$ would be constant for all t. This line of reasoning can be extended to the case where $h_x(t)/h_{x=0}(t)$ is constant over t but varies with values of the variable x. The form of the covariance between the ratio of hazards and x is often assumed to be exponential:

$$\frac{h_x(t)}{h_{x=0}(t)} = e^{\beta x}$$

where the intercept is necessarily zero (since the ratio of hazards is 1 when $x = 0$). Analogous continuous-time models for categorical outcomes without absorbing boundaries are also available (cf. Karlin & Taylor, 1981).

While biomedical researchers are generally familiar with continuous-time models for events, they are less aware of continuous-time dynamic models for continuous variables. As with the hazard model, we begin by assuming that change in $y(t)$ is determined by its own level and that the relationship is deterministic:

$$\frac{dy(t)}{dt} = \alpha_1 + \alpha_3 y(t) \tag{26}$$

where the coefficients are unknown constants. The fact that the coefficients do not vary with time prescribes $y(t)$ to a linear functional form, since (26) implies that

$$y(t) = \alpha_0 e^{\alpha_3 t} - \frac{\alpha_1}{\alpha_3} \tag{27}$$

where α_0 is the constant obtained when integrating (26). When $\alpha_3 < 0$, (27) implies that $y(t)$ approaches $-\alpha_1/\alpha_3$ as $t \to \infty$. The rapidity with which $y(t)$ approaches this equilibrium point is a function of the magnitude of α_3. Thus this equation appears attractive as a building block for a continuous-time model in which the impact of a causal variable takes place through time.

It turns out that (26) is a convenient building block for a continuous-time model that can be estimated with panel data. It can be shown, for example, that if (26) is expanded to a two-variable system

$$\frac{dy}{dt} = \alpha_1 + \alpha_2 x(t) + \alpha_3 y(t) \quad \text{for } t \geqslant 0 \tag{28}$$

$$\frac{dx}{dt} = \beta_j \qquad \text{for } t_j \leqslant t < t_{j+1}$$

where the t_j correspond to discrete measurement times, then the following discrete-time linear model

$$y_t = a_1 + a_2 x_{t-1} + a_3 y_{t-1} + a_4(x_t - x_{t-1}) \tag{29}$$

can be used to estimate the parameters of (28); the coefficients α_j in (28) are functions of the coefficients a_j in (29). In Chapter 3 such models are extended to the stochastic case and their application is demonstrated.

Unidirectional and Reciprocal Systems

A major advantage of dynamic models is that they provide the opportunity to specify reciprocal systems. We shall here consider a discrete-time system for continuous variables. (Continuous-time models with reciprocal effects are treated in Chapter 3.)

A reciprocal discrete-time model may be specified as an extension of the unidirectional model in (24). That is, we consider the case where each of two (or more) variables can influence one another. Such a model is specified in the empirical example at the end of this section, where y_t is a function of x_t and y_{t-1}, and x_t is a function of y_t and x_{t-1}. The discrete-time aspect of this model stems from its assumption that reciprocal adjustments of x to change in y, and of y to change in x, occur at the time of measurement. The process of adjustment to change occurring between $t = 0$ and $t = 1$ can be described for the deterministic case as follows: The observed values y_{i1} and x_{i1} are presumed to result from an iterative reciprocal adjustment process

$$y_{i1}^{j+1} = \alpha_1 x_{i1}^j + \alpha_2 y_{i0} \qquad x_{i1}^{j+1} = \beta_1 y_{i1}^{j+1} + \beta_2 x_{i0}$$

where j indexes iterations ($j = 1, \ldots, \infty$); the iterative sequence begins with $x_{i1}^1 = \beta_2 x_{i0}$ and iterates until y and x equilibrate (i.e., $y^j = y^{j+1}$ and $x^j = x^{j+1}$); an equivalent result occurs if the iterations begin with $y_{i1}^1 = \alpha_2 y_{i0}$.

Now, to generalize, suppose that a system involves reciprocal effects between two random variables y and x such that

$$y_{it} = \alpha_t + \alpha_1 x_{it} + \alpha_2 y_{i,t-1} + \zeta_{yit}$$

$$x_{it} = \beta_t + \beta_1 y_{it} + \beta_2 x_{i,t-1} + \zeta_{xit}$$

where

$$E(\zeta_{xit}) = E(\zeta_{yit}) = E(\zeta_{yit} y_{i,t-1}) = E(\zeta_{xit} y_{i,t-1})$$

$$= E(\zeta_{yit} x_{i,t-1}) = E(\zeta_{xit} x_{i,t-1}) = 0$$

Estimation of α_1 assuming that $\beta_1 = 0$ and $E(\zeta_{yit} x_{it}) = 0$ leads to a biased estimate if $\beta_1 \neq 0$.

Although the above discrete-time model may be an acceptable approximation in some circumstances, most reciprocal biologic systems are presumed to produce mutual adjustment through continuous time. For example, an increase in dietary consumption of energy would be expected to lead to a gradual increase in body weight through time. As noted, an equation model with more realistic time-related characteristics is the continuous-time differential equation, and it can be extended to the reciprocal case. A discussion of such models, together with software for estimation, is provided in Chapter 3.

For a discussion of dynamic reciprocal models for categorical variables, see Karlin and Taylor (1981).

Empirical Example

Consider an extension of the model in equation (24) to include an effect of blood pressure (η) on relative weight (x):

$$\eta_{it} = \alpha_t + \lambda_t \alpha_i + \alpha_1 x_{it} + \alpha_2 \eta_{i,t-1} + \zeta_{\eta it}$$

$$x_{it} = \beta_t + \gamma_t \beta_i + \beta_1 \eta_{it} + \beta_2 x_{i,t-1} + \zeta_{xit}$$

where the term $\beta_1 \eta_{it}$ has been added to the model in (24). The addition of this term allows the two variables to affect each other in a reciprocal manner. This is a discrete-time model; thus the model hypothesizes that a change in either variable between examinations comes to equilibrium with the other variable with instantaneous reciprocal adjustments. The ML estimates are as follows:

$$\hat{\alpha}_1 = .243 \ (.052) \qquad \hat{\alpha}_2 = .334 \ (.040)$$

$$\hat{\beta}_1 = -.106 \ (.039) \qquad \hat{\beta}_2 = .581 \ (.032)$$

where the association between x_{it} and α_i is negative ($\hat{\rho} = -.17$), and the association between η_{it} and β_i is positive ($\hat{\rho} = .35$). This result suggests that relative weight has a positive effect on blood pressure (α_1), whereas blood pressure has a small negative impact on relative weight (β_1). This latter effect could be an artifact of misspecification; only two variables have been incorporated in the model. If the modified random-effects structure is replaced by an autoregressive pattern among the disturbances, the estimates of reciprocal effects are both positive ($\hat{\alpha}_1 = .19 \ (.04)$; $\hat{\beta}_1 = .06 \ (.02)$. Note that the preponderant direction of influence is from RW to SBP with either assumption about the disturbance structure. This finding suggests the potential utility of such models to provide clues concerning causal direction when experiments have yet to be conducted, or when it is not feasible to perform experiments among humans. The validity of the coefficients depends, of course, on the correctness of the model specifications. And such models necessarily involve numerous untested assumptions. In the foregoing model, for example, numerous potentially important variables have not been included in the model.

ESTIMATION SUMMARY

All of the examples of continuous-variable models described in this overview were estimated with the software package LISREL (Jöreskog & Sorbom, 1988). They could also be computed with EQS (Bentler, 1985; see also Chapter 6 in this volume) with the LINCS routine in the flexible package GAUSS (Aptech Systems, 1988) or with the CALIS routine in SAS. These are packages for estimating structural equation models with errors in variables (measurement errors) and errors in equations (disturbances). The model was outlined at the beginning of the section "Statistical Models for Longitudinal Data"; see equations (6a) and (6b). The following applies to the estimation of covariance structures ($\underline{\alpha} = 0$ in [6b], and $\underline{\tau} = \mu_y$ in [6a]). Extension to include mean structures is straightforward.

Three methods of estimation are described here: (1) generalized least squares, (2) multivariate normal maximum likelihood, and (3) weighted least squares. We begin by defining two matrices:

$\underline{S}$ = the observed ($p \times p$) sample covariance matrix of the measured variables.

$\hat{\underline{\Sigma}}$ = the ($p \times p$) covariance matrix of the measured variables implied by the estimates of the parameters of the model.

1a. *Generalized least squares (GLS).* The fit function for GLS is

$$F = \text{tr}[(\underline{I} - \underline{S}^{-1}\hat{\underline{\Sigma}})^2]$$

where *tr* indicates the trace of a matrix and $\underline{I}$ is an identity matrix. In this instance F is a weighted function of the sums of squares of all the elements of $(\underline{S} - \Sigma)$; the weights are obtained from the inverse of $\underline{S}$. Minimization of F yields estimates of model parameters according to Aitken's (1934–1935) generalized least squares principle (Jöreskog & Goldberger, 1972).

1b. *Ordinary least squares (OLS).* OLS is a special case of GLS where the regression model is just identified and disturbances are presumed uncorrelated with one another and with the predictor variables.

2. *Maximum likelihood(ML).* The fit function for multivariate normal ML is

$$F = \log[\det(\hat{\underline{\Sigma}})] - \log[\det(\underline{S})] + \text{tr}(\underline{S}\hat{\underline{\Sigma}}^{-1}) - p$$

where *det* indicates the determinant of a square matrix and p is the number of measured variables. If the assumption of normality holds, the ML estimators are asymptotically efficient and best asymptotically normal (BAN). In general, then, estimators will be close to population values in large samples. In addition, the estimators are functions of minimal sufficient statistics, and are thus minimum-variance estimators when they are unbiased.

3. *Weighted least squares (WLS).* The fit function for WLS is

$$F = (\underline{s} - \hat{\underline{\sigma}})'W^{-1}(\underline{s} - \hat{\underline{\sigma}})$$

where $\underline{s}$ is a vector formed from the lower diagonal and diagonal elements of $\underline{S}$ and $\hat{\underline{\sigma}}$ is similarly derived from $\hat{\underline{\Sigma}}$. If the measured variables are multivariate normal, $\underline{W}$ can be defined to yield GLS estimates (or ML estimates if $\underline{s}$ is iteratively replaced by estimates of $\underline{\sigma}$). However, Browne (1984) has shown that an alternative-weight matrix yields "asymptotically distribution free GLS estimators":

$$w_{gh,ij} = m_{ghij} - s_{gh}s_{ij}$$

where

$$m_{ghij} = \left(\frac{1}{N}\right) \sum_{a=1}^{N} (z_{ag} - \bar{z}_g)(z_{ah} - \bar{z}_h)(z_{ai} - \bar{z}_i)(z_{aj} - \bar{z}_j)$$

are the fourth-order central moments. Asymptotically correct chi-squares and standard errors are available under very mild assumptions concerning the multivariate distribution of the continuous variables. Jöreskog and Sorbom (1988) have extended this estimation scheme to the case where variables are ordinal or censored, utilizing a probit form of the model. This approach allows estimation of a very general class of models. When the assumption of multivariate normality holds, the GLS and ML estimates have similar asymptotic properties.

A goodness of fit χ^2 is obtained as follows:

$$\chi^2 = (N - 1)F_m \qquad df = \frac{p(p + 1)}{2} - r$$

where N is the number of persons in the observed sample, F_m is the minimum value of the fit function, p is the number of measured variables, and r is the number of independent parameters to be estimated. This statistic tests the null hypothesis that the specified model is correct. Acceptance of the null hypothesis does not, of course, indicate that the model is correct. Rather it indicates that the data are an insufficient basis for rejecting the model; numerous alternative models will also be consistent with the same data. Furthermore, rejection of the model is likely when sample sizes are large (since even minor misspecifications will produce lack of fit). The goodness of fit χ^2 is most useful, then, for comparing alternative models, rather than for judging the fit of a particular model.

The generality of the model in (6a) and (6b), together with the desirable properties of the available estimators, provides longitudinal researchers with a flexible tool for analysis of longitudinal data. Markedly nonnormal data and ordinal probit models for categorical variables can be handled with WLS. Maximum likelihood or WLS estimates with incomplete data can be obtained by defining subgroups in terms of patterns of missing data (Allison, 1987); parameters are then constrained equal across groups. These models can also incorporate multiple measures of variables to adjust estimates for measurement error.

The types of models that cannot be handled by software for structural equation models include variable-coefficient models where the variable slopes involve regression on a variable other than time of measurement. The proportional-hazards model also requires specialized software, but it is widely available in general statistical packages.

A final approach to estimation that requires special software is the use of empirical Bayes estimators (see Chapter 13; Fearn, 1975). Bayes estimators of variances may be unbiased when ML estimators are biased (Harville, 1977), while they generally retain the desirable properties of consistency and asymptotic efficiency. Laird and Ware (1982) have described a procedure using the EM algorithm to obtain empirical Bayes estimates in two-stage models with variable slopes.

Estimation of the fixed-effects model with dummy variables for individual or time effects, or both, is a convenient approach in some circumstances. The OLS estimators of α (intercept), α_i (individual effects), and β (slope) are then best linear-unbiased estimators (BLUE). When sample size is large, subtracting time series means and then computing least-squares estimates avoids the inclusion of prohibitive numbers of dummy variables. However, the resulting estimator of β, while unbiased, is consistent only as $N \to \infty$; the estimator of α is consistent only as $T \to \infty$.

When the individual effects α_i are presumed random and uncorrelated with the predictor variable, the OLS estimator of β is not BLUE in finite samples. Rather the GLS estimator is BLUE. The ML estimator in this instance is asymptotically efficient. As previously noted, however, the assumption of zero correlation between α_i and x_i is usually unwarranted. If we allow α_i and x_i to correlate, the GLS, OLS, and ML estimators converge in static models with continuous variables. (For a discussion of the asymptotic efficiencies of alternative estimators for fixed- or random-effects dynamic models, variable-coefficient models, and categorical variable models, see Anderson and Hsaio, 1981, and Hsaio, 1986.)

Two promising approaches to estimation of general models for longitudinal data are discussed in Chapters 8 and 15. Moulton, Zeger, and Liang in Chapter 8 expand generalized linear models to the longitudinal case, and Arminger and Kuster in Chapter 15 expand the multivariate probit model. Some problems remain with these general approaches, but a solution for these problems and the development of practical software is now in sight.

REFERENCES

Aitken AC (1934–1935). "On least squares and the linear combination of observations." *Proceedings of the Royal Society of Edinburgh* 55: 42–48.

Allison PD (1987). "Estimation of linear models with incomplete data." in Clogg C. (ed), *Sociological Methodology*. San Francisco, Jossey-Bass, pp. 71–103.

Amemiya T (1984). "Tobit models: A survey." *Journal of Econometrics* 24: 3–61.

Anderson TW, Hsaio C (1981). "Estimation of dynamic models with error components." *Journal of the American Statistical Association* 76: 598–606.

Aptech Systems (1988). "The GAUSS System Version 2.0." Kent, Wash., Aptech Systems.

Azen SP, Guilder MV, Hill MA (1989). "Estimation of parameters and missing values under a regression model with non-normally distributed and non-randomly incomplete data." *Statistics in Medicine* 8: 217–228.

Beale EML, Little RJA (1975). "Missing values in multivariate analysis." *Journal of the Royal Statistical Society* B37: 121–145.

Bentler PM (1985). *Theory and Implementation of EQS: A Structural Equations Program.* Los Angeles, BMDP Statistical Software.

Blomqvist N (1977). "On the relation between change and initial value." *Journal of the American Statistical Association* 72: 746–749.

Box GEP, Jenkins GM. (1970). *Time Series Analysis: Forecasting and Control.* San Francisco, Holden-Day.

Browne, MW (1984). "Asymptotically distribution-free methods for the analysis of covariance structures." *British Journal of Mathematical and Statistical Psychology* 37: 62–83.

Carter RL, Yang MCK (1986). "Large-sample inference in random coefficient regression models." *Communications in Statistics—Theory and Methods* 8: 2507–2526.

Cochran WG, Cox GM (1957). *Experimental Designs.* 2nd ed. New York, Wiley.

Cochran WG, Rubin DB (1973). "Controlling bias in observational studies: A review." *Sankhya* 35: 417–446.

Cohen JE, Singer B (1979). "Malaria in Nigeria: Constrained continuous-time Markov models for discrete-time longitudinal data on human mixed-species infections." In Levin S (ed), *Mathematical Models in Biology*, Vol. 12. Providence, R.I., American Mathematical Society.

Cook N, Ware JH (1983). "Design and analysis methods for longitudinal research." *Annual Review of Public Health* 4: 1–23.

Cook TD, Campbell DT (eds) (1979). *Quasi-experimentation.* Chicago, Rand McNally.

Cox DR (1972). "Regression models and life tables." *Journal of the Royal Statistical Society* 34B: 269–276.

Cox DR (1981). "Statistical analysis of time series: Some recent developments." *Scandinavian Journal of Statistics* 8: 93–115.

Dawber TR (1980). *The Framingham Heart Study.* Cambridge, Mass., Harvard University Press.

Diem JE, Liukkonen JR. (1988). "A comparative study of three methods for analysing longitudinal pulmonary function data." *Statistics in Medicine* 7: 19–28.

Diggle PJ (1988). "An approach to the analysis of repeated measurements." *Biometrics* 44: 959–972.

Dixon WJ (ed.) (1983). *BMDP Statistical Software.* Berkeley, University of California Press.

Duncan GJ, Kalton G (1987). "Issues of design and analysis of surveys across time." *International Statistical Review* 55: 97–117.

Dwyer JH (1984). "The excluded variable problem in nonrandomized control group designs." *Evaluation Review* 8: 559–572.

Dwyer JH, Mackinnon D, Pentzm A, et al. (1989). "Estimating intervention effects in longitudinal studies." *American Journal of Epidemiology* 130: 781–795.

Fearn T (1975). "A Bayesian approach to growth curves." *Biometrika* 62: 89–100.

Fuller WA (1980). "Properties of some estimators for the errors-in-variables model." *Annals of Statistics* 8: 407–422.

Ghosh M, Grizzle JE, Pranab KS (1973). "Nonparametric methods in longitudinal studies." *Journal of the American Statistical Association* 68: 29–36.

Giesbrecht FG, Burns JC (1985). "Two stage analysis based on a mixed model: Large sample asymptotic theory and small sample simulation results." *Biometrics* 41: 477–486.

Goldstein H (1979). *The Design and Analysis of Longitudinal Studies.* London, Academic Press.

Grizzle JE, Allen DM (1969). "Analysis of growth and dose response curves." *Biometrics* 25: 357–361.

Harville DA (1977). "Maximum likelihood approaches to variance component estimation and to related problems." *Journal of the American Statistical Association* 72: 320–340.

Hausman JA, Wise D (1979). "Attrition bias in experimental and panel data: The Gary Income Maintenance Experiment." *Econometrica* 47: 455–473.

Heckman JJ (1981), "Statistical models for discrete panel data." in Mansk CF, McFadden D (eds), *Structural Analysis of Discrete Data with Econometric Applications.* Cambridge, Mass., MIT Press, pp. 114–178.

Hsaio C (1986). *Analysis of Panel Data.* Cambridge, Cambridge University Press.

Hui SL (1984). "Curve fitting for repeated measurements made at irregular time points." *Biometrics* 40: 691–697.

Jolicoeur P, Pointier J, Pernin MO, Sempe M (1988). "A lifetime asymptotic growth curve for human height." *Biometrics* 44: 995–1004.

Jöreskog KG (1970a). "A general method for analysis of covariance structures." *Biometrika* 57: 239–251.

Jöreskog KG (1970b). "Estimation and testing of simplex models." *British Journal of Mathematical and Statistical Psychology* 23: 121–145.

Jöreskog KG, Goldberger AS (1972). "Factor analysis by generalized least squares." *Psychometrika* 37: 243–250.

Jöreskog KG, Sorböm D (1988). *LISREL 7: A Guide to the Program and Applications.* Chicago, SPSS.

Karlin S, Taylor HM (1981). *A Second Course in Stochastic Processes.* New York, Academic Press.

Kauffman H (1987). "Regression models for nonstationary categorical time series: Asymptotic estimation theory." *Annals of Statistics* 15: 79–98.

Kleinbaum, DG (1973). "A generalization of the growth curve model which allows missing data." *Journal of Multivariate Analysis* 3: 117–124.

Knuiman MW, Speed TP (1988). "Incorporating prior information into the analysis of contingency tables." *Biometrics* 44: 1061–1072.

Koch GG, Amara IA, Stokes ME, Gillings DB (1980). "Some views on parametric and nonparametric analysis for repeated measurements and selected bibliography." *International Statistical Review* 48: 249–265.

Laird NM, Ware JH (1982). "Random-effects models for longitudinal data." *Biometrics* 38: 963–974.

Lange N, Laird NM (1989). "The effect of covariance structure on variance estimation in balanced growth-curve models with random parameters." *Journal of the American Statistical Association* 84: 241–247.

Lauer RL, Clarke WR, Beaglehole R (1984). "Level, trend and variability of blood pressure during childhood: The Muscatine Study." *Circulation* 69: 242–249.

Little RJA (1988). "A test of missing completely at random for multivariate data with missing values," *Journal of the American Statistical Association* 83:1198–1202.

Little RJA, Rubin DB. (1987). *Statistical Analysis with Missing Data.* New York, Wiley.

McCullagh P, Nelder JA (1983). *Generalized Linear Models.* London, Chapman and Hall.

Mundlak Y (1978). "On the pooling of time series and cross section data." *Econometrica* 46:69–85.

Muthen B (1979). "A structural probit model with latent variables." *Journal of the American Statistical Association* 74:807–811.

Nesselroade JR, Baltes PB (eds.) (1979). *Longitudinal Research in the Study of Behavior and Development,* New York, Academic Press.

Plewis I (1985). *Analyzing Change: Measurement and Explanation Using Longitudinal Data.* Chichester, England, Wiley.

Potthoff RR, Roy SN (1964). "A generalized multivariate analysis of variance model for growth curve problems." *Biometrika* 51:313–326.

Prentice RL (1988). "Correlated binary regression with covariates specific to each binary observation." *Biometrics* 44:1033–1048.

Rao CR (1965). "The theory of least squares when the parameters are stochastic and its application to the analysis of growth curves." *Biometrika* 52:447–458.

Reinsel G (1984). "Estimation and prediction in a multivariate random-effects generalized linear model." *Journal of the American Statistical Association* 79:406–414.

Reinsel G (1985). "Mean squared error properties of empirical Bayes estimators in a multivariate random-effects general linear model." *Journal of the American Statistical Association* 80:642–650.

Royall RM (1986). "Model robust inference using maximum likelihood estimators." *International Statistical Review* 54:221–226.

Stanek EJ, Diehl SR (1988). "Growth curve models of repeated binary response." *Biometrics* 44:973–984.

Stefanski LA (1985). "The effects of measurement error on parameter estimation." *Biometrika* 72:583–592.

Stiratelli R, Laird N, Ware JH (1984). "Random-effect models for serial observations with binary response." *Biometrics* 40: 961–971.

Strenio JF, Weisberg HI, Bryk AS (1983). "Empirical Bayes estimation of individual growth curve parameters and their relationship to covariates." *Biometrics* 39:71–86.

Thomas DC (1981). "General relative risk models for survival time and matched case-control analysis." *Biometrics* 37:673–686.

Vacek PM, Mickey RM, Bell DY (1989). "Application of a two stage random effects model to longitudinal pulmonary function data from sarcoidosis patients." *Statistics in Medicine* 8:189–200.

Verbyla AP, Venables WN (1988). "An extension of the growth curve model." *Biometrika* 75:129–138.

Vonesh EF, Carter RL (1987). "Efficient inference for random coefficient growth curve models with unbalanced data." *Biometrics* 43:617–628.

Ware JH (1985). "Linear models for the analysis of longitudinal studies." *American Statistician* 39: 95–101.

Ware JH, Lipsitz S, Speizer FE (1988). "Issues in the analysis of repeated categorical outcomes." *Statistics in Medicine* 7:95–107.

White H (1982). "Maximum likelihood estimation of misspecified models." *Econometrika* 50: 1–25.

Wishart J (1938). "Growth-rate determinations in nutrition studies with Bacon Pig, and their analyses." *Biometrics* 30:16–28.

Wu MC, Kusek JW (eds.) (1988). "Methods for analyzing repeated measurements." *Statistics in Medicine* 7:11–362.

Zeger SL (1988). "A regression model for time series of counts." *Biometrika* 75: 621–629.

Zeger SL, Liang K-Y, Albert PS (1988). "Models for longitudinal data: A generalized estimating equation approach." *Biometrics* 44:1049–1060.

Zeger SL, Qaqish B (1988). "Markov regression models for time series: A quasi-likelihood approach." *Biometrics* 44:1019–1032.

2

Considerations in the Design of Longitudinal Surveys of Health

LESTER CURTIN AND MANNING FEINLEIB

Survey organizations have traditionally been involved in the design and analysis of cross-sectional surveys. The National Center for Health Statistics (NCHS), for example, conducts many national cross-sectional health surveys. Some surveys, like the National Hospital Discharge Survey or the National Nursing Home Survey, are related to health care facilities. Other surveys are record based, in which the sampling frame is a set of administrative records; an example is the National Mortality Followback Survey, based on death certificates. Still other surveys, such as the National Health Interview Survey (NHIS) and the National Health and Nutrition Examination Survey (NHANES), are "population-based" surveys in which individuals or households of individuals are the final sample units.

National population-based surveys are conducted annually or on a periodic basis. When different individuals are sampled at each time point, the periodic surveys are called *repeated cross-sectional surveys*. The NHIS, for example, is conducted every year with a new sample of individuals selected each year. Trends over time in such data can be examined, but the trends must be analyzed with the constraint of the survey data being from different individuals at each time point.

As long as analytic requirements for survey data are limited to single point-in-time estimates or measures of aggregate change, cross-sectional surveys are appropriate. However, health issues and analytic uses of national health data have been changing. There is increasing demand for the measurement of individual change over time, for the investigation of risk factors in the development of disease, for the determination and targeting of high-risk groups, and for the examination of the impact of health intervention programs. For these types of survey objectives, longitudinal data are needed.

The term *longitudinal* merely implies measurement over time. A single-point-in-time cross-sectional survey could collect retrospective histories, and thus give longitudinal data. However, *longitudinal surveys* are usually thought to be prospective in nature. Data from prospective surveys may be of better quality than retrospective data in that retrospective data suffer from recall bias and reference frame problems.

The usefulness of prospective longitudinal health data has been demonstrated, in part, by such epidemiologic studies as Framingham (Gordon, Sorlie, & Kannel, 1971), the Six Cities study (Ferris et al., 1983), the Muscatine study (Clarke et al., 1978), and others. These studies are primarily community-based studies with relatively narrow study objectives; their results may not be applicable to the general population. For nationally representative estimates, large-scale prospective health surveys are required.

There are two basic designs for collecting prospective longitudinal data: the repeated cross-sectional and the panel survey. Repeated cross-sectional surveys can give prospective longitudinal data, but as already noted, the data are for a different collection of sample persons at each time point. Thus some types of longitudinal objectives cannot be met. In a panel survey individuals are sampled at the initial time point and are then repeatedly observed or interviewed over time. Panel surveys may not be appropriate for some types of cross-sectional survey objectives.

Leaving aside cost and operational considerations, a decision between these two basic survey designs often depends on the relative importance of the possible survey objectives. Seven types of health survey objectives are briefly examined in the next section, from the viewpoint of which survey design is most appropriate for each type of objective.

RELATION OF SURVEY OBJECTIVES
TO SURVEY DESIGN

One of the first steps in the design of a survey is development of a formal statement of the analytic requirements, that is, the survey's objectives. When some of these objectives are longitudinal, a decision framework, such as that by Duncan and Kalton (1987), is helpful in determining the basic design. The Duncan and Kalton framework can be used to compare the advantages and disadvantages of different design options in meeting specific survey objectives. The basic design options considered by Duncan and Kalton for a survey over time are: a series of repeated cross-sectional surveys, a long-term panel survey, a rotating-panel survey, and a split-panel survey. When the survey objectives are narrow in scope and well defined, the Duncan and Kalton framework can lead to an appropriate design decision.

Objectives for a national health survey are usually well defined but are not narrow in scope. Rather they tend to have multiple objectives covering a wide range of analytic goals. Historically, one of the most important survey objectives for the NCHS has been the ability to make national prevalence estimates for health and nutrition variables. For example, a survey may be targeted to estimate the prevalence of certain chronic conditions, the number of bed days of disability, or the proportion of the U.S. population with an elevated serum cholesterol level. A repeated cross-sectional survey, such as the National Health

Interview Survey, can be designed to be representative of the current target population and can thus provide national prevalence estimates for each point in time. A panel survey is not quite as appropriate due to problems of a changing population, attrition bias, and panel conditioning. (Because of their importance, sources of panel bias will be discussed separately in the section "Implications of Split-Panel Design for Survey Bias.")

A different consideration exists if long-term recall periods are needed to provide basic estimates. A single cross-sectional survey is not appropriate for such estimates due to measurement problems. This type of survey objective is best met with a short-term panel design, with multiple data collection points within a one-year time period. Each point estimate can be based on a short recall period, and the individual point estimates aggregated to form annual estimates. An example of this type of short-term panel survey is the National Medical Care Utilization and Expenditure Survey (Bonham, 1983).

A third type of health survey objective is to provide estimates of the prevalence of relatively rare acute and chronic disease outcomes. A single cross-sectional survey does not provide enough sample to estimate rare events, but a series of repeated, independent cross-sectional surveys is an excellent means for cumulating samples over time. For example, several years of NHIS data can be combined to estimate relatively rare health events or for relatively small subdomains, such as Hispanics (Trevino & Moss, 1984). One drawback of the repeated cross-sectional survey is that there is no means to detect the telescoping of events for acute disease outcomes. A panel survey does provide for bounded recall periods to detect the telescoping of events, but because the same individuals are observed at each time point, a pure panel study cannot accumulate sample over time.

The first three types of survey objectives just discussed are prevalence-type objectives. In the past, national health surveys have been designed specifically to meet only prevalence objectives. Now survey data are used with increasing frequency to meet other analytic objectives. The next four types of survey objectives are analytic in nature and, in particular, address the measurement of change over time.

Change over time can be categorized into aggregate (or net) change and individual (or gross) change. Aggregate change refers to differences between subgroups of the target population or differences over time for a specific subgroup. An example of an aggregate change is the change in the proportion of women with high blood pressure between two points in time.

Either a panel survey or a repeated cross-sectional survey can be used for monitoring aggregate changes in prevalence estimates over time. A deciding factor in the basic design decision may be the consideration of the changing nature of the target population over time. Repeated, independent cross-sectional surveys automatically take population changes into account because a new representative design is used at each time point. However, in determining aggregate change, repeated cross-sectional estimates combine the effects of changing values and the changing population. For a panel survey there is a need to define some mechanism for taking population change into account. Otherwise the later waves of data may not be representative of the current population. In a panel survey, however, the variance of the estimated change is reduced by positive correlation between data collected on the same individuals at various time points (Cook & Ware, 1983). Thus, while either type of survey is adequate, the panel survey, when sources of bias can be controlled, is more efficient than a series of cross-sectional surveys in that a smaller sample size is needed to meet a specified level of precision for the estimated change.

Similarly, either a repeated cross-sectional or a panel survey can be used to determine subdomain and geographic differences in health variables. When such differences are measured within a time period, the survey design considerations are the same as those for any cross-sectional survey. When the differences are to be examined over time, the choice of a basic survey design depends on whether the sources of bias in panel survey may be considerable for the specific differences of interest and whether aggregate or individual change is to be measured.

The decision between selection of a cross-sectional or a panel design is less problematic when the survey objective is to measure individual changes in health and nutrition status. An example of individual change would be to estimate the number of women who exhibit a decrease in their blood pressure level between two time points. Because different individuals are measured at different time points, repeated cross-sectional surveys do not allow for any measurement of individual change, whereas panel surveys are obviously well suited for this purpose.

The final analytic objective is concerned with examination of risk factors for specified disease outcomes. If retrospective data collection for risk factors is adequate, or if the only interest is in determining the current presence or absence of risk factors for a known disease outcome, then cross-sectional data are adequate. Panel data are required if a survey objective is to determine the prevalence of a disease at baseline, to measure the initial risk factors, and then to examine the initial noncases for future development of that disease.

For these seven types of survey objectives, the "best" design decision is summarized in Table 2-1. Some health survey objectives, such as measurement of individual change, can be met only by a panel survey.But at later waves (time points) of the survey, a pure panel survey would be inappropriate for some cross-sectional objectives. For example, suppose a health examination survey is required to estimate the proportion of the U.S. population with undiagnosed hypertension. Clearly, in a panel survey the proportion of the population with *undiagnosed* hypertension could not be estimated at the second time point. It would appear then that a survey design that is best suited to meet the multiple objectives of national health surveys would be some combination of a cross-sectional and panel survey, that is, some type of split-panel design.

THE SPLIT-PANEL DESIGN

Split-panel design is a term used by Kish (1981) to describe a combination of a cross-sectional design and a panel design. There can be many variations of a split-panel design (as indicated by Kish, 1983). Table 2-2 summarizes three

Table 2–1. Survey objectives and basic design decision

Survey objective	Survey design
Annual prevalence estimates	Cross-sectional
Prevalence of measures requiring long-term recall periods	Short-term panel
Prevalence of rare diseases outcomes	Aggregated data from a series of cross-sectional
Aggregate change in health status	Panel or cross-sectional
Individual change	Panel
Subdomain and geographic comparisons	Panel or cross-sectional
Examination of risk factors	Panel or cross-sectional

examples: a simple design, a design maximizing the panel aspects, and one type of intermediate split-panel design.

In a simple split-panel design, only the first cross-sectional cohort is followed over time, and a new, independent representative survey of individuals is selected at each time point. The sample at the initial time point could be designed as a single cross-sectional sample or as two independent cross-sectional samples. For example, at the initial time point two samples of 10,000 persons each could be selected. One of these samples forms the panel to be followed over time and the other sample is observed at the initial time only. Alternatively, only one sample of 10,000 might be taken and that sample would form the panel. Then at the second time point, observations could be taken on a new sample of 10,000 persons as well as on all of the initial panel members who can be found and will respond. At the later time points, part of each new cross-sectional sample could be used to "freshen" the initial panel to replace those sample persons lost through attrition or to reduce the effect of panel conditioning.

A number of alternatives exist for the split-panel design if it is desired to follow *each* new cross-sectional sample as new panels. For the example of an intermediate design, the initial time point has two independent cross-sectional samples, each one nationally representative. One cross-sectional survey is considered to be the panel survey, and that sample is followed through some time intervals. In the particular example in Table 2-2, each new cross-sectional cohort is followed for only two time points.

The most demanding split-panel design, from the viewpoint of operations

Table 2–2. Types of split panel designs

Time point	Simple split panel	Split panel with rotating panels	Split panel with maximum overlap
1	C_1, P_1	C_1, C_2, P_1	P_1
2	C_2, P_1	C_2, C_3, P_1	P_1, P_2
3	C_3, P_1	C_3, C_4, P_1	P_1, P_2, P_3
4	C_4, P_1	C_4, C_5, P_1	P_1, P_2, P_3, P_4

and cost, is a design in which each new cross-sectional sample is used as the baseline for a panel survey and *all* cohorts are followed in successive time intervals. For this type of design, a major operational and cost problem is the accumulation of the total sample over time. As a hypothetical example, consider Table 2-3 for a series of health surveys. In this example there is assumed to be a relatively large amount of attrition due to death, longitudinal nonresponse, and loss to follow-up. Even so, a survey of 10,000 at time 1 would grow to a survey of 25,000 by time 3. By time 6, over 125,000 observations would have been recorded for the entire collection of samples. Consider the implications if 30,000 (as in the NHANES II survey) or 100,000 (as in the NHIS survey) individuals were sampled in each new cohort; the survey costs for tracking the panel members, for data collection, and for processing the data would be immense.

In the preceding example of a split-panel design, each panel was assumed to be the complete, new cross-sectional sample. One obvious alternative design would be to select only a subsample of each new cross-sectional sample to form new panels to be followed over time. This would reduce the operational costs because a smaller number of sample persons would be accumulated over time. The design of such longitudinal subsamples would have to be done with great care for national surveys, otherwise some potential analytic uses of the longitudinal data could be eliminated.

IMPLICATIONS OF SPLIT-PANEL DESIGN FOR SURVEY BIAS

The split-panel design can be used to meet all of the seven survey objectives listed earlier. It is also clear from previous discussion that the split-panel design may be very appropriate for reducing one of the problems inherent in a pure-panel design. Namely, in a split-panel survey sources of bias in the panel component may be eliminated, controlled, or at least examined. This section briefly looks at bias resulting from panel attrition, a changing population over time, and panel conditioning.

Table 2–3. Maximum available yearly and total sample sizes for maximum overlap split-panel design

Cohort	Time 1	Time 2	Time 3	Time 4	Time 5	Time 6	Total cohort observations by time 6
1	10,000	8,000	5,000	2,000	500	0	25,500
2	—	10,000	8,000	5,000	2,000	500	25,500
3	—	—	10,000	8,000	5,000	2,000	25,000
4	—	—	—	10,000	8,000	5,000	23,000
5	—	—	—	—	10,000	8,000	18,000
6	—	—	—	—	—	10,000	10,000
Total	10,000	18,000	23,000	25,000	25,500	25,500	127,000

Panel Attrition

In panel surveys, attrition results from those responding at the first time point and not responding at later time points. As stated by Lehnen and Koch (1974), "the major statistical shortcoming of panel designs . . . is the inability to control attrition in the original sample when administering subsequent interviews." Besides attrition from death, disinterest, and failure to locate, attrition also results from data processing as inconsistent data are eliminated by use of quality control checks. Attrition may lead to biased estimates; the extent of bias is related to two factors.

The first factor is the proportion of nonresponse at each time point. The decrease in panel response rates over time is particularly important because if nonresponse is high initially, the overall response rate for later waves of data collection, with additional between-wave attrition, will soon become quite low, perhaps to the point that the issue of potential bias becomes overwhelming. For example, in a health examination survey with 75-percent response at the initial time point and 90-percent response of the same people at the second time point, the overall response rate at the second time point will be only 68 percent. Similarly, if response is 90 percent between the second and third wave, the overall response rate will be 61 percent for the third time point of data collection. With each wave of data collection the panel becomes smaller and possibly more selected.

The second factor contributing to attrition bias is the magnitude of the differences between those who remain in the panel and those who are lost to follow-up. If these two groups are not different and attrition can be considered random, simple adjustments to survey estimation procedures can be used without the potential for bias. If attrition is not at random, the possibility of panel bias exists and the panel may not remain representative over time.

A particular problem occurs when the attrition mechanism is related to the analytic variable of interest. In a sample of adolescents on intelligence variables, Labouvie, Bartsch, Nesselroade, and Baltes (1974) found that the response behavior of adolescents was correlated with the initial measurement of intellectual functioning. They concluded that the relation of attrition to the variable of analytic interest seriously jeopardized the external validity of that panel design. As a further example, Seigler and Botwinick (1979) reported on a twenty-year panel study of aging and adult intelligence. Those initially superior on first testing were more likely to remain in the study and showed little decline in intelligence with age. The results from later waves of the study could not be generalized to the population of all older persons.

A similar problem is present in health surveys where sample persons lost to follow-up may be atypical for mobility, social class, and health. In several investigations of potential panel bias, those nonrespondents in later waves were compared with all initial respondents and found to have higher rates of intellectual impairment (Schaie, Labouvie, & Barrett, 1975; Seigler & Botwinick, 1979); lower socioeconomic status and poorer physical health (Goudy, 1976, 1985; Powers & Bultena, 1972; Streib, 1966). Norris (1985) also found that the healthier the initial respondents, for both physical and psychologic measures of well being, the longer they stayed in the study.

These investigations compared all initial respondents with all later nonrespondents. The potential for nonresponse or attrition bias actually varies by reason for nonresponse. Thus in a panel survey there is a need to distinguish between subject loss due to selective survival and subject loss due to selective drop-out (Seigler, McCarty, & Logue, 1982). Again, types of panel attrition considered are those deceased, those found but not responding at later time points, and those who could not be located at later time points.

In a panel study of the aged, Norris (1985) found that the deceased were not a source of bias and the panel was still representative of the surviving cohort. Norris (1985) also found that those located but disinterested in continuing in the study did not differ significantly from the respondents. Dohrenwend and Dohrenwend (1968) also found that the disinterested or refusers posed little threat to representativeness of sample.

Other types of attrition do seem to be selective. Of particular interest in a health survey are the disabled or partially disabled. Norris (1985) found the disabled similar to the deceased in characteristics. In general, those "not found" seem to contribute more to attrition bias than those who refuse follow-up interviews.

Although attrition bias is a major concern for longitudinal health surveys, only a limited number of survey design options are available for reducing such bias. Response at the initial time point can be increased by increasing the number of persons selected per household. This, however, has implications for the precision of the survey estimates in that it tends to increase the variance of survey estimates. For a pure-panel design, attrition effects may be minimized by increasing the initial sample size of those groups most likely to drop out. For a split-panel design, the new cross-sectional sample can be used to bring the panel up to size with random replacement at later waves.

No matter how intensive the effort or how many resources expended, there will always be some degree of nonresponse. After the problem has been minimized through design and operational considerations, nonresponse is handled through estimation and analytic techniques. Techniques for weighting and imputation adjustment of survey data are well documented in the literature (Kalton, 1983; Little, 1982) and are discussed for panel surveys as well (Kalton, 1986; Little, 1985). As an alternative to weighting or imputation, data can be treated as missing data in the application of specific analytic methods (for example, Little & Rubin, 1987; Rubin, 1987).

Changing Target Population over Time

For population-based surveys, the target population (sample universe) is usually the civilian, noninstitutionalized population of the United States. The changing composition of the target population over time is due to changes in those considered in-scope for the survey (transitions into or out of the military or institutions), deaths, in-migration, and out-migration. An obvious problem arises in panel surveys when the target population is changing over time. Because the panel is selected at the first time point, the representativeness of the panel relative to the current population becomes more questionable as time goes on.

This problem is discussed by Judkins, et al. (1984) for panel surveys. One solution is to consider the population at the initial time point as a cohort; the cohort at the later time points is considered to represent only the original target population. An alternative solution is to allow for additions and deletions from the target universe. Here the split-panel design has a decided advantage over a pure-panel design. At each time point, the new cross-sectional component can be designed to be representative of the current target population. The estimates from the panel component can then be compared with estimates from the new cross-sectional component to examine changes due to the changing population, and some of the new sample can be added to the longitudinal cohort to make the panel representative of the current population.

Panel Effects (Conditioning)

Another source of bias in panel studies is *conditioning* of the panel, that is, respondents being asked certain questions at the initial time point may affect their responses at later time points. This is particularly true in attitudinal and educational surveys. Sobol (1959) found that repeated interviewing may cause changes in attitudes and also panel attrition. Some panel members become more pessimistic and tend to drop out; the remaining members then provide more optimistic responses than a random sample. In educational surveys it has been surmised that age-related longitudinal increases in intelligence variables could be due mainly to retest effects (Baltes, 1968; Campbell & Stanley, 1963: Labouvie et al., 1974; Schaie, 1965, 1973).

For health surveys, conditioning effects may also be present. When sample persons are interviewed about personal health practices and risk factors, they may subsequently change their health practices. McFall (1977) discovered that, during a period in which smoking habits were monitored, subjects who felt uncomfortable about their smoking habit smoked fewer cigarettes. As another example, consider the problem of a panel survey, with an examination component, that has the goal of estimating the proportion of persons in the nation with elevated cholesterol levels. Some individuals, such as those with elevated cholesterol levels on initial examination, might be motivated to participate in passive intervention measures, such as change in diet. If this were to occur, the later waves of the panel would no longer be representative of the target population. The panel survey could measure the intervention effect of diet, or the proportion of persons who initiate intervention measures once diagnosed, but could no longer measure the national distribution of persons with elevated levels of cholesterol.

With a split-panel design, the survey can be specifically designed to measure panel effects. The new cross-sectional component provides a control group at later times so that the panel can be compared with the new random sample by using identical questions at the same calendar period. If there is evidence of panel conditioning, only the new cross-sectional component would be used to estimate national prevalence distributions.

CONSIDERATIONS IN THE DESIGN OF SPLIT-PANEL SURVEYS

For a split-panel survey, the survey at the initial time point can be designed as any cross-sectional survey, with the additional consideration that the sample design must be adequate to meet the longitudinal analytic objectives. The panel component can consist of either a subsample or the entire cohort sampled at the first time point. The first consideration, however, is the design of the survey at the initial time point.

For population-based surveys, it is not cost effective to take a simple random sample of the U.S. population. The sampling units would be geographically scattered and the data collection costs would be considerable. To reduce survey costs, data collection must be restricted to a limited number of areas selected to form a representative sample of the entire country. For major national surveys, the sample design is thus likely to be a multistage probability design, with stratification and clustering at various stages.

When estimates are based on such complex probability samples, their variances are often quite different from those of survey estimates based on simple random samples of the same size. Compared with simple random sampling, stratification can help reduce variability, while clustering and unequal selection probabilities can increase variability. In designing multistage surveys it is useful to have a measure of the relative change in variability due to the complex design; such a measure is the *design effect* (Kish, 1965).

As developed by Kish, the design effect, or DEFF, is defined the sampling variance for the complex survey estimate divided by the hypothetical variance of that same estimate, as if the estimate had been based on a simple random sample of the same size. That is

$$ \text{DEFF} = \frac{\text{var(complex)}}{\text{var(simple random sample)}} $$

The term *DEFT* is used for the ratio of standard errors, so that DEFT is the square root of DEFF. In general, complex multistage survey design effects are greater than 1 due to the clustering of the household sample and to differential weighting (that is, unequal probability sampling). Table 2-4 illustrates several examples of DEFTs for the NHANES II survey. For NHANES II, the DEFTs are somewhat different for the selected health variables shown. Also, the design effect is greater for survey estimates for the total population, aged 6 through 74 years, than for individual age groups because there are fewer persons per cluster in individual age groups.

For consideration of multistage probability design options, design-effect models can be used to determine expected design effects for each proposed

Table 2-4. Example of design effects (DEFT) for survey estimates

Age (years)	Decayed, missing, and filled teeth	Systolic blood pressure	Calories
6–74	2.03	2.21	2.94
6–17	1.54	2.23	2.03
18–24	1.77	1.49	1.58
25–34	1.83	1.52	1.57
35–44	1.56	1.54	1.58
45–54	1.16	1.78	1.45
55–64	1.22	1.18	1.43
65–74	1.28	1.80	1.81

Source: Landis et al. (1982), Table 10.

sample design option. A simple design-effect model for a one-stage cluster design is given by

$$DEFF = (1 + m\rho)$$

where m is the average cluster size and ρ is the intracluster correlation coefficient (Cochran, 1977). Similar types of expected design-effect models are important in determining the contribution to the overall sampling error of each stage in a multistage, cross-sectional survey design and in deciding on the final design for selection of sample persons.

Selection of Sample Persons

In any survey, an important consideration is determination of the analytic subdomains of interest and the minimum sample size required for each subdomain. Again, for the initial time point in a split-panel survey, the statistical issues for minimum sample size are similar to those for any cross-sectional design. These statistical issues include requirements for the precision of estimates, the necessary significance levels and power for comparisons (both within and between time points), and the ability to estimate sampling errors.

Sample size requirements for comparisons (simple hypothesis testing) tend to be larger than those for precision of simple prevalence estimates. For example, a sample size of 300 may be required to estimate a certain prevalence rate for a specified subdomain, but a sample size of 1000 may be needed to detect a difference between the prevalence rates for two subdomains. Thus, when only prevalence considerations are used to set sample size, analysts may later find it impossible to detect subdomain differences with any degree of statistical accuracy. If it is known beforehand, in the design stage of the survey, that a major survey objective is the detection of aggregate differences over time or aggregate differences between subdomains, then the minimum sample size required for hypothesis testing should be used in determining the sample size requirements.

If simple random sampling is assumed, the minimum sample size for an analytic subdomain can be determined by methods described in many textbooks (for example, Levy & Lemeshow, 1980, for precision and Fleiss, 1981, for hypothesis testing). The expected design effect can then be used to inflate a simple random sample size to obtain a quick approximation of the desired sample size for the complex survey. Suppose a design-effect model indicates an expected DEFF of 1.5 for a particular multistage design. Further, suppose that the assumption of a simple random sample implies that a minimum of 500 sample persons is required. Then the required sample size for the multistage survey would be 750 persons.

Once the minimum sample size for an analytic subdomain is determined, the survey planner can investigate design options, in connection with cost models, for optimal designs that leads to the most efficient selection of the desired number of sample persons. Final design decisions for the selection of sample persons might include the specification of the analytic subdomains of interest, the size of the household clusters, variables to be used in stratification of primary sampling units (PSUs), and the age-sex specific sampling fractions. The usual design considerations and optimization procedures for a cross-sectional survey are outlined in many standard textbooks (for example, Cochran, 1977; Kish, 1965).

PSU Selection

One additional design consideration is important for analytic surveys: The survey design must allow for accurate assessment of sampling variability for the survey estimates. Although design-effect models are used to approximate the "true" sampling error in the design stage of a survey, once the survey has been completed the practical problem is the actual estimation of the sampling errors. Exact variance equations for many survey estimates are not available, and approximations are usually needed. Complex survey variance approximations are often based on first-order Taylor series approximations (Tepping 1968; Woodruff, 1971) or replication methods, such as balanced repeated replication or jackknife approaches (Kish & Frankel, 1977; McCarthy, 1966). Variance estimation techniques for complex survey estimates are reviewed in Rao (1975), Rust (1985) and Wolter (1985).

Because of the need for approximations to estimate sampling errors, a major design decision for a survey involves the number of strata and the number of PSUs selected per stratum. Under suitable conditions, variability of survey estimates is reduced when 1 PSU is selected per stratum. However, for estimating variances based on complex survey data, many of the approximations require 2 PSUs to be selected per stratum. If a survey is designed with 1 PSU per stratum, then pseudostrata with 2 PSUs per stratum must be formed and the design efficiency of 1 PSU per stratum is lost in the variance estimation process.

In addition, the stability of the survey variance estimates is related to the number of PSUs with sample observations (Kish, Groves, & Krotki, 1976). Because of geographic clustering, there may be only a limited number of PSUs with a sufficient number of sample observations for, say, an analytic subdomain such as Black men aged 20 through 29 years. In this case, not only will variance estimates be imprecise, but analytic methods for survey data may be affected. For example, it is known that the Wald statistic, commonly used for categorical data analysis of survey data (Koch, Freeman, & Freeman, 1975; Koch & Lemeshow, 1972; Landis et al., 1982), does not perform well when the variance estimator is not stable (Thomas & Rao, 1984, 1985). Thus, for the purpose of variance estimation and analysis of the survey data, an important design consideration is not only the selection of PSUs to get a *total* sample size by subdomain, but also the *distribution* of that sample across PSUs.

Sampling for Time Points

For panel surveys, time points as well as individuals are sampled. Cook and Ware (1983) called this "sampling for occasions" and "sampling for persons." The determination of the spacing of time points in a panel survey requires knowledge of type of statistical method to be used, such as comparison of relative risks, regression analysis, or survival analysis. For these types of analyses, intermediate intervals of data collection as well as the endpoints are often required, and the design must consider the relationship between available sample size, the lengths of the follow-up intervals (frequency of measurement), and the overall duration of the longitudinal component. For each analytic method many factors may be involved, namely, significance levels, statistical power, relative variance (and covariance) for a number of variables, the proportion exposed to each risk factor, annual incidence rates for each disease, cumulative attrition rates, and time-interval nonresponse rates. In addition, the estimation procedures for coefficients in analytic models do not lend themselves to a simple solution for the expected sample size and duration. Here, some research for clinical trials and follow-up studies may be applied to sample surveys.

For regression analysis, Schesselman (1973a, 1973b) has examined the issue of sample size and sample time points in some detail and his results may be useful in planning data collection intervals for panel surveys. Palta and McHugh (1979, 1980) have examined the sample size and duration needed for follow-up (cohort) studies when there is a certain amount of sample lost to follow-up. For survival analysis, Schoenfeld (1983) examined sample sizes needed for Cox regression (proportional hazard) models, while Palta and Amini (1985) have looked at sample sizes needed for a stratified design in the presence of covariates. Taulbee and Symons (1983) have also examined the sample sizes needed for survival analysis in the presence of covariates. In addition, this problem has been considered by Schesselman (1982) for case control studies.

The complex problems in considerations of necessary time points for a panel survey can be illustrated by the comparatively simple example of determining the minimum sample size and duration for detecting relative risks. Relative risk is defined as the ratio of the cumulative incidence rate in the population exposed to a risk factor to the cumulative incidence rate in the population unexposed to the risk factor. To examine relative risks over time, only the first and last measurements are needed, so that sample size and the survey's duration are factors, but the intermediate intervals of measurement are not a factor.

With some simplifying assumptions, the determination of significant relative risk is very similar to the determination of significant difference between the two proportions (Bryant & Morgenstein, 1987). Given a functional form for the cumulative incidence rate, say an exponential function, Bryant and Morgenstein developed an equation that can be used to examine the relationship among relative risk, sample size, and duration for specified levels of significance, power, incidence rate of those exposed, and proportion of the population exposed.

In the following examples, from Bryant and Morgenstein (1987), it is assumed that the stated significance level should be 95 percent ($\alpha = 0.05$) and the significance test performed with 80 percent power ($\beta = 0.2$). Further, assume that half (0.5) of the population is exposed to the risk of developing a certain disease condition and that this disease has an annual incidence rate of 5 per 10,000 population (0.0005). This incidence rate is similar to the incidence rate for lung cancer among women aged 45 through 54 years in the United States. Suppose, due to expected incidence rates, design, and cost considerations that a maximum sample size of 1000 persons is possible. Under these conditions, the survey could detect a relative risk of 5.76 in ten years and a relative risk of 3.86 in twenty years.

Smaller relative risks could be detected if the survey had a larger sample size or if the disease condition had a higher incidence rate. Thus consider an incidence rate of 100 per 10,000 population; this is similar to the incidence rate for coronary heart disease in women aged 55 through 64 years in the United States. If the sample size and other considerations in the previous example remained unchanged, a relative risk of 1.64 could be detected after ten years and a relative risk of 1.42 could be detected after twenty years.

As an alternative, given a desired relative risk to be detected at each duration, the minimum required sample size can be determined. With the same exposure and significance assumptions as in the previous example, suppose the survey objective is to detect a relative risk of 1.64 in ten years. For a disease with an annual incidence rate of 27 per 10,000 population, a sample size of 4800 would be needed. Similarly, to detect a relative risk of 1.6 in twenty years but with an annual incidence rate of 54 per 10,000 population, a sample of 2300 persons would be required.

Clearly the number of possible combinations of proportion exposed in the population, disease-specific incidence rates, expected relative risks, and possible durations makes the determination of any single sample size nearly impossible. It may be best to use the sample size as determined from the descriptive objectives (precision of estimates and simple hypothesis testing) and then examine, for each specific application, the required durations needed to detect a specified relative risk. This also may become a decision mechanism for determining the final content in the health survey, since such a calculation would indicate the feasibility of fulfilling a survey objective for any disease component. Again, the issue of determining sample size and duration for detecting relative risks, while complex, is relatively simple compared with the problem of determining the sample size, number of intermediate intervals, and total duration that would be required for a regression analysis of prospective survey data.

SUMMARY

This discussion of general considerations in the design of longitudinal surveys of health has focused on the use of the survey's analytic objectives to determine the basic survey design. Although some types of longitudinal objectives can be met by either cross-sectional or pure-panel surveys, other survey objectives can be met by only one of the two basic designs. For national health surveys, which are multipurpose in nature, the split-panel survey provides a design that can meet a wide variety of survey objectives.

A split-panel design has two components. The panel component can be used to measure individual change over time, to measure components of individual change, to provide the means to measure the frequency and timing of events occurring in a given time period, and to measure aggregate change over time. An advantage of a prospective-panel survey is that such a survey allows for increased precision of estimates of aggregate change by eliminating individual variation through repeated measurements on the same individuals. The independent cross-sectional component at each time point can be compared with the panel component to determine possible nonresponse bias (both internal and external), attrition and panel effects, and the effect of changing population. The split-panel design is particularly advantageous if these effects are minimized so that the data for the two components can be combined for more precise estimates for a single point in time.

Because the panel component will get smaller over time, a critical issue for the prospective part of the split-panel survey is that the survey design and the survey operations must maximize response for initial examination and minimize attrition thereafter. From an operations standpoint, this is addressed by having intensive follow-ups, minimizing respondent burden, encouraging continued participation, and generally expending resources in an effort to increase response. Past studies have indicated that persons who *refuse* to participate are generally similar to participants, but the different determinants of the *non-available* sample persons may result in differential bias of the remaining panel sample. This implies that, to best allocate follow-up resources, follow-up efforts should focus on disabled and the hard to find. In addition, the new cross-sectional sample can be used to add members to "freshen" the panel sample.

In the split-panel survey, the design considerations at the initial time point are similar to those for any cross-sectional survey. The design of the initial survey requires specification of minimum sample size and the sample selection mechanism to attain that sample size. Sample size is often determined as the minimum number needed to meet specified levels of precision or specified levels of aggregate differences that can be detected. If a multistage design is used, an expected design effect must be known.

When an initial sample is used as a cohort in a split-panel survey, an additional consideration is that the initial sample size must be adequate to meet the longitudinal analytic objectives. For the panel component, there is a need to determine sample size, number and spacing of time intervals, and total duration. In a multipurpose national survey each disease condition can give rise to different sample sizes and required time intervals. For the panel portion of the survey, the specific longitudinal objectives must be individually examined to see if the initial cross-sectional sample size is sufficient to meet the longitudinal needs within a desired period of survey duration. For some specific objectives, the sample size in the initial cohort may not be sufficient. That is, if cost limitations imply a maximum sample size, then the concepts of detectable differences over time can be used as a decision mechanism for survey content.

The split-panel design is extremely flexible. At each time point there are actually two or more surveys. The first time point can be used as a single national sample or as several national samples. For example, the National Health Interview Survey is designed as four independent national samples for each year. One or more of these independent samples can be considered as a panel for later follow-up.

For later time points, the split-panel survey will provide a new cross-sectional component and allow for reinterview of some or all of those persons initially selected. Furthermore, the cross-sectional samples at each time interval could also be considered as panels for later follow-up. Thus, the split-panel design is especially advantageous for health surveys in which there is continuous change in data needs and survey objectives as health issues evolve over time.

REFERENCES

Baltes PB (1968). "Longitudinal and cross-sectional sequences in the study of age and generation effects." *Human Development* 11:145–171.

Bonham GS (1983). *Procedures and Questionnaires of the National Medical Care Utilization and Expenditures Survey.*" *National Medical Care Utilization and Expenditures Survey, Series A, Methodological Report No. 1*, National Center for Health Statistics, DHHS Pub. No. 83-20001. Washington, D.C., Government Printing Office.

Bryant E, Morgenstein DR (1987). "Sample size determination for longitudinal surveys." *Proceedings of the Section on Survey Research Methods*, Washington, D.C., *American Statistical Association*, pp. 189–193.

Cambell DT, Stanley JC (1963). "Experimental and quasi-experimental designs for Research on teaching," in Gage NL (ed), *Handbook on Research on Teaching*. Chicago, Rand McNally.

Clarke WR, Schrott HG, Leaverton PE, Connor WE, Lauer RM (1978). "Tracking of blood lipids and blood pressures in school age children: The Muscatine study." *Circulation* 58:626–634.

Cochran WG (1977). *Sampling Techniques*, 3rd Ed. New York, Wiley.

Cook NR, Ware JH (1983). "Design and analysis methods for longitudinal research." *Annual Review of Public Health* 4:1–23.

Dohrenwend BS, Dohrenwend BP (1968). "Sources of refusal in surveys." *Public Opinion Quarterly* 32:74–83.

Duncan GJ, Kalton G (1987). "Issues of design and analysis of surveys across time." *International Statistical Review* 55:97–117.

Ferris BG Jr, Dockery DW, Ware JH, Speizer FE, Spiro R III (1983). "The six-city study: Examples of problems in analysis of the data." *Environmental Health Perspectives* 52:115–123.

Fleiss JR (1981) *Statistical Methods for Rates and Proportions.* New York, Wiley.

Gordon T, Sorlie P, Kannel WB (1971). *Coronary Heart Disease, Atherothrombotic Brain Infarction, Intermittent Claudication—A Multivariate Analysis of Some Factors*

Goudy WJ (1976). "Nonresponse effects on relationships between variables." *Public Opinion Quarterly* 40:360–369.

Goudy WJ (1985). "Sample attrition and multivariate analysis in the retirement history study." *Journal of Geronltology* 40: 358–367.

Judkins D, Hubble D, Dorsch J, McMillen D, Ernst L (1984). "Weighting of persons for SIPP longitudinal tabulations." *Proceedings of Survey Research Methods,* Washington, D.C., *American Statistical Association,* pp 676–681.

Kalton G. (1983. *Compensating for Missing Survey Data.* Ann Arbor, Survey Research Center, University of Michigan.

Kalton G (1986). "Handling wave nonresponse in panel surveys." *Journal of Official Statistics* 2:303–314.

Kish L (1965). *Survey Sampling.* New York, Wiley.

Kish L (1981). "Split panel designs." *Survey Methods Newsletter,* Social and Community Planning Research, London.

Kish L (1983). "Data collection for details over space and time," in Wright T (ed), *Statistical Methods and the Improvement of Data Quality,* Orlando, Academic Press, pp 73–84.

Kish L, Frankel M (1974). "Inference from complex surveys." *Journal of the Royal Statistical Society B* 36:1–37.

Kish L, Groves RM, Krotki KP (1976). *Sampling Errors for Fertility Surveys* Occasional Paper, no. 17. London, World Fertility Survey.

Koch GG, Freeman DH, Freeman JL (1975). "Strategies in the multivariate analysis of data from complex surveys." *International Statistical Review* 43:59–78.

Koch GG, Lemeshow S (1972). "An application of multivariate analysis to complex sample survey data." *Journal of the American Statistical Association* 67:780–782.

Labouvie EW, Bartsch TW, Nesselroade JR, Baltes PB (1974). "On the internal and external validity of simple longitudinal designs." *Child Development* 45:282–290.

Landis J, Lepkowski J, Eklund S, Stehouwer S (1982). *A Statistical Methodology for Analyzing Data from a Complex Survey, the First National Health and Nutrition Examination Survey,* Vital and Health Statistics, Series 2, No. 92, DHHS Pub. No. 82-1366. Washington, D.C., Government Printing Office.

Lehnen RG, Koch GG (1974). "Analyzing panel data with uncontrolled attrition." *Public Opinion Quarterly* 38:40–56.

Levy PS, Lemeshow SL (1980). *Sampling for Health Professionals.* Belmont, Calif., Lifetime Learning Publications.

Little RJA (1982). "Models for nonresponse in sample surveys." *Journal of the American Statistical Association* 77:237–250.

Little RJA (1985). "Nonresponse adjustments in longitudinal surveys: Models for categorical data." *Bulletin of the International Statistical Institute* 15.1:1–15.

Little RJA, Rubin DB (1987). *Statistical Analysis with Missing Data.* New York, Wiley.

McCarthy PJ (1966). *Replication: An Approach to the Analysis of Data from complex surveys.* Vital and Health Statistics, Series 2, No. 14. Department of Health, Education, and Welfare. Washington, D.C., Government Printing Office.

McFall RM (1977). "Parameters of self-monitoring," In Stewart RM (ed), *Behavioral Management: Strategies, Techniques and Outcome*. New York, Bruner-Mazel.

Norris FH (1985). "Characteristics of older nonrespondents over five waves of a panel study." *Journal of Gerontology* 40:627–636.

Palta M, Amini SB (1985). "Consideration of covariates and stratification in sample size determination for survival time studies." *Journal of Chronic Disease* 38:801–809.

Palta M, McHugh R (1979). "Adjusting for loss to followup in sample size determination for cohort studies." *Journal of Chronic Disease* 32:315–326.

Palta M, McHugh R (1980). "Planning the size of a cohort study in the presence of both losses to followup and noncompliance." *Journal of Chronic Disease* 33:501–512.

Powers EA, Bultena GC (1972). "Characteristics of deceased dropouts in longitudinal research." *Journal of Gerontology* 27:530–535.

Rao JNK (1975). "Unbiased variance estimation for multistage designs." *Sankya C* 37:133–139.

Related to Their Incidence: Framingham Study, 16-year Follow-up. Washington, D.C., Government Printing Office.

Rubin DB (1987). *Multiple Imputation for Nonresponse in Surveys*. New York, Wiley.

Rust K (1985). "Variance estimation for complex estimators in sample surveys." *Journal of Official Statistics* 1:381–397.

Schaie KW (1965). "A general model for the study of developmental problems." *Psychological Bulletin* 64:92–107.

Schaie KW (1973). "Methodological problems in descriptive development research on adulthood and aging. In Nesselroade, JR, Reese HW (eds), *Life Span Developmental Psychology: Methodological Issues*. New York, Academic Press.

Schaie KW, Labouvie G, Barrett T (1975). "Selective attrition effects in a fourteen-year study of adult intelligence." *Journal of Gerontology* 28:328–334.

Schesselman JJ (1973a). "Planning a longitudinal study. I. Sample size determination." *Journal of Chronic Disease* 26:553–560.

Schesselman JJ (1973b). "Planning a longitudinal study. II. Frequency of measurement and study duration." *Journal of Chronic Disease* 26:561–570.

Schesselman JJ (1982). *Case Control Studies, Design, Conduct, Analysis*. New York, Oxford University Press.

Schoenfeld DA (1983). "The asymptotic properties of nonparametric test for comparing survival distributions." *Biometrika* 86:316–319.

Seigler I, Botwinick J (1979). "A long-term longitudinal study of intellectual ability of older adults: The matter of selective subject attrition." *Journal of Gerontology* 34:242–245.

Seigler I, McCarty S, Logue P (1982). "Wechsler memory scale scores, selective attrition, and distance from death." *Journal of Gerontology* 37:176–181.

Sobol MG (1959). "Panel mortality and panel bias." *Journal of the American Statistical Association* 54:52–68.

Streib GF (1966). "Participants and drop-outs in a longitudinal study." *Journal of Gerontology* 21:200–209.

Taulbee JD, Symons MJ (1983). "Sample size and duration for cohort studies of survival time with covariables." *Biometrics* 39:351–360.

Tepping BJ (1968). "Variance estimation in complex surveys." *Proceedings of the Social Statistics Section, Washington, D.C., American Statistical Association*, pp 11–18.

Thomas DR, Rao JNK (1984). *A Monte Carlo Study of Exact Levels for Chi-square Goodness-of-fit Statistics Under Cluster Sampling*. Technical Report, no. 35. Ottawa, Canada, Carleton University/University of Ottawa, Laboratory for Research in Statistics and Probability.

Thomas DR, Rao JNK (1985). "On the power of some goodness-of-fit tests under cluster sampling." Technical Report 66. In *Analysis of Categorical Data from Sample Surveys: A Collection of Five Papers.* Ottawa, Canada, Carleton University/University of Ottawa, Laboratory for Research in Statistics and Probability, pp 57–82.

Trevino FM, Moss AJ (1984). *Health Indicators for Hispanic, Black and White Americans.* Vital and Health Statistics, Series 10, No. 148. National Center for Health Statistics DHHS Pub. No. (PHS) 84-1576. Washington, D.C., Government Printing Office.

Wolter KM (1985). *Introduction to Variance Estimation.* New York, Springer-Verlag.

Woodruff RS (1971). "A simple method for approximating the variance of a complicated estimate." *Journal of the American Statistical Association* 66: 411–414.

I
Models for Continuous Variables

3

Differential Equation Models for Longitudinal Data
Application: Blood Pressure and Relative Weight

JAMES DWYER

A model for interpreting longitudinal data in terms of continuous-time differential equations, rather than in terms of discrete-time "integrated" equations, has two advantages. The first derives from the fact that researchers construe most biologic processes they study as continuous time–continuous state space processes; thus continuous time models are more realistic and interpretable tools of study. The second is that the parameters of the differential form of the model are more "fundamental" in that they are invariant over studies with differing time intervals between examinations.

The most complex differential equation (DE) model to be discussed in this chapter allows investigation of temporal asymmetries among variables. This means that the directionality of a relation (i.e., the extent to which X predicts change in Y, and Y predicts change in X) can be explored.

Applications of DEs with negative feedback to panel data have thus far been quite limited. Most applications of these models in biology have been to time series such as growth data (Sandland & McGilchrist, 1979), and in epidemiology to time series data from epidemics (Ackerman, Elveback, & Fox, 1984; Bartlett, 1960). Applications to *panel data* are primarily found in economics (cf. Bergstrom & Wymer, 1976) and sociology (Coleman, 1968).

This chapter is restricted to models for continuous variables measured in continuous time, although analogous models for categorical variables in discrete time were the historical precursors of the continuous-state-space–continuous-time stochastic models (cf. Karlin & Taylor, 1981). These continuous equations are known as *diffusions*, since they are derived from models of the diffusion of particles through a permeable membrane.

After a review of several types of deterministic and stochastic DEs, a stochastic DE is fit to blood pressure and relative weight data from the Framingham Heart Study. A two-step method of estimation is described. The first step involves maximum likelihood estimation of the integrated form of the model, assuming multivariate normality. The second step uses the estimates of parameters and their covariances from the first step to estimate the parameters of the DE by the delta method. The conclusion from this example analysis is that elevated relative weight is a precursor of elevated blood pressure rather than vice versa.

NOMENCLATURE

An *ordinary* differential equation (DE) involves a dependent variable $Y(t)$ that is a function of a single variable (e.g., time or age); a *partial* DE expresses change in Y as a function of several variables. The *order* of a DE refers to the highest order derivative included in the equation. The *degree* of a DE is the power to which the highest order derivative in the equation is raised. A DE is said to be *linear* if all derivatives of the dependent variable, and the dependent variable itself, are of the first degree. A linear DE is thus of the form

$$\psi(t) = f_n(t)\frac{d^n y}{dt^n} + f_{n-1}(t)\frac{d^{n-1}y}{dt^{n-1}} + \cdots + f_1(t)\frac{dy}{dt} + f_0(t)y$$

where $d^n y/dt^n$ denotes the nth derivative of y with respect to t. Finally, a linear DE is *homogeneous* if $\psi(t)$ is defined to be zero. As an example,

$$\frac{dy}{dt} = \frac{\psi(t)}{f_1(t)} - \frac{f_0(t)}{f_1(t)}y = g_1(t) + g_2(t)y$$

is a nonhomogeneous (if $g_1(t) \neq 0$), first-order, ordinary linear DE of the first degree. It is models of this type that will be the focus of this chapter.

An additional distinction is made between *deterministic* and *stochastic* DEs. A stochastic continuous-time process $y(t)$ includes a component, say $B(t)$, that is Gaussian in some sense. The derivative of this process, dB/dt, is then the stochastic component of a stochastic DE—which is often referred to as *white noise*. Precise specification of such a continuous process in continuous time is not straightforward. Considerable attention has been given to such equations as models of *Brownian motion*.

The *solution equation* of a DE expresses the dependent variable as a function of independent variables that does not involve derivatives. For example, if $dY/dt = \beta$, then the general solution equation is obtained by integration $Y(t) = \alpha + \beta t$. If $dY/dt = \beta Y$, then $Y(t) = e^{\alpha + \beta t}$ is the general solution. Solution equations are also referred to as *integrated equations*. The *particular* solution is distinguished from the general solution (or primitive) by solving for the integration constant in terms of a particular value of the independent variable. Thus a particular solution of $dY/dt = \beta$ is given by

$$Y(t) = Y(t_0) + \beta(t - t_0)$$

and a particular solution of $dY/dt = \beta Y$ is given by

$$Y(t) = Y(t_0)e^{\beta(t - t_0)}$$

where the integration constant α is defined at $t = t_0$.

DETERMINISTIC DIFFERENTIAL EQUATIONS WITHOUT FEEDBACK

The most general deterministic DE to be considered here is of the form

$$\frac{dy}{dt} = g_1(t) + g_2(t)y(t) \tag{1}$$

where $y(t)$ is a continuous function of time and neither $g_1(t)$ nor $g_2(t)$ involves a stochastic component. The reason for choosing this form is that it is somewhat flexible, and yet its solution is readily obtained. The solution equation is given by

$$e^{-G_2(t)t}y(t) = \int g_1(t)e^{-G_2(t)t}dt \tag{2}$$

where $G_2(t) = \int g_2(t)dt$. Some deterministic cases of (1) that will be discussed in this chapter are outlined in Table 3-1. The cases where $g_2(t)$ is zero do not involve feedback, and these are the models considered in this section. The solution equations following from such models yield regression models for panel data that are static (or unconditional). In contrast, when $g_2(t)$ is a constant, the implied regression models for panel data are dynamic (or conditional); these models are considered in the next section.

Uniform Change

One of the simplest DEs is a nonhomogeneous equation with $g_1(t) = \alpha_1$ and $g_2(t) = 0$:

$$\frac{dY}{dt} = \alpha_1 \tag{3}$$

where dY/dt is the first derivative of Y with respect to time, and α_1 is constant through time. The first derivative is the slope of the function $Y(t)$ at time t: the instantaneous rate of change in Y per unit time (e.g., millimeters of mercury per year for blood pressure, BP). Blood pressure, for example, may then be modeled as a deterministic function of time (or age):

$$BP(t) = \alpha_0 + \alpha_1 t \tag{4}$$

where the solution equation (4) is obtained from the DE (3) by integration. This model states that the *rate* of change in BP (or time trend α_1) is uniform (invariant) over t and thus independent of t, whereas the *level* of BP at time t—$BP(t)$—is entirely a function of t and the level at t_0. In fact, however, we know from longitudinal ovservation of BP that such a model violates several known characteristics of BP development:

1. BP does not increase at the same rate in all persons.
2. BP does not increase without bound as age increases, but can come to an equilibrium.

Table 3–1. Deterministic linear differential equations and corresponding solution equations for panel data

General form: $dY/dt = g_1(t) + g_2(t) \cdot Y(t)$

Special case 1: $g_2(t) = 0$

1A. $g_1(t) = 0$

$$Y(t) = \alpha_0$$

1B. $g_1(t) = \alpha_1$

$$Y(t) = \alpha_0 + \alpha_1 t = Y(t_0) + \alpha_1(t - t_0)$$

1C. $g_1(t) = \alpha_1 + \alpha_2 t$

$$Y(t) = \alpha_0 + \alpha_1 t + \left(\frac{\alpha_2}{2}\right)t^2 = Y(t_0) + \alpha_1(t - t_0)$$
$$+ \left(\frac{\alpha_2}{2}\right)(t^2 - t_0^2)$$

1D. $g_1(t) = \alpha_1 + \alpha_2 X(t)$

if $\dfrac{dX}{dt} = \beta_1$ and $X(t) = \beta_0' + \beta_1 t$, then

$$Y(t) = \alpha_0 + \alpha_1 t + \frac{\alpha_2 t[X(t) + X(t_0)]}{2}$$
$$= Y(t_0) + \alpha_1(t - t_0) + \frac{\alpha_2(t - t_0)[X(t) + X(t_0)]}{2}$$

Special case 2: $g_2(t) = \alpha_3$

2A. $g_1(t) = 0$

$$Y(t) = \left(\frac{1}{\alpha_3}\right) e^{\alpha_0 + \alpha_3 t} = Y(t_0)e^{\alpha_3(t - t_0)}$$

2B. $g_1(t) = \alpha_1$

$$Y(t) = \alpha_0 e^{\alpha_3 t} - \frac{\alpha_1}{\alpha_3} = e^{\alpha_3 \Delta t} Y(t_0) - \left(\frac{\alpha_1}{\alpha_3}\right)(1 - e^{\alpha_3 \Delta t})$$

2D. $g_1(t) = \alpha_1 + \alpha_2 X(t)$

if $\dfrac{dX}{dt} = \beta_0 + \beta_1 t$, then

$$Y(t) = a_0 + a_1 X(t_0) + a_2 Y(t_0) + a_3[X(t) - X(t_0)]$$

if $\dfrac{dX}{dt} = \beta_1 + \beta_3 X$ and $X(t) = \beta_0 e^{\beta_3 t} - \dfrac{\beta_1}{\beta_3}$, then

$$Y(t) = a_0 + a_1 X(t_0) + a_2 Y(t_0)$$

if $\dfrac{dX}{dt} = \beta_1 + \beta_2 Y + \beta_3 X$, then

$$Y(t) = a_0 + a_1 X(t_0) + a_2 Y(t_0)$$
$$X(t) = b_0 + b_1 Y(t_0) + b_2 X(t_0)$$

or

$$Y(t) - Y(t_0) = a_0 + a_1 X(t_0) + (a_2 - 1)Y(t_0)$$
$$X(t) - X(t_0) = b_0 + b_1 Y(t_0) + (b_2 - 1)X(t_0)$$

3. BP is not a linear function of age over the entire life span.
4. BP as measured with a sphygmomanometer and stethoscope is subject to apparently random variability that could not be accounted for in such a simple deterministic model.

However, before one develops more elaborate process models that attempt to incorporate what is known about BP, it is instructive to see how observed data could be used to assess the model in equation (3). First suppose that only two waves of observation are collected at age t_1 and age t_2. Then, solving for α_0 in equation (4) when $t = t_1$ and substituting, equation (4) can be rewritten as

$$BP(t_2) = BP(t_1) + \alpha_1(t_2 - t_1)$$

or

$$BP(t_2) - BP(t_1) = \alpha_1(t_2 - t_1)$$

The fit of this model with longitudinally observed BP for a sample of persons could be assessed by regressing the change in BP on change in t:

$$BP_i(t_2) - BP_i(t_1) = a_0 + a_1(t_2 - t_1) + \zeta_i \qquad (5)$$

with the constraint that the intercept a_0 is zero and the variance, var(ζ), and mean, E(ζ), of the residuals across persons are zero. If the model fits the data well, $\hat{a}_1$ would be an estimate of α_1 in model equation (5). Alternatively, ζ could be considered random error in the measurement of ΔBP; in this instance there would be no "test" of the model. Note that if t_1 and t_2 are 1 time unit apart for all cases (say ages 13 and 14), then α_1 is simply the difference between the expected values of BP at the two ages.

Equations (3) and (4) are the crucial depictions of the model. Equation (3) depicts how the model explains change in BP over continuous time, and equation (4) depicts how the model explains change in BP between two discrete points in time. Since panel studies involve measurement at discrete points in time, translation of a continuous-time process model into relations among observations at discrete points in time is central. Thus derivation of the form of equations analogous to (4) will be the primary focus of this chapter, since these equations inform us how we can interpret observed change between discrete points in time. In the instance of the simple uniform-change model in equation (3), this translation is trivial. But such is not the case in more realistic process models.

If BP is observed at more than two points in time, the uniform-change model in equation (3) predicts that each pair of scores for a single case, divided by the time change, is equal to α_1. These time series observations would then be related to time as in equation (4). The linear time trend in BP would again be reflected in the coefficient α_1. The test of the fit of the model would be based on the similarity of the time trends across cases, since the model predicts that they will be identical:

$$BP(t_3) - BP(t_2) = \alpha_1(t_3 - t_2)$$
$$BP(t_2) - BP(t_1) = \alpha_1(t_2 - t_1)$$

or

$$\mathrm{BP}(t_j)_i = \alpha_0 + \alpha_1 t_{ij}$$

where $\mathrm{BP}(t_j)_i$ is the observed BP at time t_j for the ith person, t_{ij} is the age of the ith person at time t_j. This model can be extended to incorporate interindividual differences in intercept or slope by incorporating random effects into the model:

$$\mathrm{BP}(t_j)_i = (\alpha_0 + \alpha_i) + (a + \alpha_i)t_{ij}$$

where we then have the differential model defined for individual members of the population $(dY_i/dt = \alpha + \alpha_i)$.

Time-Dependent Rate of Change

The uniform-change model in equation (3) specifies that the rate of change is independent of time. A DE model in which the rate of change is a function of time is the polynomial

$$\frac{d(\mathrm{BP})}{dt} = \alpha_1 + \alpha_2 t + \alpha_3 t^2 + \cdots$$

The solution equation is then

$$\mathrm{BP}(t) = \alpha_0 + \alpha_1 t + \frac{\alpha_2}{2}t^2 + \frac{\alpha_3}{3}t^3 + \cdots$$

or

$$\mathrm{BP}(t_2) = \mathrm{BP}(t_1) + \alpha_1(t_2 - t_1) + \frac{\alpha_2}{2}(t_2^2 - t_1^2)$$

(Note that the last term does not involve the square of the time difference but the difference of the squared times.) In the case of a first-order polynomial DE, the solution equation may be written

$$\mathrm{BP}(t) = \alpha_0 + \left(\alpha_1 + \frac{\alpha_2 t}{2}\right)t$$

where it is clear that the rate of change in BP with respect to time $[\alpha_1 + (\alpha_2/2)t]$ is itself a function of time.

Another differential equation employing a nonlinear function of t is that in which the rate of change in BP is an exponential function of time:

$$\frac{d(\mathrm{BP})}{dt} = \alpha_1 e^{\alpha_2 t}$$

where e indicates the Naperian base number ($2.718\ldots$). If α_2 is less than zero, this model implies that the rate of change approaches zero as t approaches infinity. Thus a model of this form has the advantage that it does not predict unbounded change as time (or age) progresses. Furthermore, it has an additional important property, which can be seen by integrating to obtain the solution equation

$$BP(t) = \alpha_0 + \frac{\alpha_1}{\alpha_2} e^{\alpha_2 t}$$

If we now multiply the solution equation by α_2 we have

$$\alpha_2 BP(t) = \alpha_0 \alpha_2 + \alpha_1 e^{\alpha_2 t}$$

which implies that

$$\frac{d(BP)}{dt} = -(\alpha_0 \alpha_2) + \alpha_2 BP(t)$$

That is, the rate of change in BP is a function of the level of BP itself. When a differential equation model is specified such that the derivative is a function of the level of the dependent variable, this aspect of the model is sometimes termed *feedback*, since the level feeds back to change the rate of change. In fact, then, $g_2(t) = \alpha_2$ in equation (1) when the rate of change is assumed to be an exponential function of time. We will return to this model when considering models where g_2 is a constant (next section).

Exogenous Influence

To this point we have assumed that $Y(t)$ was a direct function of time. We now extend the DE to the case where dY/dt is a function of $X(t)$, such that $Y(X(t), t)$ is still a function of t, but indirectly. A simple DE is then

$$\frac{dY}{dt} = \alpha_1 + \alpha_2 X(t) \tag{6}$$

where

$$\int dY = \int [\alpha_1 + \alpha_2 X(t)] dt \;\Rightarrow\; Y(t) - Y(t_0) = \alpha_1 t + \int_{t_0}^{t} \alpha_2(\tau) d\tau$$

If we now assume that change in X is uniform with respect to time

$$\frac{dX}{dt} = \beta_1 \;\Rightarrow\; X(t) = \beta_0 + \beta_1 t \tag{7}$$

then equation (6) can be rewritten as

$$\frac{dY}{dt} = \alpha_1 + \alpha_2(\beta_0 + \beta_1 t)$$

The solution to (6) is then

$$Y(t) = \alpha_0 + (\alpha_1 + \beta_0 \alpha_2)t + \left(\frac{\beta_1 \alpha_2}{2}\right) t_2 \tag{8}$$

$$= \alpha_0 + \left[\alpha_1 + \alpha_2 \left(\frac{X(t) + X(t_0)}{2}\right)\right] t$$

The particular solution with α_0 defined at $Y(t_0)$ is then

$$Y(t) = Y(t_0) + (\alpha_1 + \beta_0\alpha_2)(t - t_0) + \frac{\beta_1\alpha_2}{2}(t^2 - t_0^2)$$

Regrouping terms yields

$$Y(t) - Y(t_0) = \alpha_1(t - t_0) + \alpha_2\left[\beta_0(t - t_0) + \frac{\beta_1}{2}(t + t_0)(t - t_0)\right]$$

$$= \Delta t\left[\alpha_1 + \alpha_2\left(\frac{X(t) + X(t_0)}{2}\right)\right] \tag{9}$$

since $[X(t) + X(t_0)]/2 = \beta_0 + (\beta_1/2)(t + t_0)$, and $\Delta t = (t - t_0)$. Thus the solution (9) to the system of equations (6) and (7) indicates that change in Y per unit time between t_0 and t should be linearly related to the mean of X at the two points in time. Equations (6) and (7) define a continuous-time model, whereas (9) is the discrete-time solution implied by the continuous-time model.

The integrated equation (9) can be extended to the analysis of panel data by assuming individual variation in the parameters of (7):

$$\frac{dY_i}{dt} = \alpha_1 + \alpha_2 X_i(t)$$

$$\frac{dX_i}{dt} = \beta_{1i} \Rightarrow X_i(t) = \beta_{0i} + \beta_{1i}t$$

where i indexes members of a population in which the parameters in equation (6) are invariant across members. In the case of two measurement points, t_0 and t_1, equation (9) implies the regression equation

$$Y_i(t_1) - Y_i(t_0) = \Delta t\left[\alpha_1 + \alpha_2\left(\frac{X_i(t_1) + X(t_0)}{2}\right)\right] + \zeta_i$$

where ζ_i is random measurement error in ΔY. Generalizing to more than two time points yields the regression model

$$Y_i(t_j) - Y_i(t_{j-1}) = (t_j - t_{j-1})\left[\alpha_1 + \alpha_2\left(\frac{X_i(t_j) + X(t_{j-1})}{2}\right)\right] + \eta_i + \zeta_{ij}$$

where η_i is a random effect for individuals with $E(\eta_i) = 0$ and $E\{\eta_i[X_i(t_j) + X(t_{j-1})]/2\}$ possibly nonzero. If the number of measurement points is sufficient, heterogeneity in the parameters of (6) could also be added to the model.

It is clear from equation (8) that $Y(t)$ increases or decreases without bound. This assumption was also made for $X(t)$. Such model may be suitable for short-term approximations of biologic or social systems, but it is unlikely to be a realistic model of such a system. Living systems tend to equilibrate more often than they explode or collapse.

A Reciprocal Effects Model

The models considered thus far assume that the direction of influence, or the temporal precedence, between two variables is unidirectional and known (i.e., from X to Y rather than from Y to X). An alternative assumption is that influences are reciprocal. For example,

$$\frac{dY(t)}{dt} = \alpha_1 + \alpha_2 X(t) \Rightarrow Y(t) = \alpha_1 t + \alpha_2 \int X(t)dt$$

$$\frac{dX(t)}{dt} = \beta_1 + \beta_2 Y(t) \Rightarrow X(t) = \beta_1 t + \beta_2 \int Y(t)dt$$

The solution of this type of model is more complex. If $\beta_1 = \alpha_1 = 0$ and $\beta_2 = \alpha_2$, then a solution is given by

$$Y(t) = e^{\beta_2 t} \qquad X(t) = e^{\beta_2 t}$$

since $Y(t) = \beta_2 \int X(t)dt \Rightarrow Y(t) = \beta_2^2 \int [\int Y(t)dt]dt$ (since $X(t) = \beta_2 \int Y(t)dt$). Notes that the reciprocal model, with the specified constraints, is equivalent to the negative feedback model obtained previously ("Exogenous Influence"). For this process, $Y(t)$ and $X(t)$ increase without bound if $\beta_2 > 0$, and they collapse to zero if $\beta_2 < 0$.

If we again assume that β_1 and β_2 are zero, and constrain $\beta_2 \alpha_2 = -1$, then

$$Y(t) = \frac{-1}{\beta_2} \cos(\beta_2 \alpha_2 t) \qquad X(t) = \sin(\beta_2 \alpha_2 t)$$

yields a solution, since

$$\beta_2 \alpha_2 \int\int \sin(\beta_2 \alpha_2 t)dt\, dt = \frac{-1}{\beta_2 \alpha_2} \sin(\beta_2 \alpha_2 t)$$

These equations describe a process in which $Y(t)$ and $X(t)$ oscillate about zero, and about one another, as t increases. An interesting aspect of this model is demonstrated by the case where $\beta_2 < 0$ and $\alpha_2 > 0$. In this instance the sine wave $X(t)$ "leads" the cosine wave $Y(t)$ through time.

DETERMINISTIC DIFFERENTIAL EQUATIONS WITH FEEDBACK

The deterministic DEs considered to this point have the disadvantage that they describe processes that explode, collapse, or cycle. In contrast, the addition of a feedback term to the DE yields systems that equilibrate. Some simple cases of such models are described in this section.

Linear Feedback

The addition of feedback to the model in (1) is achieved most simply by setting $g_2(t) = \alpha_3$ (see Table 3-1):

$$\frac{dY}{dt} = \alpha_3 Y(t)$$

A solution to this equation is obtained by recalling that the exponential function is one where the function is equal to its own slope. Thus

$$Y(t) = e^{\gamma_0 + \alpha_3 Y(t)} \Rightarrow \frac{dY}{dt} = \alpha_3 e^{\gamma_0 + \alpha_3 Y(t)} = \alpha_3 Y(t)$$

where $Y(t)$ explodes if $\alpha_3 > 0$, but $Y(t)$ equilibrates to zero if $\alpha_3 < 0$. A feedback model that equilibrates is then referred to as a "negative feedback" model. The particular solution is given by

$$Y(t) = e^{\ln[Y(t_0)] - \alpha_3 Y(t_0) + \alpha_3 Y(t)} = Y(t_0) e^{\alpha_3[Y(t) - Y(t_0)]}$$

where γ_0 is defined at t_0. This feedback model can be extended to include equilibration to a level other than zero (e.g., μ):

$$\frac{dY}{dt} = \alpha_1 + \alpha_3 Y(t) = \alpha_3[Y(t) - \mu]$$

where $\mu = -\alpha_1/\alpha_3$. This is equivalent to the specification in equation (1) that $g_1(t)$ is the constant α_1. The solution (from [2]) is then

$$Y(t) = \alpha_0 e^{\alpha_3 t} - \frac{\alpha_1}{\alpha_3}$$

where

$$Y(t) = e^{\alpha_3 \Delta t} Y(t_0) - \frac{\alpha_1}{\alpha_3}(1 - e^{\alpha_3 \Delta t})$$

$$= \mu + e^{\alpha_3 \Delta t}[Y(t_0) - \mu] \tag{10}$$

when α_0 is defined at t_0, and $\Delta t = t - t_0$ (ignoring γ_0). It is clear from (10) that this simple feedback model brings $Y(t)$ to the equilibrium point $-(\alpha_1/\alpha_3)$ as Δt increases when $\alpha_3 < 0$. Given the lack of stability of the system if $\alpha_3 > 0$, α_3 in (10) is often replaced by $-\alpha_3$, and α_3 is constrained to be positive.

Logistic Feedback

Although the linear feedback model is the simplest feedback model, the model applied most widely to time series growth data is the logistic. It has been applied in many areas, including growth in body dimensions and the growth of population size.

The logistic is a nonlinear DE with quadratic feedback. It is of the following general form:

$$\frac{dY}{dt} = \alpha_1 Y + \alpha_2 Y^2$$

However, the logistic DE is usually parameterized as

$$\frac{dY}{dt} = (\gamma_1 - Y)\gamma_2 Y$$

where Y is the characteristic that is growing and γ_1 is the asymptote of that growth. Note that as Y approaches γ_1, the derivative approaches zero—meaning that Y is constant (at equilibrium) after an initial growth period. It can then be shown (cf. Steen, 1955) that

$$Y(t) = \frac{\gamma_1}{1 + e^{-\gamma_1(\gamma_0 + \gamma_2 t)}}$$

is the solution equation of the logistic DE. The negative feedback incorporated into this logistic growth curve is typical of the assumptions made when modeling biological systems that grow to a state of equilibrium with no subsequent growth. Several analogous, but somewhat simpler, models are developed below.

Interestingly, the discrete-time–continuous-space analog of the logistic model

$$Y_t = (\gamma_1 - Y_t)Y_{t-1}\gamma_2$$

is a potentially chaotic model (Feigenbaum, 1978). When $\gamma_1 = 1$, Y_t becomes nonperiodic and unpredictable (without perfect measurement) as γ_2 approaches 3.56994.... Thus such simple models offer the prospect of modeling nonperiodic processes—that have heretofore been treated as stochastic—with deterministic equation systems. Chaotic models are discussed briefly in the section "Chaotic Processes."

Exogenous Influence

The logical extension of the simple feedback model involves including an exogenous determinant of dY/dt in (1) by including an $X(t)$ in $g_1(t)$:

$$\frac{dY}{dt} = \alpha_1 + \alpha_2 X(t) + \alpha_3 Y(t) \tag{11}$$

The solution equation is then obtained from

$$e^{-\alpha_3 t} Y(t) = \int [\alpha_1 + \alpha_2 X(t)]e^{-\alpha_3 t} dt \tag{12}$$

or

$$Y(t) = \int_0^t [\alpha_1 + \alpha_2 X(\tau)]e^{\alpha_3(t-\tau)} d\tau$$

An explicit form of equation (12), however, requires an explicit specification of $X(t)$. Following Coleman (1968), we consider two cases for $X(t)$: uniform change and negative feedback.

Uniform Change

Assuming uniform change with respect to time for $X(t)$ means that the rate of change in X is a constant. The two-equation DE is then specified as

$$\frac{dY(t)}{dt} = \alpha_1 + \alpha_2 X(t) + \alpha_3 Y(t) \tag{13a}$$

$$\frac{dX}{dt} = \beta_1 \quad [\Rightarrow X(t) = \beta_0 + \beta_1 t] \tag{13b}$$

which implies that

$$\frac{dY}{dt} = \alpha_1 + \alpha_2(\beta_0 + \beta_1 t) + \alpha_3 Y$$

To obtain a solution to equation (13a) we apply equation (2) with

$$p(t) = -\alpha_3 \implies P(t) = a_0 - \alpha_3 t$$

$$q(t) = \alpha_1 + \alpha_2(\beta_0 + \beta_1 t)$$

By substitution,

$$e^{a_0 - \alpha_3 t} Y(t) = \int e^{a_0 - \alpha_3 t} [\alpha_1 + \alpha_2(\beta_0 + \beta_1 t)] dt$$

$$= \alpha_1 \int e^{a_0 - \alpha_3 t} dt + \alpha_2 \beta_0 \int e^{a_0 - \alpha_3 t} dt + \alpha_2 \beta_1 \int t e^{a_0 - \alpha_3 t} dt$$

$$= C - \frac{\alpha_1}{\alpha_3} e^{a_0 - \alpha_3 t} - \frac{\alpha_2 \beta_0}{\alpha_3} e^{a_0 - \alpha_3 t} - \frac{\alpha_2 \beta_1}{\alpha_3^2} (\alpha_3 t + 1) e^{a_0 - \alpha_3 t}$$

The integration constant C can then be removed by fixing it at time $t = t_0$:

$$C_{t0} = e^{a_0 - \alpha_3 t_0} Y(t_0) + \frac{\alpha_1}{\alpha_3} e^{a_0 - \alpha_3 t_0} + \frac{\alpha_2 \beta_0}{\alpha_3} e^{a_0 - \alpha_3 t_0}$$

$$+ \frac{\alpha_2 \beta_1}{\alpha_3^2} (\alpha_3 t_0 + 1) e^{a_0 - \alpha_3 t_0}$$

$$\Rightarrow e^{a_0 - \alpha_3 t} Y(t) = e^{a_0 - \alpha_3 t_0} Y(t_0) + \frac{\alpha_1}{\alpha_3} e^{a_0 - \alpha_3 t_0} + \frac{\alpha_2 \beta_0}{\alpha_3} e^{a_0 - \alpha_3 t_0}$$

$$+ \frac{\alpha_2 \beta_1}{\alpha_3^2} (\alpha_3 t_0 + 1) e^{a_0 - \alpha_3 t_0}$$

$$- \frac{\alpha_1}{\alpha_3} e^{a_0 - \alpha_3 t} - \frac{\alpha_2 \beta_0}{\alpha_3} e^{a_0 - \alpha_3 t} - \frac{\alpha_2 \beta_1}{\alpha_3^2} (\alpha_3 t + 1) e^{a_0 - \alpha_3 t}$$

$$\Rightarrow Y(t) = e^{\alpha_3(t-t_0)} Y(t_0) + \frac{\alpha_1}{\alpha_3} e^{\alpha_3(t-t_0)} + \frac{\alpha_2\beta_0}{\alpha_3} e^{\alpha_3(t-t_0)}$$

$$+ \frac{\alpha_2\beta_1}{\alpha_3^2} (\alpha_3 t_0 + 1) e^{\alpha_3(t-t_0)}$$

$$- \frac{\alpha_1}{\alpha_3} - \frac{\alpha_2\beta_0}{\alpha_3} - \frac{\alpha_2\beta_1}{\alpha_3^2} (\alpha_3 t + 1)$$

$$= \frac{\alpha_1}{\alpha_3} (e^{\alpha_3(t-t_0)} - 1) + e^{\alpha_3(t-t_0)} Y(t_0) + \frac{\alpha_2\beta_0}{\alpha_3} (e^{\alpha_3(t-t_0)} - 1)$$

$$+ \frac{\alpha_2\beta_1}{\alpha_3^2} (e^{\alpha_3(t-t_0)} - 1) + \frac{\alpha_2\beta_1}{\alpha_3^2} \alpha_3 t_0 e^{\alpha_3(t-t_0)}$$

$$- \frac{\alpha_2\beta_1}{\alpha_3^2} \alpha_3 t$$

$$= \frac{\alpha_1}{\alpha_3} (e^{\alpha_3(t-t_0)} - 1) + e^{\alpha_3(t-t_0)} Y(t_0) + \left(\frac{\alpha_2}{\alpha_3}\right) e^{\alpha_3(t-t_0)} - 1) X(t_0)$$

$$+ [X(t) - X(t_0)] \frac{\alpha_2}{\alpha_3^2} \left[\frac{(e^{\alpha_3(t-t_0)} - 1) + \alpha_3 t_0 e^{\alpha_3(t-t_0)} - \alpha_3 t}{t - t_0} \right]$$

which simplifies to

$$Y(t) = \frac{\alpha_1}{\alpha_3} (\lambda - 1) + \lambda Y(t_0) + \frac{\alpha_2}{\alpha_3} (\lambda - 1) X(t_0)$$

$$+ \Delta X \left(\frac{\alpha_2}{\alpha_3^2}\right) \frac{(\lambda - \alpha_3 \Delta t - 1)}{\Delta t}$$

when $t_0 = 0$ and $\lambda = e^{\alpha_3(t-t_0)}$. In terms of a regression model for equally spaced panel observations, we would then have

$$Y_{it} = a_0 + a_1 X_{i,t-1} + a_2 Y_{i,t-1} + a_3(X_{it} - X_{i,t-1}) + \zeta_{it} \tag{14}$$

where

$$a_0 = (\alpha_1/\alpha_3)(\lambda - 1), \quad a_2 = \lambda, \quad a_1 = (\alpha_2/\alpha_3)(\lambda - 1),$$

and

$$a_3 = (\alpha_2/\alpha_3^2)(\lambda - \alpha_3 \Delta t - 1)/\Delta t$$

These results yield the following relations:

$$a_2 = \lambda \qquad \Rightarrow \alpha_3 = \frac{\ln(a_2)}{\Delta t}$$

$$a_0 = \frac{\alpha_1}{\alpha_3}(\lambda - 1) \Rightarrow \alpha_1 = \frac{a_0 \ln(a_2)}{(a_2 - 1)\Delta t}$$

$$a_1 = \frac{\alpha_2}{\alpha_3}(\lambda - 1) \Rightarrow \alpha_2 = \frac{a_1 \ln(a_2)}{(a_2 - 1)\Delta t}$$

where

$$a_3 = \frac{\alpha_2}{\alpha_3^2} \left[\frac{(\lambda - \alpha_3 \Delta t - 1)}{\Delta t} \right]$$

yields the testable constraint that

$$a_3 = \frac{a_1}{\Delta t} + \frac{\left[\frac{a_1 \ln(a_2)}{(a_2 - 1)\Delta t} \right]}{[\ln(a_2)/\Delta t]}$$

$$= \frac{a_1}{\ln(a_2)} + \frac{a_1}{(a_2 - 1)}$$

When applied to panel data, the regression model in (14) could be expanded to include fixed or random effects (see Chapter 1).

The model in (13) is the simplest choice for modeling the continuous time relationship between two random variables when the directionality of influence is known (X influences Y, but not vice versa), and equilibration of the X variable over the interval between observations either does not occur or is small enough to be ignored. There are two major advantages of the DE specification in (13) over the integrated form in (14). First, it is rather difficult to interpret the parameters of (14), whereas the parameters of (13) have a straightforward meaning. The DE model "makes sense" in continuous time. It is intuitively appealing in many biologic contexts to suppose that X impacts dY/dt almost instantaneously (α_2), with changes in $Y(t)$ accumulating over time and $Y(t)$ subject to negative feedback (α_3). However, interpretation of (14) without reference to (13) (i.e., interpreting (14) as a discrete-time model) leads to clearly unrealistic interpretation of a_1, for example, as the effects of X at t_0 on Y at t_1. Second, the coefficients in (14) are a function of Δt, whereas the coefficients in (13a) are independent of Δt. This means that comparisons between studies involving different observation intervals are directly comparable when in the form of equation (13), but not in the case of equation (14). In these two senses, then, the DE is the more fundamental specification of the proposed process.

Determinant with Feedback

When considering the effect of relative body weight (RW) on blood pressure, it is implausible to presume that RW is not also subject to negative feedback pressures. Thus a more useful version of the model in equation (11) allows $X(t)$ to incorporate negative feedback:

$$\frac{dY(t)}{dt} = \alpha_1 + \alpha_2 X(t) + \alpha_3 Y(t) \tag{15a}$$

$$\frac{dX(t)}{dt} = \beta_1 + \beta_3 X(t) \quad \left[\Rightarrow X(t) = \beta_0 e^{\beta_3 t} - \frac{\beta_1}{\beta_3} \right] \tag{15b}$$

Following a similar strategy to that used to obtain a solution to (13), the solution to (15) is

$$Y(t) = (1 - f_1)\frac{\alpha_1}{(-\alpha_3)} + (1 - f_1)\frac{\alpha_2\beta_1}{\alpha_3\beta_3} + (f_2 - f_1)\frac{\alpha_2\beta}{\beta_3(\beta_3 - \alpha_3)} + f_1 Y(t_0)$$

$$+ (f_2 - f_1)X(t_0)\frac{\alpha_2}{\beta_3 - \alpha_3}$$

$$X(t) = (1 - f_2)\frac{\beta_1}{(-\beta_3)} + f_2 X(t_0)$$

where

$$f_1 = e^{\alpha_3(t - t_0)} \quad \text{and} \quad f_2 = e^{\beta_3(t - t_0)}$$

Thus $Y(t)$ is a linear function of Δt and lagged values of Y and X. The solution to (15) can then be rewritten in the usual linear form as

$$Y(t) = a_0 + a_1 X(t_0) + a_2 Y(t_0) \tag{16a}$$

$$X(t) = b_0 + b_2 X(t_0) \tag{16b}$$

which is the first-order autoregressive process familiar from time series models.

The relations between coefficients of the DE in (15) and the solution equation in (16) are as follows:

$$\alpha_3 = \frac{\ln(a_2)}{\Delta t}$$

$$\beta_3 = \frac{\ln(b_2)}{\Delta t}$$

$$a_2 = a_1 \left(\frac{\beta_3 - \alpha_3}{f_2 - f_1}\right)$$

$$\alpha_1 = \left[a_0 - (1 - f_1)\frac{\alpha_2\beta_1}{\alpha_3\beta_3} - (f_2 - f_1)\frac{\alpha_2\beta_1}{\beta_3(\beta_3 - \alpha_3)}\right]\frac{-\alpha_3}{1 - f_1}$$

$$\beta_1 = \frac{-\beta_3 b_0}{1 - f_2}$$

where estimates of the coefficients in (16) can be obtained from panel data.

Reciprocal Effects

Sometimes the directionality of relations between variables is unknown, or is reciprocal. In such an instance it is useful to specify a model that allows estimation of temporal relations between changes in the two variables. In other words, do changes in one variable lead (in time) to changes in the other? This is a difficult question to answer when panel data, rather than time series data, are collected.

To address the question of temporal precedence with linear DEs, a reciprocal model can be specified:

$$\frac{dY}{dt} = \alpha_1 + \alpha_2 X + \alpha_3 Y \tag{17a}$$

$$\frac{dX}{dt} = \beta_1 + \beta_2 Y + \beta_3 X \tag{17b}$$

where α_3 and β_3 are presumed negative. It can be shown that the solution equations of this system are of the form

$$Y(t) = a_0 + a_1 X(t_0) + a_2 Y(t_0) \tag{18a}$$

$$X(t) = b_0 + b_1 Y(t_0) + b_2 X(t_0) \tag{18b}$$

or

$$Y(t) - Y(t_0) = a_0 + a_1 X(t_0) + (a_2 - 1)Y(t_0)$$

$$X(t) - X(t_0) = b_0 + b_1 Y(t_0) + (b_2 - 1)X(t_0)$$

where (18) can be estimated with panel observations.

Such reciprocal systems are of particular interest for panel observations of biologic systems when the process is stochastic. Estimation of the parameters of (18) is feasible in the stochastic case with software such as LISREL (Jöreskog & Sorbom, 1988) or EQS (Bentler, 1985). Estimates of the DE parameters and their standard errors will be discussed in the next section.

A solution to a *system* of DEs provides a more general approach to estimation. The relationship between the coefficients of the DE and the integrated equations (IEs) is best described with matrix notation. First, we rewrite the system of DEs and IEs in matrix form:

$$\text{DE:} \begin{bmatrix} \dfrac{dY}{dt} \\ \dfrac{dX}{dt} \end{bmatrix} = \underline{C} \begin{bmatrix} Y(t) \\ X(t) \end{bmatrix} \qquad \text{IE:} \begin{bmatrix} Y(t) \\ X(t) \end{bmatrix} = \underline{\Omega} \begin{bmatrix} Y(t_0) \\ X(t_0) \end{bmatrix} + \underline{\zeta}$$

or $d\underline{Y}/dt = \underline{C}\underline{Y}(t)$ and $\underline{Y}(t) = \underline{\Omega}\underline{Y}(t_0) + \underline{\zeta}$, where the number of variables in $\underline{Y}$ is arbitrary and $\underline{\Omega}$ can be estimated by regression from panel data. The above solutions of the DEs can now be depicted as follows (Tuma & Hannan, 1984):

$$\underline{\Omega} = \underline{V}e^{\lambda \Delta t}\underline{V}^{-1} \quad \text{and} \quad \underline{C} = \underline{V}\underline{\lambda}\underline{V}^{-1}$$

where $e^{\lambda \Delta t}$ is a diagonal matrix of eigenvalues of $\underline{\Omega}$ in the form $e^{\lambda \Delta t}$, $\Delta t = t - t_0$, $\underline{V}$ is a square matrix of eigenvectors of $\underline{C}$ or $\underline{\Omega}$ (Strang, 1976), and $\underline{\lambda}$ is a diagonal matrix of the eigenvalues (λ_j) of $\underline{C}$. Estimation of $\underline{C}$ is thus achieved in the following steps: $\underline{\Omega}$ is estimated by linear regression, $\underline{V}$ and $e^{\lambda \Delta t}$ are then calculated from $\underline{\Omega}$, $\underline{\lambda}$ is obtained from $e^{\lambda \delta t}$, and then $\underline{C}$ is calculated from $\underline{C} = \underline{V}\underline{\lambda}\underline{V}^{-1}$.

This solution leads to IEs for $Y(t)$ and $X(t)$ that are of the same form as those in equations (18). A program (entitled DIFFLONG) written in the GAUSS programming language (Aptech, 1988) calculates estimates of the DE from estimates of the integrated equation. The program is given in the appendix. The computation of standard errors, however, is not currently implemented in DIFFLONG, since the statistical characteristics of these estimates have not been evaluated.

STOCHASTIC DIFFERENTIAL EQUATIONS (SDEs)

Many variables in biologic systems involve apparently random fluctuations through time. This apparent randomness may arise because a process is a function of a large number of independent determinants. The standard exemplar from the physical sciences is the path of a particle descending in water; the path appears to include random "sideways" fluctuations due to numerous collisions with water molecules. Some of the simplest and mathematically most tractable stochastic models of such processes are discussed in this section. This discussion is derived from Karlin and Taylor's (1981) treatment of "diffusion processes," which may be consulted for further details.

Some of the more complex issues in SDEs are avoided by restricting consideration to linear first-order DEs and the Ornstein–Uhlenbeck process. In particular, the alternative solutions available (known as the Ito and Stratonovich solutions) are equivalent in these simple cases.

Brownian Motion

One approach to modeling a stochastic temporal process $Y(t)$ stems from the study of Brownian motion. To understand Brownian motion it is useful to consider its analog in discrete time and space: the random walk.

The Random Walk

The simplest discrete-time–discrete-space stochastic process is the "random walk." An example is the process $\{X_t; t = 0, 1, \ldots\}$ such that

$$\mathrm{pr}[X_t = x \pm 1 \mid X_{t-1} = x] = .5 \pm (\alpha - .5)$$

where $0 < \alpha < 1$. If $\alpha = .5$, X_t will wander up and down without bound, but its expected value does not change with time. If $\alpha > .5 \, (\alpha < .5)$, X_t will tend to drift downward (upward). Note that the random walk is essentially unstable and may drift to $+\infty$ or $-\infty$ as $t \to \infty$.

Continuous-Time–Continuous-Space Random Walk

A continuous-time and continuous-state-space analog of the random walk with $\alpha = .5$ is unidimensional Brownian motion $\{B(t); t \geq 0\}$. Brownian motion is defined as a continuous-time stochastic process with the following properties:

1. $B(t + \Delta t) - B(t)$ is independent of $B(t)$.
2. $B(t + \Delta t) - B(t)$ depends on Δt, but is homogeneous wrt t.
3. $\lim_{\Delta t \downarrow 0} \{ \text{pr}[\,|\,B(t + \Delta t) - B(t)\,| > \varepsilon]/\Delta t \} = 0$.

The third property implies that $B(t)$ is continuous. The Markov property of Brownian motion is implied by the independent increments of $B(t)$. The mean and variance of change in $B(t)$ are linear functions of time:

$$E[B(t) - B(0)] = \mu t$$

$$\text{var}[B(t) - B(0)] = \sigma^2 t$$

where $\mu = 0$ and $\sigma = 1$ define *standardized* Brownian motion. However, $B(t)$ is neither differentiable nor bounded. The limit

$$\lim_{\Delta t \downarrow 0} \frac{1}{\Delta t} \text{var}(\Delta B)$$

is finite, but $\lim_{\Delta t \to 0} \text{var}(\Delta B/\Delta t)$ is not.

The most desirable property of Brownian motion is the normal distribution of $\zeta(t) = B(t + \Delta t) - B(t)$:

$$\text{pr}[\kappa_0 < \zeta(t) < \kappa_1] = \int_{\kappa_0}^{\kappa_1} (2\pi\sigma^2)^{-.5} e^{-\tau^2/2\sigma^2} d\tau$$

for all t [note that $\text{var}(B(t))$ increases with t, but $\text{var}(\zeta(t))$ does not]. An approximation to Brownian motion is depicted in Figure 3-1. This time path was generated with a discrete-time–continuous-space process with small intervals between time points. As $\Delta t \downarrow 0$, such a process approaches Brownian motion.

Notice in Figure 3-1 that $Y(t)$ tends to increase in variance with time. Brownian motion is clearly not stationary. Rather the system tends to expand. This is analogous to the notion of entropy in thermodynamics. However, biologic systems usually equilibrate or return to some sort of steady state after being perturbed. The Ornstein–Uhlenbeck (OU) process is a modification of Brownian motion that is more suited to the modeling of such processes.

Brownian Motion with Negative Feedback (Ornstein–Uhlenbeck Process)

Ehrenfest Diffusion Model

To understand the OU process it is useful to specify its discrete-time–discrete-space analog. A simple discrete-time model that involves negative feedback toward an equilibrium point is the Ehrenfest model of diffusion between two containers of equal size separated by a permeable membrane. The process $\{X_t;\ t = 0, 1, 2, \ldots\}$ is defined by

$$\text{pr}[X_t = x \pm 1 \,|\, X_{t-1} = x] = .5 \pm \frac{N - x}{2N}$$

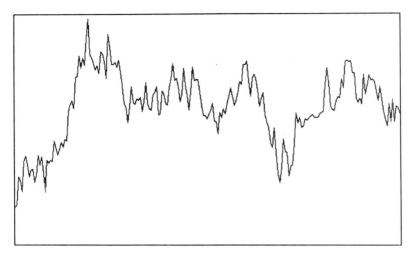

Figure 3-1. Discrete-time approximation of the time path of a continuous-time Gaussian process [standardized Brownian motion with infinitesimal parameters $\mu(x, t) = 0$ and $\sigma^2(x, t) = 1$].

where X_t is the number of particles in the first container at time t and $2N$ is the number of particles in both containers. Note that $0 \leqslant X_t \leqslant 2N$, and that the expected direction of movement is related to x. If $X_{t-1} > N$, then $(X_t - X_{t-1})$ is more likely downward than upward. Furthermore, as X_t increases above N the probability of downward movement increases. Such models are appropriate for biological processes involving equilibrating processes such as the behavior of ions in solutions separated by a permeable membrane.

Continuous-Time-Continuous-Space Diffusion

A continuous-time–continuous-space analog of the Ehrenfest model is the OU process $\{X(t); t \geqslant 0\}$. This process is the solution of the following stochastic differential equation (SDE):

$$\frac{dX(t)}{dt} = -\alpha X(t) + \sigma \frac{dB(t)}{dt}$$

where $\alpha > 0$ and $B(t)$ is Brownian motion with infinitesimal variance σ^2. The expected value of $X(t + \Delta t)$ is given by

$$E[X(t + \Delta t) \,|\, X(t) = x] = xe^{-\alpha \Delta t}$$

The variance of $X(t + \Delta t)$ is then

$$\text{var}[X(t + \Delta t) \,|\, X(t) = x] = \frac{(1 - e^{-2\alpha \Delta t})\sigma^2}{2\alpha}$$

which converges to $\sigma^2/2\alpha$ as Δt increases. The covariance of $X(t)$ and $X(s)$, $s < t$, is

$$E[X(t)X(s)] = \sigma^2 e^{-\alpha(t-s)}\left(\frac{e^{2\alpha s} - 1}{2\alpha}\right)$$

which decays to zero as t increases relative to s; it also increases to an asymptote for fixed $(t - s)$ as t increases.

An OU process is depicted in Figure 3-2. Note that the OU process is distinguished from Brownian motion (Figure 3-1) by its tendency to return to the equilibrium level. The OU process, then, is a reasonable building block for stochastic DEs. The OU process also provides a rationale for the negative feedback form of DE models. Without negative feedback, a Gaussian process such as Brownian motion is unstable. If all the reciprocal relations between variables are adequately specified, then a system may not require this sort of "black box" negative feedback. However, practical observational studies of systems are unlikely to involve sufficient knowledge or measurement to eliminate the need for negative feedback to achieve a realistic model of equilibrating biologic processes.

Chaotic Processes

One of the more interesting developments in continuous-time DEs is that of chaotic nonlinear systems. These models stem from the work of Lorenz (1963, 1984), who used a simple system of homogeneous equations to model three

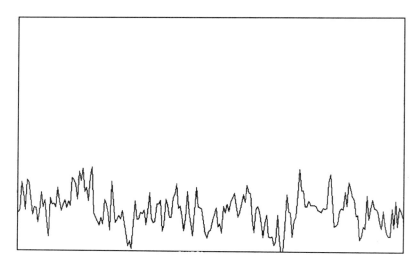

Figure 3–2. Discrete-time approximation of the continuous-time path of an Ornstein-Uhlenbeck process $dX/dt = -\beta X + \sigma\, dB/dt$ driven by white noise [with $\beta = .3$, $\mu(x, t) = 0$, and $\sigma^2(x, t) = 1$].

variables descriptive of weather conditions:

$$\frac{dX}{dt} = \alpha_1 X + \alpha_2 Y + \alpha_3 Z$$

$$\frac{dY}{dt} = \beta_1 X + \beta_2 Y + \beta_3 Z - YZ$$

$$\frac{dZ}{dt} = \gamma_1 X + \gamma_2 Y + \gamma_3 Z + XY$$

where the product terms YZ and XY introduce nonlinearity to the system. Assigning the following values to the coefficients yields a chaotic system: $-\alpha_1 = \alpha_2 = 10$, $\alpha_3 = 0$; $\beta_1 = 26$, $\beta_2 = -1$, $\beta_3 = 0$; $\gamma_1 = \gamma_2 = 0$, $\gamma_3 = -8/3$. The intriguing aspect of such a *deterministic* system is that $X(t)$ is apparently nonperiodic and, in the absence of perfect measurement, unpredictable beyond a short period of time. However, in contrast to Brownian motion or the OU process, regularity is found in the phase space $[dt(t)/dt$ versus $X(t)]$. The orderly pattern in the phase space is called the *Lorenz attractor*. Whether these models will have application to the processes studied by biomedical researchers remains to be seen (cf. Olsen, Truty, & Schaffer, 1988; Rogers, Yang, & Yip, 1986).

Estimating a System of SDEs

Point estimates of a system of deterministic DEs were described in the section "Deterministic Differential Equation with Feedback." Estimation in the stochastic case is described here. These derivations, developed by Wymer (1972), apply the delta method to the estimation of SDE parameters and their standard errors from corresponding estimates of the integrated equations.

In the notation of Wymer (1972), a system of SDEs is specified as

$$D^r y(t) = \sum_{k=1}^{r} A_k D^{k-1} y(t) + Bz(t) + u(t) \tag{19}$$

where D is an operator for some form of stochastic differentiation, $y(t)$ is a vector of n endogenous variables, $z(t)$ is a vector of m exogenous variables, $u(t)$ is a vector of n unobserved disturbances, the matrices A_k are of order n, and B is an $(n \times m)$ matrix. This may be reduced to the first-order system

$$Dy^*(t) = A^* y^*(t) + B^* z(t) + u^*(t)$$

where $y^*(t)$ is an $(rn \times 1)$ vector.

If we assume a first-order system (i.e., $r = 1$), the equation system (19) is simply

$$Dy(t) = Ay(t) + Bz(t) + u(t)$$

where $Dy(t)$ is a stochastic version of $dy(t)/dt$.

It is assumed that $u(t)$ is generated by a stationary process with constant spectral density Ω so that the integral

$$\zeta(t) = \int_0^t u(s)ds$$

is such that $\zeta(t)$ is a homogeneous random process with uncorrelated increments. However, $\zeta(t)$ is then nondifferentiable, so $u(t)$ cannot be rigorously defined. Thus equation system (19) may be respecified as

$$\frac{dy(t)}{dt} = Ay(t) + Bz(t) + \frac{d\zeta(t)}{dt} \tag{20}$$

where $u(t)$ is replaced by the mean square differential of the process $\zeta(t)$. The disturbance process may then be rigorously defined by using the Stieltjies integral

$$\xi(t) = \int_{-\infty}^t e^{-As}d\zeta(s)$$

where it can be shown that $\xi(t)$ is continuous and differentiable in the mean square.

If we assume that the system is first order, the solution to (20) is then

$$y(t) = e^{At}y(0) + \int_0^t e^{A(t-\theta)}Bz(\theta)d\theta + \int_0^t e^{A(t-\theta)}d\zeta(\theta) \tag{21}$$

or

$$y(t) = e^{A\delta}y(t-\delta) + \int_0^\delta e^{As}Bz(t-s)ds - \int_0^\delta e^{As}d\zeta(t-s)$$

where δ is the time interval between observations.

To estimate A and B, consider the discrete regression model

$$y_t = A^+y_{t-1} + B^+Mz_t + w_t$$

where $M = (1 + L)/2$ and $Lz_t = z_{t-1}$. It can then be shown (Wymer, 1972) that

$$A = H\Lambda H^{-1} \tag{22}$$

where the canonical form of $A^+ = P = H^{-1}A^+H = H^{-1}e^{\delta A}H$ (H is a matrix whose columns are the eigenvectors of A^+ (and A), P is a diagonal matrix of eigenvalues of A^+, and $\Lambda = \log(P)/\delta$ is a diagonal matrix of eigenvalues of A). An estimate of A is then obtained by substituting sample estimates of H and Λ into (22). Estimates of B are obtained as in Arminger (1986).

We are now concerned with the sampling variance of $\hat{A} = \text{var}(\hat{A})$. First we rewrite $\hat{A}$ as a column vector where rows of $\hat{A}$ are transposed and stacked to form $\hat{a}$. It can then be shown (Wymer, 1972) that

$$\text{var}(\hat{A}) = (H' \circ H^{-1})'[\Lambda\bar{P}\bar{K} \, \text{var}(\hat{a}^+)\bar{K}'\bar{P}\Lambda + \text{var}(\hat{\lambda})]$$

$$\times (H' \circ H^{-1}) \tag{23}$$

and

$$\text{var}(\hat{\lambda}) = (P^{-1} \circ I) \, \text{var}(\hat{p})(P^{-1} \circ I) \tag{24}$$

$$\text{var}(\hat{p}) = \bar{K} \, \text{var}(\hat{a}^{+})\bar{K}' \tag{25}$$

where $\circ$ is the Kroenecker product; $\bar{P}$ is such that each diagonal element is the inverse of the corresponding element in $(I \circ P) - (P \circ I)$ for nonzero elements and otherwise zero, where P is the canonical form of $A^{+}(=H^{-1}A^{+}H)$; $\bar{K} \stackrel{c}{=} (H^{-1} \circ H')$ where the equality holds only for the rows of $\bar{K}$ corresponding to nonzero elements of p, and the rows of $\bar{K}$ corresponding to zero elements of p are zero; $\bar{K} \stackrel{c}{=} (H^{-1} \circ H')$ where the equality holds only for the rows of $\bar{K}$ corresponding to zero elements of p, and the rows of $\bar{K}$ corresponding to nonzero elements of p are zero; and p is the vector form of P. The estimate of var($\hat{a}$) is then obtained by substituting sample estimates of the matrices on the right side of equations (23–25).

This approach to estimation is demonstrated in the following section and is implemented in the DIFFLONG program (see the appendix).

EXAMPLE ANALYSIS

The relationship between relative weight and systolic blood pressure in the Framingham Heart Study (see Chapter 1) may be addressed with a system of SDEs. The underlying assumption is that each variable operates as a diffusion process. That is, each variable moves through time in a manner analogous to shifts in concentration between permeable membrane. Changes in blood pressure, for example, occur both because of the impact of other systematic variables (such as relative weight) and because of a large number of factors whose sum may be considered stochastic. The negative feedback model for blood pressure has considerable biologic rationale (Guyton, 1977).

The covariances of SBP and RW across the first six examinations for men aged 34 through 38 at baseline are presented in Table 1-1 of Chapter 1.

The SDE is specified as follows:

$$\frac{d(\text{BP})}{dt} = \alpha_1 + \alpha_2 \text{RW} + \alpha_3 \text{BP} + \alpha_4 \eta + \frac{d\zeta^{\text{BP}}}{dt} \tag{26}$$

$$\frac{d(\text{RW})}{dt} = \beta_1 + \beta_2 \text{BP} + \beta_3 \text{RW} + \beta_4 \xi + \frac{d\zeta^{\text{RW}}}{dt}$$

$$\frac{d\eta}{dt} = \gamma_1 \eta + \frac{d\zeta^{\eta}}{dt}$$

$$\frac{d\xi}{dt} = \gamma_2 \xi + \frac{d\zeta^{\xi}}{dt}$$

where $d\zeta/dt$ indicates the derivative of Brownian motion (and thus each equation includes an Ornstein–Uhlenbeck stochastic process). Given this specification for the unmeasured random effects η and ξ, they will be first-order autoregressive in the solution equations. The measured variable BP in equations (26) is a latent variable in a measurement model (see Chapter 1) of the form

$$BP_{ijt} = \lambda_{10} + BP_{it} + \varepsilon_{ijt}$$

where BP_{ijt} is the jth measurement of SBP ($j = 1, 2$) at the tth examination ($t = 1, \ldots, 6$) for the ith case in the sample ($i = 1, \ldots, 596$); ε is a random measurement error with expected value of zero for (all i, j, and t) and variance σ_{jt}^2 for all i. The variables BP_{it} are then error-free latent variables in equations (27). The solution equations (integrated equations) are then specified as

$$BP_t = a_0 + a_1 RW_{t-1} + a_2 BP_{t-1} + \eta_{t-1} + \zeta_t^{BP} \qquad (27)$$

$$RW_t = b_0 + b_1 BP_{t-1} + b_2 RW_{t-1} + \xi_{t-1} + \zeta_t^{RW}$$

$$\eta_t = g_1 \eta_{t-1} + \zeta_t^{\eta}$$

$$\xi_t = g_2 \xi_{t-1} + \zeta_t^{\xi}$$

for $t = 2, 3, \ldots, 6$. The parameters of equations (27) can then be estimated by maximum likelihood (Jöreskog & Sorbom, 1988; Lee & Jennrich, 1984). The disturbances (ζ) are assumed to be uncorrelated with one another, normally distributed, and with constant variance over time (except at baseline). The random effects are allowed to correlate with both RW and BP and with one another and are thus analogous to fixed effects.

Given the two-year interval between examinations in the Framingham study, it is likely that the parameters a_2 and b_2 will be small and close to zero. This is the case, since both variables are known to change within weeks, or even days, in response to experimental manipulations. To increase the precision of estimates of these parameters, then, the constraints $a_2 > 0$, $b_2 > 0$, and $b_2/a_2 = 2$ were incorporated into the estimation procedure. The latter constraint derives from the *a priori* assumption that BP adjusts to change more rapidly than RW. The choice of 2 for the ratio of coefficients is arbitrary and should be subjected to sensitivity analysis.

The resulting estimates of crucial parameters in equations (27) are as follows:

$$RW \rightarrow BP: \quad \hat{a}_1 = .131 \ (.060) \qquad \hat{a}_2 = .060 \ (.075)$$

$$BP \rightarrow RW: \quad \hat{b}_1 = .007 \ (.015) \qquad \hat{b}_2 = .120 \ (.075)$$

$$\hat{g}_1 = .976 \ (.014) \qquad \hat{g}_2 = .989 \ (.005)$$

where estimated standard errors are given in parentheses. Note that $\hat{a}_1$ is considerably larger than $\hat{b}_1$. The latter is close to zero. This asymmetry is indicative that change in RW leads change in BP (or that change in BP lags behind change in RW—even though the SDE in (26) does not involve lagged effects).

This asymmetry is better seen in terms of the parameters of the SDE. Using DIFFLONG (see the appendix), we find that

$$\hat{\alpha}_2 = 1.58 \qquad \hat{\alpha}_3 = -2.90$$

$$\hat{\beta}_2 = 0.08 \qquad \hat{\beta}_3 = -2.17$$

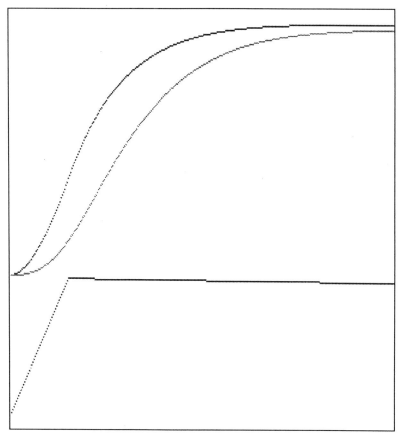

Figure 3-3. Simulated depiction of blood pressure response (middle line) to an increase in relative weight (to line) induced by a stepped increase in ξ (bottom line). See model in equation (26).

These coefficients are for the lag of two years between observations. If we divide these estimates by 2, they are then in the metric of years. The parameters of the SDE are invariant with lag between observations, but they are a function of the time metric chosen.

The response of BP to a change in RW, according to the obtained estimates of the model in (26), is then depicted in Figure 3-3. An increase in RW (top line) is induced by a stepped increase in ξ (bottom line). Such an increase in RW might be induced by an increase in dietary intake of energy. Note that the change in RW "leads" the change in BP (middle line). In contrast, inducing a change in BP via a stepped increase in η (Figure 3-4) is not followed by an increase in RW (middle line). This characteristic of the estimated model is, of course, consistent with what has been found in experimental studies of the response of BP to manipulated RW (Palgi et al., 1985; Tuck et al., 1981).

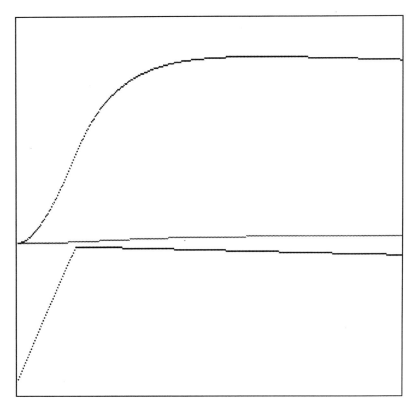

Figure 3-4. Simulated depiction of relative weight response (middle line) to an increase in blood pressure (to line) induced by a stepped increase in η (bottom line).

These results suggest the potential utility of SDEs for the analysis of temporal relations with panel data. In many instances, however, the rate of adjustment of variables will produce fairly complete adjustment in time intervals considerably shorter than the interval between panel examinations. In this instance, precise estimates of adjustment parameters will require large samples. Future work on SDEs for panel data should focus on issues of statistical power and evaluation of proposed estimates of standard errors. The results reported here, however, are encouraging in that the direction of influence known to operate was correctly detected.

Appendix

A program in the GAUSS programming language (Aptech Systems, 1988) to estimate the parameters of a stochastic differential equation model with negative feedback (cf equation 26) from estimates of an autoregressive linear regression model (cf equation 27).

```
/*DIFFLONG: A program to calculate the parameters
of differential equation models for longitudinal data by
David P. MacKinnon, James H. Dwyer, and Gerhard Arminger*/

@INPUT@

/*Insert the number of endogenous variables*/p=2;
/*Insert the matrix of integrated model parameters
relating endogenous
variables from the LISREL Beta matrix here.*/
Let bhs[2, 2] = .060  .131
               .007  .120;

@CALCULATIONS@

@Calculation of the A parameters@
clear god, godi, godr;
z=eig(bhs,"god");
col=z[.,1];
zero=zeros(p,p);
d=diagrv(zero,col);
/*Test if the eigenvectors and eigenvalues satisfy
the characteristic equation. */left=bhs*godr; right=godr*d;
zchar=left-right;
qhat=zeros(p,p);
teg=z[.,1];
hhat=godr;
lhat=ln(teg);
lhat=diagrv(qhat,lhat);
ahat=hhat*lhat*inv(hhat);

@OUTPUT@

Format /ml/rd 8,4;
"This matrix must equal zero to satisfy the
characteristic equation";zchar;
"Bhs matrix";bhs;
"Eigenvalues of the bhs matrix";d;
"Imaginary eigenvectors of the bhs matrix";godi;
"Real eigenvectors of the bhs matrix";godr;
"A parameter matrix"; ahat;
```

REFERENCES

Ackerman E, Elveback LR, Fox JP (1984). *Simulation of Infectious Disease Epidemics.* Springfield, Ill., Charles C. Thomas.

Aptech Systems (1988). "The Gauss System, Version 2.0." Kent, Wash., Aptech Systems.

Arminger G (1986). "Linear stochastic differential equation models for panel data with unobserved variables" *Sociological Methodology*, 187–212.

Bartlett MS (1960). *Stochastic Population Models in Ecology and Epidemiology.* New York, Wiley.

Bentler PM (1985). *Theory and Implementation of EQS: A Structural Equations Program.* Los Angeles, BMDP Statistical Software.

Bergstrom AR, Wymer CR (1976). "A model of disequilibrium neoclassical growth and its application to the United Kingdom." In Bergstrom AR (ed), *Statistical Inference in Continuous Time Economic Models.* New York, American Elsevier, pp 81–96.

Coleman JS (1968). "Mathematical models of change." In Blalock H, Blalock M (eds), *Methodology in Social Research.* New York, McGraw-Hill.

Feigenbaum MJ (1978). "Qualitative universality for a class of nonlinear transformations." *Journal of Statistical Physics* 19:25–52.

Guyton AC (1977). "An overall analysis of cardiovascular regulation." *Anesthesiology and Analgesia* 56:761–778.

Jöreskog KG, Sorbom D (1988). *LISREL 7: A Guide to the Program and Applications.* Chicago, Statistical Package for the Social Sciences.

Karlin S, Taylor HM (1981). *A Second Course in Stochastic Processes.* New York, Academic Press.

Lee SY, Jennrich RI (1984). "The analysis of structural equation models by means of derivative free nonlinear least squares." *Psychometrika* 49:521–528.

Lorenz EN (1963). "Deterministic non-periodic flow." *Journal of Atmospheric Science* 20:130–141.

Lorenz EN (1984). "The local structure of a chaotic attractor in four dimensions." *Physica* 13D:90–104.

Olsen LF, Truty GL, Schaffer WM (1988). "Oscillations and chaos in epidemics: A nonlinear dynamic study of six childhood diseases in Copenhagen, Denmark." *Theoretical Population Biology* 33:344–370.

Palgi A, Read JL, Greenberg I, Hoefer MA, Bistrian BR, Blackburn GL (1985). "Multidisciplinary treatment of obesity with a protein-sparing modified fast: Results in 668 outpatients." *American Journal of Public Health* 75:1190–1194.

Rogers TD, Yang ZC, Yip LW (1986). "Complete chaos in a simple epidemiological model." *Journal of Mathematical Biology* 23:263–268.

Sandland RL, McGilchrist CA (1979). "Stochastic growth curve analysis." *Biometrics* 35:255–271.

Steen FH (1955). *Differential Equations.* New York, Ginn.

Strang G (1976). *Linear Algebra and Its Applications.* New York, Academic Press.

Tuck ML, Sowers J, Dornfield L, et al. (1981). "The effect of weight reduction on blood pressure, plasma renin activity, and plasma aldosterone levels in obese patients." *New England Journal of Medicine* 304:930–937.

Tuma NB, Hannan MT (1984). *Social Dynamics.* New York, Academic Press.

Wymer CR (1972). "Econometric estimation of stochastic differential equation systems." *Econometrica* 40:565–577.

4

Unconditional Linear Models for Analysis of Longitudinal Data

CHRISTINE WATERNAUX AND JAMES WARE

This chapter describes the use of unconditional models of change in the analysis of longitudinal data. By unconditional models we mean that $E(Y_{ij})$, the expected outcome for the ith subject at the jth occasion, is modeled as a linear function of time and "within-" and "between-subject" covariates. These covariates may represent risk factors (e.g., exposure) or potential confounders (e.g., sociodemographic factors). Conditional models, on the other hand, express the expected outcome on the jth occasion as a function of previous observed outcomes: $Y_{i,j-1}, \ldots, Y_{i,j-k}$.

Unconditional models are used here as a data-analytic tool for a prospective longitudinal study of the effect of environmental lead on cognitive development. A cohort of 214 children exposed to low and moderate amounts of lead have been followed since birth and examined semiannually. Prenatal and postnatal exposure to lead is determined by blood lead concentrations, and cognitive development is measured by the score on the Bayley Scales of Infant Development. Two types of unconditional models are described and compared: general multivariate models and random-effects models. In both approaches the study hypotheses (relationship between lead exposure and scores on cognitive tests) are expressed as a sequence of linear models. The estimates of the regression coefficients associated with the lead exposure variables and their standard errors yield important findings about the temporal relationships between lead exposure and cognitive development. Because of the presence of missing data (mostly as a result of attrition), special estimation methods need to be implemented. For the general multivariate model, iterative weighted least-squares methods are used. For the random-effects model, restricted maximum likelihood methods are used. Methods for the analyses of residuals, influence analysis, and outlier detection techniques, necessary for the assessment of the goodness of fit and appropriateness of the models, are also discussed. We begin by briefly describing the longitudinal study used to illustrate the methods.

THE BOSTON LEAD STUDY

Between April 1979 and April 1981, umbilical cord blood lead concentrations of approximately 10,000 newborns at Brigham and Women's Hospital (97% of all births in the hospital) were measured. Infants were assigned to "High Lead" (greater than 10 μg/dl), "Mid Lead" (between 6 and 7 μg/dl) and "Low Lead" (less than 3 μg/dl) groups. A random sample of 214 infants drawn from these three groups was enrolled in a longitudinal study requiring semiannual measurement of blood lead concentrations and of mental and psychomotor development (Bellinger et al., 1984). Demographics, prenatal data, and perinatal data were recorded at enrollment. Infants and their families were subsequently evaluated when the infants were 6, 12, and 18 months of age. On each occasion a battery of developmental assessments was administered and blood lead concentration was measured. This chapter focuses on a single response, the Mental Development Index (MDI) of the Bayley Scales of Infant Development (Bayley, 1969). To correct for known effects of socioeconomic and perinatal factors on development, the Bayley scores at each age were adjusted, using ordinary least-squares regression methods, for the effects of gestational age at birth, score on the HOME scale (measuring the quality of the rearing environment), ethnic group, and a measure of parent-child interaction. The adjusted scores (MDIA), that is, the residuals from the regression of Bayley scores on the relevant covariates at each examination age, were used in subsequent analyses. The mean MDIA scores and blood lead concentrations for each group at each age of examination are displayed in Table 4-1.

Table 4-1. Mean blood concentrations (μg/dl) and mean mental development index (adjusted) (MDIA) scores ($\pm$ SEM) in three cord blood lead groups

Age group	Low	Mid	High	All
Birth				
Blood lead	1.73 $\pm$ 0.08	6.48 $\pm$ 0.04	14.00 $\pm$ 0.37	7.06 $\pm$ 0.40
	($N = 76$)	($N = 74$)	($N = 64$)	($N = 214$)
6 months				
Blood lead	4.66 $\pm$ 0.50	7.10 $\pm$ 1.10	7.07 $\pm$ 1.18	6.23 $\pm$ 0.55
MDIA6[a]	2.5 $\pm$ 1.3	−0.3 $\pm$ 1.2	−2.6 $\pm$ 1.2	0 $\pm$ 0.22
	($N = 76$)	($N = 74$)	($N = 64$)	($N = 214$)
12 months				
Blood lead	5.87 $\pm$ 0.61	8.49 $\pm$ 0.93	8.90 $\pm$ 0.83	7.64 $\pm$ 0.51
MDIA12[a]	1.3 $\pm$ 1.4	2.2 $\pm$ 1.5	−4.1 $\pm$ 1.6	0 $\pm$ 0.9
	($N = 72$)	($N = 72$)	($N = 61$)	($N = 205$)
18 months				
Blood lead	6.75 $\pm$ 7.00	8.43 $\pm$ 1.05	7.56 $\pm$ 0.77	7.55 $\pm$ 0.43
MDIA18[b]	0.8 $\pm$ 1.16	2.0 $\pm$ 2.0	−3.1 $\pm$ 2.0	0 $\pm$ 1.0
	($N = 68$)	($N = 60$)	($N = 56$)	($N = 184$)

[a]Adjusted for gestational age and score on the HOME scale at 6 months of age.
[b]Adjusted for gestational age, ethnic group, and score on the HOME scale at 16 months of age.

The analyses presented here address the following scientific questions:

1. Are cord blood lead concentrations associated with developmental level, as measured by fitted MDIA score at 6 months of age?
2. Are cord blood lead concentrations associated with rate of development, as measured by changes in the MDIA score between 6 and 18 months of age?
3. Is lead exposure during infancy associated with level or rate of change of MDIA score?

Three measures of lead exposure during infancy were considered. To reduce skewness, each blood lead measurement was expressed as the natural logarithm of 1 plus the blood lead concentration. These values are denoted by PBB6, PBB12, and PBB18. We first investigated whether blood lead levels at a given examination were associated with the rate of subsequent cognitive development. We also considered a measure of cumulative exposure, CUMPBB, defined as the sum of these transformed values at all examinations up to and including that at which an MDIA was measured. Thus, CUMPBB is a time-varying covariate and may require up to three values for each participant.

MODELING AND ESTIMATION

Unconditional Linear Models

The family of unconditional models presented here is a generalization of ordinary least-squares regression methods. The mean vector $\mu_i = E[Y_i]$ is modeled in a very general fashion using a linear function of risk factors, grouping variables, age, dummy variables, and interactions. This allows for the same flexibility as in ordinary least-squares regression. The covariance structure is modeled independently of the mean vector. The investigator may choose to estimate an arbitrary (unconstrained) covariance structure, as with general multivariate models, or to assume specific covariance structure, as with longitudinal random-effect models or autoregressive models. The choice of the covariance structure, however, will affect the estimation procedures and the estimate of α.

Specifically, each individual i ($i = 1, \ldots, m$) is observed on n_i occasions and the observed responses for the individual i's are arranged as an $n_i \times 1$ vector denoted by Y_i. We assume that Y_i arises from the linear model.

$$Y_i = X_i\alpha + r_i \tag{1}$$

where X_i is the "design" matrix for the ith individual, α is a $p \times 1$ vector of unknown parameters, and r_i is the vector of random deviations from the model (errors) with a multivariate normal distribution $N(0, \Sigma_i)$. The r_i's are assumed to be independently distributed ($i = 1, \ldots, m$). The unknown parameters α model the relationship of response to risk factors and/or confounders, as shown below. The covariance matrix Σ_i accounts for the correlations of responses within the ith individual.

This representation (1) allows for unbalanced designs. When each subject is observed at the same n occasions and no observations are missing, the design is *balanced on time*. Methods for analyzing balanced data have been well developed in the literature. The design matrix will generally include between- and within-subject (time-invariant and time-varying) covariates. When X_i does not depend on i, the design is *completely balanced*.

Modeling the Mean Value

In the Boston Lead Study, models for the mean vectors were developed on the basis of previous knowledge and were designed to test specific hypotheses about the temporal relationship of lead exposure to MDI scores. All models considered here assume that the expected response varies linearly with age with a slope and an intercept that may depend on covariates. The three questions set out previously can be expressed as models in which the lead exposure variables modify the intercept and slope (growth rate) as follows:

$$\mu_i = X_i\alpha \quad (i = 1, \ldots, m) \tag{2}$$

where α denotes the $p \times 1$ vector of unknown parameters to be estimated and X_i denotes the $n_i \times p$ design matrix for the ith child. Thus, X_i includes main effects for age and risk factors of interest, as well as interaction terms with age and covariates affecting the rate of growth. If the ith child does not have an MDIA score at the jth occasion, for example, then $n_i = 2$ and X_i has only two rows.

We consider four models for the expected response, all of which are special cases of (2). The simplest model (I) assumes that cord blood lead concentration affects the child's MDIA level but not the child's rate of growth. If LO_i and MID_i are indicator variables for the Low and Mid Lead groups, and AGE_{ij} is the age of the ith child at the jth occasion, the expected MDIA score is given by

Model I

$$\mu_{ij} = \alpha_0 + \alpha_1 LO_i + \alpha_2 MID_i + \alpha_3 AGE_{ij} \quad (j = 1, \ldots, n_i; i = 1, \ldots, m)$$

We code age as 0, 1, and 2 at 6, 12, and 18 months, so that α_0 represents the expected MDIA score at 6 months in the High Lead group. The parameters α_1 and α_2 represent the differences in expected MDIA scores of the Low and the Mid Lead groups relative to the High Lead group at all ages, and α_3 represents the slope of the linear time trend in all three lead groups.

To test the hypothesis that prenatal lead exposure may also affect growth rate, we add the interactions of age with the group indicators:

Model II

$$\mu_{ij} = \alpha_0 + \alpha_1 LO_i + \alpha_2 MID_i + \alpha_3 AGE_{ij} + \alpha_4 LO_i * AGE_{ij} + \alpha_5 MID_i * AGE_{ij}$$

where α_4 and α_5 represent the differences in slopes between the Low and High Lead groups and the Mid and High Lead groups.

Models that allow the expected MDIA response to depend on postnatal lead exposure can again be formulated as special cases of (2). We consider two measures of postnatal exposure:

Model III

$$\mu_{ij} = \alpha_0 + \alpha_1 LO_i + \alpha_2 MID_i + \alpha_3 AGE_{ij} + \alpha_4 CUMPBB_{ij}$$

where $CUMPBB_{ij}$ is the cumulative lead exposure of the ith child at the jth occasion as defined earlier, and

Model IV

$$\mu_{ij} = \alpha_0 + \alpha_1 LO_i + \alpha_2 MID_i + \alpha_3 AGE_{ij} + \alpha_4 AGE_{ij} * PBB6_i$$

Model III posits that the expected MDIA score is affected both by prenatal (cord blood) and postnatal lead exposure; prenatal lead exposure determines a constant offset (α_1 or α_2), while postnatal exposure affects both current and future levels, hence rate of development. Model IV implies that prenatal exposure affects initial MDIA level, whereas early postnatal exposure affects rate of growth.

Modeling the Covariance Structure

Many different models could be proposed for the covariance matrix Σ_i. Choosing among them involves consideration of goodness of fit, feasibility, and other issues discussed at the end of this section. We review three types of covariance structure we have found useful in biomedical applications: an arbitrary covariance structure, a variance-components decomposition of the error structure using random effects, and an autoregressive structure. Although mean vector and covariance structure are modeled independently, the choice of a covariance structure has implications for the estimation of α.

If Σ_i were known, then the maximum likelihood (ML) estimate for α under multivariate normality would be the weighted estimator

$$\alpha_{GLS} = \left(\sum_{i=1}^{m} X_i^T W_i X_i \right)^{-1} \left[\sum_{i=1}^{m} X_i^T W_i X_i \right]$$

where $W_i = (\Sigma_i)^{-1}$. This is Aitken's (1935) generalized least-squares (GLS) estimator; it is best linear unbiased for α.

For unknown Σ_i, if one estimates Σ_i by maximum likelihood (assuming a multivariate normal distribution for the Y_i's) and substitutes $W_i = (\Sigma_i)^{-1}$ for W_i, then (α_{GLS}, Σ) are the joint maximum likelihood estimates and

$$\left(\sum_{i=1}^{m} X_i^T W_i X_i \right)^{-1}$$

is a consistent estimator of the variance of α_{GLS}.

Arbitrary Covariance Structure

In our example, since each child is measured on at most three occasions common to all children, it is feasible to allow an arbitrary (3×3) covariance structure, Σ, for the response vector. Then, when observations are missing, the covariance matrix for the ith individual is obtained by deleting appropriate rows and columns of Σ.

Estimation Procedure. For the general multivariate model, the results reported here are based on a three-step approximation to the ML estimator, called the GLS,1 estimator by Freedman and Peters (1984). We first set $W_i = I$ and calculate the ordinary least-squares (OLS) estimate α_{OLS}, then compute each element of the sample covariance matrix from all possible pairs of scalar residuals from the vectors $Y_i - X_i\alpha_{OLS}$. The GLS estimator, α_{GLS}, is obtained by substituting $(S_i)^{-1}$ for W_i. The estimate S_i can be refined by successively reestimating α and Σ, and maximum likelihood estimates can be obtained by applying the EM algorithm (see below) to the residuals from the current GLS fit to update Σ (Beale & Little, 1975; Ware & de Gruttola, 1985). On the other hand, estimating a general covariance structure is not always feasible. The approach is attractive even when observations are missing or the design is moderately unbalanced across individuals (Kleinbaum, 1973). However, if n_i is large or if the times of observations vary over individuals, more parsimonious models for Σ must be considered.

Longitudinal Random-Effect Models

With longitudinal random-effect (LRE) models proposed by Laird and Ware (1982), the random deviation r_{ij} is further decomposed into two parts corresponding to within- and between-subject variance components:

$$r_i = Z_i B_i + \varepsilon_i \qquad (3)$$

where Z_i is an $(n_i \times q)$ known "design" matrix, B_i is a $q \times 1$ vector of child-specific random effects, and ε_i is an $(n_i \times 1)$ vector of deviations (errors) from the model. We assume that the B_i's have a multivariate normal distribution $N(O, D)$, that the ε_i's have a multivariate normal distribution $N(O, R_i)$, and that the B_i's and the ε_i's are independently distributed. Although one might consider correlated errors, that is, var $\varepsilon_i = R_i$, we assume here conditional independence for the errors: var $\varepsilon_i = \sigma^2 I$.

The number of random effects, q, determines the complexity of the covariance structure for the response, var Y_i, since (3) implies that

$$\Sigma_i = Z_i D Z_i^T + \sigma^2 I \qquad (4)$$

In the simplest case, one may set $q = 1$ and Z_i to be a column of 1's, so that

$$r_{ij} = B_{i1} + \varepsilon_{ij} \quad (j = 1, \ldots, n_i)$$

This is the well-known case of the "repeated measurements" design, which assumes an equicorrelation structure for Σ_i:

$$\text{var } Y_{ij} = \delta + \sigma^2 \quad (j = 1, \ldots, n_i; i = 1, \ldots, m)$$

$$\text{corr}(Y_{ij}, Y_{ik}) = \frac{\delta}{\delta + \sigma^2} \quad (j, k = 1, \ldots, n_i; j \neq k)$$

In our example we choose to use a linear combination of two random effects

$$r_{ij} = B_{i1} + B_{i2}a_{ij} + \varepsilon_{ij} \quad (j = 1, \ldots, n_i)$$

where a_{ij} denotes the age of the ith child at the jth occasion. For a child with $n_i = 3$ observations, the first column of the Z_i matrix is then $(1\ 1\ 1)^T$, and the second column is $(0\ 1\ 2)^T$. (Recall that we code age as 0, 1, and 2 for 6, 12, and 18 months.) The two random effects are then a random intercept and random slope (in a plot of MDIA scores against age) that can be interpreted as the ith child's deviations from the population slope and intercept.

Since we have at most three observations per child, the use of three random effects would result in overparametrization. We note that the LRE model with two random effects is more parsimonious than the multivariate model with unconstrained covariance matrix. In the first case we estimate four variance components parameters: σ^2, and three parameters for the covariance matrix D of the B_i's: d_{11}, d_{12}, and d_{22}. The general covariance structure for 3×3 multivariate distributions requires the estimation of six parameters.

More complex parametrization of the covariance structure might allow the Z_i matrix to depend both on polynomials in a_{ij}, on other grouping variables such as gender, and on interactions of the time variable with these grouping variables. Note, however, that in the formulation proposed by Laird and Ware, the columns of Z_i matrix must be a subset of the columns of the X_i matrix.

Estimation Method. LRE models are not amenable to conventional estimation methods such as maximum likelihood or least-squares estimation, because the dimensionality of the parameter space that includes the subject-related parameters (the random effects) increases with the sample size. In this case, the accepted approach is maximum likelihood estimation in the marginal distribution, that is, in the distribution that is obtained by integrating over the assumed distribution of the subject-related effects. We consider a modified approach of the restricted maximum likelihood estimation (REML) method discussed by Harville (1977), which maximizes the likelihood obtained by simultaneously integrating over the random effects and the location parameters α, the latter with respect to a flat prior distribution.

Laird (1982) and Laird and Ware (1982) noted that REML estimates of the variance components can be computed via the EM algorithm proposed by Dempster, Laird, and Rubin (1977). The EM algorithm is a two-step iterative algorithm for estimating unknown parameters when data are incomplete. At the E (expectation) step, estimates of the sufficient statistics with missing observations are calculated by setting these statistics equal to their expected values, conditional on the observed data. At the M (maximization) step, the maximum likelihood estimates of the parameters are derived. A suitable initial estimate of the parameters is used to start the procedure, and one alternates between the E step and the M step until changes in the computed estimates become smaller than a prespecified value. If the model belongs to the exponential family, the EM algorithm will always converge, albeit sometimes slowly.

In the case of LRE models, the unobservable subject-related effects are treated as missing data. The method allows estimation of the parameters even with unbalanced designs. Laird and Ware (1982) showed the interpretation of the REML estimates of the subject-related effects as empirical Bayes estimates, since they are estimates of the mean of the posterior distribution of these effects conditional on the observed data. As such they enjoy optimal statistical properties: empirical Bayes estimates have minimum mean-square error when integration is done over the distribution of subject-related effects (Lindley & Smith, 1972; Morris, 1983). In this sense, the empirical Bayes estimate of a subject-related parameter is, on the average, closer to the true value of the parameter than any other estimator.

Formulas for the estimate of the EB residuals and their variances are given in Laird and Ware (1982).

Autoregressive Structure

Although we do not illustrate their use here, models with first-order autoregressive error structure have special advantages in the longitudinal setting (Louis & Spiro, 1986). When the design is balanced on time, let

$$r_{ij} = pr_{i,j-1} + u_{ij}$$

where u_{ij} has mean 0, has variance σ^2, and is independent of r. Then we can write the regression model as

$$Y_{i1} = X_{i1}\alpha + r_{i1}$$
$$Y_{ij} - pY_{i,j-1} = (X_{ij} - pX_{i,j-1})\alpha + (r_{ij} - pr_{i,j-1}) \qquad j \geq 2$$

This representation shows the close relationship between the first-order autoregressive model and analysis of successive differences. Whereas the successive differences are correlated, the differences $Y_{ij} - pY_{i,j-1}$ are not. Louis and Spiro (1986) suggested an estimation procedure for the first-order model. Their iteratively reweighted least-squares procedure uses the working estimate of α to update the estimates of p and σ^2 through regression of

$$Y_{ij} - X_{ij}^T\hat{\alpha} \qquad \text{on} \qquad Y_{i,j-1} - X_{i,j-1}^T\hat{\alpha}$$

Although this approach extends directly to higher order autoregressive models, more complex models may be more difficult to interpret. The first-order model also has special advantages in residual analysis, as we discuss subsequently. Extensions to autoregressive moving-average structure require fundamentally different estimation procedures than those discussed by Louis and Spiro.

Choosing a Model for the Covariance Matrix

Given the many possible specifications for the covariance structure, the analyst faces a choice among these possibilities for a specific application. The choice should be based on several considerations. The overriding consideration, of course, is feasibility. In particular, if the number of replicates per individual is large or if the design is highly unbalanced in time, the assumption of an unconstrained covariance matrix requires the estimation of many nuisance parameters and is therefore impractical. With the random-effects and autoregressive models, the number of covariance parameters does not increase with the number of observations per individual. When the intervals between successive observations vary, however, the natural first-order autoregressive model has autocorrelation p^{dt}, where dt is the interval length. Existing software for autoregressive models often does not allow this extension.

Goodness of fit is also a consideration. Since Aitken's estimator uses the weighting function, $(S_i)^{-1}$, the estimate of α will depend on the model for Σ. The estimator will be consistent even when the model is misspecified, however, and for relatively short series of repeated observations it tends to be insensitive to the model used in estimating Σ. The estimated covariance matrix for α will depend more directly on Σ, particularly for elements of α that measure change over time and are, therefore, estimated by contrasts between repeated observations on individuals. Zeger et al. (1985) have shown that the estimated covariance matrix for parameters of the marginal distribution of Y is insensitive to the assumed form of the covariance matrix, including the assumption that the successive observations are uncorrelated. As we shall see, both the general covariance structure and the random-effects structure provide good fit to the covariance matrix of successive observations of cognitive status in the Boston Lead Study, whereas the first-order autoregressive model, which implies constant variance over time, does not.

A final consideration is ease of implementation. None of the methods we have proposed can be implemented using standard software, except for completely balanced and complete data sets. Thus, special programs must be written to perform the matrix calculations. These calculations are quite simple, especially for the GLS estimator, but the programs are complicated by the need to consider all patterns of missing observations. The GLS estimater has, in our experience, performed well with a single iteration. When previous analyses have provided good estimates for the variance parameters, the random-effects and first-order autoregressive estimators can also be used without iteration.

EXAMPLE

Table 4-2 displays the estimates of the regression coefficients for models I through IV and their standard errors using the RE, GLS, and OLS regression methods. The estimate of the covariance matrix D of the random effects is also shown. The estimates obtained with the GLS and RE methods differ by less than 10 percent except in Model II, where some shifting between the main effects and the interaction terms involving cord blood group is seen. Good agreement would be expected, since the random-effects model gives good fit to the unconstrained covariance matrix (Table 4-3).

All four models provide clear evidence of the association between prenatal exposure to lead and MDIA score at all three ages. Children in the Low and Mid Lead groups score on average 5 ± 1.5 and 4 ± 1.5, points, respectively, higher than those in the High Lead group. Cord blood lead category does not seem to affect substantially the slopes of the mean growth curves in the three lead groups; 95-percent confidence intervals from Model II for the differences in

Table 4–2. Longitudinal random-effect (LRE), generalized least-squares (GLS), and ordinary least-squares (OLS) estimates of the regression coefficients $\pm$ SE of models I–IV

	LRE	GLS	OLS
Model I (N = 603)			
Intercept	-3.18 ± 1.14	-3.23 ± 1.18	-3.30 ± 1.11
AGE	-0.04 ± 0.61	-0.03 ± 0.63	0.01 ± 0.63
LO	5.13 ± 1.45	5.10 ± 1.44	4.84 ± 1.26
MID	4.02 ± 1.46	3.88 ± 1.45	4.55 ± 1.27
D Matrix	$29.02 \; -3.8$	NA	NA
	$-3.8 \;\; 27.9$	NA	NA
Model II (N = 603)			
Intercept	-2.95 ± 1.29	-2.88 ± 1.35	-3.01 ± 1.43
AGE	-0.45 ± 1.11	-0.52 ± 1.16	-0.29 ± 1.14
LO	5.27 ± 1.76	5.17 ± 1.76	5.36 ± 1.95
MID	3.18 ± 1.71	2.82 ± 1.77	3.18 ± 1.96
LO*AGE	-0.22 ± 1.50	-0.12 ± 1.55	-0.54 ± 1.55
MID*AGE	1.33 ± 1.53	1.59 ± 1.58	1.46 ± 1.58
D Matrix	$29.2 \;\; -3.8$	NA	NA
	$-3.8 \;\;\; 27.9$	NA	NA
Model III (N = 551)			
Intercept	-3.02 ± 1.97	-2.91 ± 1.43	-2.78 ± 1.32
AGE	0.85 ± 1.08	0.82 ± 1.09	1.40 ± 0.98
LO	5.93 ± 1.48	5.74 ± 1.46	5.61 ± 1.29
MID	3.96 ± 1.50	3.71 ± 1.48	4.59 ± 1.32
CUMPBB	-0.45 ± 0.47	-0.45 ± 0.47	-0.69 ± 0.39
D Matrix	$29.1 \;\; -4.8$	NA	NA
	$-4.8 \;\;\; 29.0$	NA	NA
Model IV (N = 571)			
Intercept	-3.64 ± 1.16	-3.56 ± 1.16	-3.75 ± 1.12
AGE	1.86 ± 1.12	1.78 ± 1.13	2.03 ± 0.98
LO	5.86 ± 1.47	5.73 ± 1.45	5.50 ± 1.27
MID	4.11 ± 1.49	3.84 ± 1.47	4.64 ± 1.29
AGE*PBB6	-1.20 ± 0.59	-1.17 ± 0.59	-1.27 ± 0.47
D Matrix	$28.6 \;\; -3.9$	NA	NA
	$-3.9 \;\;\; 27.1$	NA	NA

Table 4–3. Estimated Σ_i for children with three observations

Generalized least-squares structure			Random-effects structure		
109.3	30.1	8.5	118.0	24.7	20.9
(0.23[a])	150.5	69.7	(0.19)	137.4	71.3
(0.06)	(0.40)	202.6	(0.13)	(0.42)	211.1

[a]Corresponding correlation coefficients.

BASIS FOR CLASSIFICATION

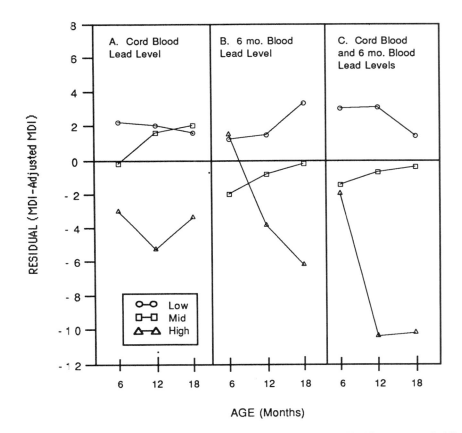

Figure 4-1.   Mean mental development index (Adjusted) (MDIA) scores at 6, 12, and 18 months of age for children in the Low, Mid, and High Lead groups (1A), for children with low, moderate, and high blood lead concentrations at 6 months (1B), and for children in the Low Lead group with low blood lead at 6 months. Children in the Mid Lead group with moderate blood lead at 6 months, and children in the High Lead group with high blood lead at 6 months (1C).

the slopes are $(-3.2, 2.7)$ and $(-1.7, 4.5)$. On the other hand, Model IV indicates that the slopes correlated positively with 6-month blood lead concentrations. The 12- and 18-month MDIA scores of children with higher blood lead levels at 6 months of age show a sharp decline relative to those of children with little or no lead in the blood at 6 months (Figure 4-1B). Figure 4-2 plots the expected MDIA score given by Model IV for six hypothetical individuals. Finally, we see little evidence for an effect of cumulative blood lead exposure on MDIA score. The estimated coefficient (and SE) for CUMPBB is $-.45 \pm .47$. Other analyses,

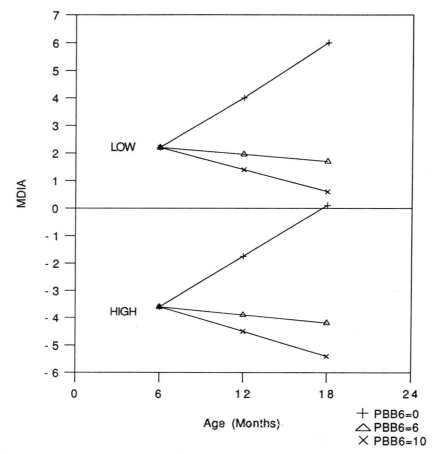

Figure 4–2. Predicted mental development index (adjusted) (MDIA) scores at 6, 12, and 18 months of age from Model IV for children in the Low and High Lead groups with six-month blood lead concentrations equal to 0, 6, and 10 μg/dl.

not shown, failed to show evidence of a relation between other measures of postnatal lead and the slope of later scores.

The OLS estimates of regression coefficients are usually close to the RE and GLS estimates. One notable exception is the coefficient of AGE in Model III, which differs by about 0.5 standard error from the estimates given by the multivariate methods. The estimated standard errors, however, are less concordant. In particular, the standard errors of the regression coefficients of the lead group indicators are, except in Model II, approximately 20 percent lower with the OLS method.

Random-effects and general multivariate linear models have thus allowed a more comprehensive investigation of the effect of blood lead concentrations than simpler univariate methods would. The analyses show, in particular, that the developing brain appears to be more vulnerable prenatally than postnatally to the adverse effects of low-level lead exposure.

RESIDUAL ANALYSES

The regression perspective provided in this chapter suggests a natural generalization of residual analyses for the longitudinal setting. As in ordinary least-squares regression analysis, residuals should be helpful for identifying outliers, assessing goodness of fit, and suggesting ways of improving the model. For instance, plots of the residuals of a preliminary model against predictors (or candidate predictors) should indicate the need for reexpressing or adding variables in the regression equation. This feature is particularly critical here, since model fitting is both time consuming and expensive.

The residuals, $u_i = (Y_i - X_i\alpha)$, from a generalized least-squares regression fit are correlated and are not orthogonal to the columns of the design matrix $X = (X_1^T \mid \ldots \mid X_m^T)^T$ in the Euclidean norm, since

$$\Sigma u_i^T W_i X_i^T = 0$$

Thus, standard bivariate plots may suggest that the u_i's are correlated with the predictors in X_i. One can, however, find linear combinations of the residuals that mimic the residuals in OLS using any decomposition of the $n_i \times n_i$ matrix Σ_i such that $\hat{\Sigma}_i = L_i^T L_i$. Let L be the $N \times N$ block diagonal matrix with the L_i's on the diagonal. The $N \times 1$ vector Lu is orthogonal to the columns of the matrix LX. Standard residual analyses for OLS regression can be applied to the residuals Lu. Possible applications include outlier detection, exploratory analysis through partial residual plots, and regression diagnostics. For the random-effects model, the L_i's are obtained from the decomposition of $\hat{\Sigma}_i = \hat{\sigma}^2 I + Z_i^T D \hat{Z}_i$. With the GLS approach, the decomposition is applied to S_i. This approach to exploratory analysis is attractive, since, in our experience, Σ_i is relatively insensitive to choice of model for the mean, μ_i.

The Cholevski decomposition $\hat{\Sigma}_i = L_i^T L_i$, where L_i is a lower triangular matrix, is particularly interesting because the residuals $L_i u_i$ have a nice interpretation as "longitudinal residuals." For a subject with $n_i = 3$, the first element of $L_i u_i$ is the standardized residual for the first observation; the second and third longitudinal residuals are standardized deviations from the conditional expectation given previous observations. For instance, the third residual is

$$(\hat{\sigma}_{3.12})^{-1}[\hat{y}_{i3} - (\hat{\mu}_{i3} | y_{i1}, y_{i2})]$$

where $(\hat{\mu}_{i3} | y_{i1}, y_{i2})$ and $\hat{\sigma}_{3.12}^2$ denote the estimates of the conditional mean and variance of y_{i3} given y_{i1} and y_{i2}.

Once a model has been selected and fitted, regression diagnostic analyses for independent observations (Belsley, Kuh, & Welsch, 1980; Cook & Weisberg, 1982) can be applied by calculating the appropriate L_i from the fitted W_i, transforming the independent and dependent variables, and "refitting" the model using a standard regression package with the desired diagnostic procedures.

LRE models allow additional types of residual analyses. The estimated random effects B_{i1} and B_{i2} are estimates of the deviation of the ith child's level and slope, respectively, from the population expected value. Thus, they can be used to identify children for whom the growth patterns depart from the average—a feature that is important to investigators of longitudinal studies.

RELATION TO OTHER METHODS

Both growth-curve and classic repeated-measures models are special cases of the family of unconditional models discussed here. The direct approach to modeling the mean value function is more flexible, however. First, individuals need not be observed at the same times or on the same number of occasions. Second, time-varying covariates can be included in the model, provided that their contribution to the expected response is linear. Finally, the representation of the expected response as a linear function of covariates allows the analyst to use modeling techniques directly analogous to those appropriate for conventional multiple regression problems.

The models described here are also closely related to the concept of tracking. Several different definitions of tracking have been proposed (Foulkes & Davis, 1981; Ware & Wu, 1981), but the most widely accepted definition is based on the notion that individuals remain at a constant percentile of the population distribution over time (McMahan, 1981). More precisely, a population is said to track with respect to an observable characteristic if, for each individual, the expected value of the deviation from the population mean remains fixed over time.

To develop a quantitative analysis of tracking, McMahan assumed that the data of interest arise from a polynomial growth curve model

$$Y_i | \alpha_i \sim N(X\alpha_i, \sigma^2 I)$$

where α_i is a $k \times 1$ vector of individual growth curve parameters and

$$\alpha_i \sim N(\alpha, A)$$

The two-stage model implies that Y_i has the marginal distribution

$$Y_i \sim N(X\alpha, XAX^T + \sigma^2 I)$$

The total variance of Y consists of between-individual variation, XAX^T, and error variance, $\sigma^2 I$. Further, the definition implies that

$$E(Y_{ij} | \alpha_i) = \mu_j + k_i \delta_j$$

where μ_j and δ_j are the population mean and interindividual standard deviation at time j. The k_i is constant for the ith individual and $E(k_i) = 0$, $\mathrm{var}(k_i) = 1$ in the population. This can be expressed in matrix terms as

$$X\alpha_i = X\alpha + k_i \delta$$

where $\delta' = (\delta_i, \ldots, \delta_p)$ and $\delta^2 = (XAX^T)_{ii}$. Hence, tracking is equivalent to a restriction on the interindividual covariance matrix, namely

$$XAX^T = \delta\delta'$$

The notion of tracking is principally of value in providing a concise description of population patterns of growth and aging. It can also be relevant to prediction of future values, provided that the data from which tracking was established include the range of ages considered in the prediction problem. It is of limited value in the study of individual characteristics and risk factors that modify patterns of change.

REFERENCES

Aitken AC (1935). "On least-squares and linear combinations of observations." *Proceedings of the Royal Society of Edinburgh* 55:42–48.

Bayley N (1969). *Bayley Scales of Infant Development*. New York, The Psychological Corporation.

Beale EML, Little RJ (1975). "Missing values in multivariate analysis." *Journal of the Royal Statistical Society*, Series B 37:129–145.

Bellinger DC, Needlemen HL, Leviton A, Waternaux CM, Rabinowitz MB, Nichols ML (1984). "Early sensory-motor development and prenatal exposure to lead." *Neurobehavioral Toxicology and Teratology* 6:387–402.

Belsley DA, Kuh E, Welsch RE (1980). *Regression Diagnostics*. New York, John Wiley.

Cook RD, Weisberg S (1982). *Residuals and Influence in Regression*. New York, Chapman and Hall.

Dempster AP, Laird NM, Rubin DB (1977). "Maximum likelihood from incomplete data via the EM algorithm." *Journal of the Royal Statistical Society*, Series B 39:1–38.

Foulkes MA, Davis CE (1981). "An index of tracking for longitudinal data." *Biometrics* 37:439–466.

Freedman DA, Peters SC (1984). "Bootstrapping a regression equation: Some empirical results." *Journal of the American Statistical Association* 79:97–106.

Harville DA (1977). "Maximum likelihood approaches to variance component estimation and to related problems." *Journal of the American Statistical Association* 72:320–340.

Kleinbaum D (1973). "A generalization of the growth curve model that allows for missing data." *Journal of Multivariate Analysis* 3:117–124.

Laird NM (1982). "Computation of variance components using the EM algorithm." *Journal of Statistical Computation and Simulation* 14:295–303.

Laird NM, Ware JH (1982). "Random-effects models for longitudinal data." *Biometrics* 38:963–974.

Lindley DV, Smith AF (1972). "Bayes estimates for the linear model." *Journal of the Royal Statistical Society*, Series B 34:1–41.

Louis TA (1984). "Estimating a population of parameter values using Bayes and empirical Bayes methods." *Journal of the American Statistical Association* 79:393–398.

Louis TA, Spiro A (1986). "Fitting first order autoregressive models with covariates." Submitted for publication.

McMahan CA (1981). "An index of tracking." *Biometrics* 37:447–455.

Morris CN (1983). "Parametric empirical Bayes inference: Theory and applications." *Journal of the American Statistical Association* 78:47–65.

Rao CR (1965). "The theory of least-squares when the parameters are stochastic and its application to the analysis of growth curves." *Biometrika* 52:447–458.

Rao CR (1975). "Simultaneous estimation of parameters in different linear models and applications to biometric problems." *Biometrics* 31:545–554.

SAS Users' Guide: Statistics (1982). Statistical Analysis System, Inc., Cary, N.C.

Ware JH (1985). "Linear models for the analysis of longitudinal studies." *The American Statistician* 39.

Ware JH, de Gruttola V (1985). "Multivariate linear models for longitudinal data: A bootstrap study of the GLS estimator." In Sen PK (ed), *Biostatistics: Statistics in Biomedical, Publis Health and Environmental Sciences* (Bernard G. Greenberg Volume). Amsterdam, Elsevier Science.

Ware JH, Wu MC (1981). "Tracking: Prediction of future values from serial measurements." *Biometrics* 37:439–446.

Zeger SL, Liang KY, Self SG (1985). "The analysis of binary longitudinal data with time-independent covariates." *Biometrika* 72:31–38.

5

Conditional Linear Models for Longitudinal Data
Application: Cigarette Smoking and Respiratory Function in Adolescents

BERNARD ROSNER AND ALVARO MUÑOZ

Longitudinal epidemiologic studies often involve collection of both outcome and exposure data at several points in time. Usually, a large number of individuals and exposure variables are available for analysis, while the number of time points for each individual is small. Some special problems encountered in modeling longitudinal data are (1) both fixed (e.g., sex) and time-dependent (e.g., height in children) covariates are available and have to be considered in the analysis, and (2) missing and/or unequally spaced visits are a frequent occurrence. One possible goal for such studies is to relate changes in outcome to either current or previous levels of exposure or to changes in exposure over time. Since the outcome values for an individual over time are likely to be correlated, it is important to note that the units that should be considered statistically independent are the collections of measurements for different individuals. Modeling the correlation structure of repeated measurements provided by specific individuals is of key importance for studying change within an individual. In particular, estimation of the correlation structure is needed if one is interested in the prediction of future outcome values given past values. Furthermore, the correlation structure provides insight into longitudinal behavior for specific individuals that is difficult to capture from cross-sectional or marginal types of analyses.

Several approaches to the analysis of longitudinal data are (1) analysis of the data cross-sectionally, (2) analysis over the total follow-up period by computation of slopes and relation of these slopes to initial exposure levels or changes in exposure, and (3) analysis over short periods of time and relation of changes in outcome to exposure levels or changes in exposure.

CROSS-SECTIONAL ANALYSIS

In the first approach, the data are analyzed cross-sectionally and the outcomes are related to current levels of exposure or previous changes in exposure. It is difficult to use such analyses to infer relationships between exposure and changes in outcome over time. Indeed, if a population has been selected for initial healthiness or initial sickness, one can reach very different conclusions regarding relationships between outcome and exposure from cross-sectional and longitudinal data. For example, a natural history study was undertaken in the Berman–Gund Laboratory at the Massachusetts Eye and Ear Infirmary (Berson et al., 1985). The study population consisted of ninety-four persons with retinitis pigmentosa, an hereditary ocular disorder often resulting in severe visual loss. Each person was seen annually for four consecutive years to assess the natural history of the disease. The key measure used to monitor such persons is the electroretinogram or ERG, which is a measure of the electrical activity in the eye. Persons are self-referred for their initial visit, and usually come to the clinic when they have already lost some visual function. Analysis of changes in ERG amplitude based on both cross-sectional (i.e., initial visit) and longitudinal data are given in Table 5-1.

For the cross-sectional analysis, a simple linear regression analysis was run relating ln(ERG amplitude) to age based on initial-visit data. The expected annual percent change was obtained from $1.0 - \exp(b)$, where b is the estimated slope of the regression line. For the longitudinal analysis, the average observed change in ln(ERG amplitude) $= \Delta$ was obtained over a three-year period and the annual rate of change was estimated from $1.0 - \exp(\Delta/3)$. Major differences were found between the two analyses: there was a 6.6 percent change in ERG amplitude per year of age based on the initial-visit data and an 18.4-percent change per year based on the average annual rate of change observed in the three-year longitudinal data. These differences have important implications in predicting degree of visual loss over long periods of time.

ANALYSIS OVER LONG PERIODS OF TIME

In the second approach, data gathered over long periods of time are analyzed by means of regression slopes to relate changes in outcome over long periods to

Table 5–1. Change in electroretinogram amplitude (30 Hz) in persons with retinitis pigmentosa

	Cross-sectional analysis[a]	Longitudinal analysis
Mean change per year (ln(ERG amplitude))	−0.068	−0.203
Annual percent change	6.6	18.4

[a]Based on initial-visit data.

either changes or levels of exposure at the time of initial assessment of the outcome variables. This method has the advantage of utilizing the longitudinal nature of the data. However, it represents an inefficient use of the data if changes in outcome are nonlinear over time. Furthermore, it is difficult to infer cause-and-effect relationships from such analyses, since the time dependence of the covariates that change over time is not considered. This could be important, for example, in looking at the relationship between cigarette smoking habit and change in pulmonary function over long periods, during which the subjects may change their smoking habit several times. In particular, this method is not useful for comparing the growth of pulmonary function in children who start smoking at a given age with growth in those who remain nonsmokers over time.

ANALYSIS OVER SHORT PERIODS OF TIME

The third approach is to relate changes in outcome to changes in exposure over short periods of time. One important point in this regard is that changes in outcome are related to previous levels through regression to the mean and possibly other factors. For this reason we choose to relate outcome to exposure, conditional on previous level or levels (Rosner et al., 1985), as presented in equation (1).

$$y_{it} = \alpha + \sum_{l=1}^{L} \gamma_l y_{i,t-l} + \sum_{j=1}^{J} \beta_j x_{ijt} + \sum_{k=1}^{K} \beta_k^* z_{ik} + e_{it} \qquad (1)$$

where $i = 1, \ldots, n$; $t = L, \ldots, T$; y_{it} = outcome for the ith individual at the tth examination; and e_{it} are statistically independent for all i, t with a common $N(0, \sigma^2)$ distribution. Note that outcome at time t is modeled as a linear function of outcome at the previous L time points; time-dependent exposure variables x_{ijt}, which could include level of exposure at any period of time at or prior to time t, such as current height, or changes in exposure at any period of time at or prior to time t, such as change in height; and fixed covariates (z_{ik}), such as sex. Some key assumptions of such a model are:

1. A linear relationship is assumed between outcome and exposure conditional on previous outcome levels over *short periods of time*.
2. The residuals (e_{it}) are assumed to be independent, normally distributed, random variables with mean 0 and variance σ^2.
3. The same relationship between outcome and exposure is assumed for each individual; this can be relaxed by the use of interaction terms.

Note that we assume linearity over short periods of time between current outcome and the exposure variables conditional on previous levels of outcome. This assumption is often not valid over the long term and is not required with this method of analysis, but is with slope analyses over long periods of time. Also we assume that the residuals are independent, normally distributed, random variables with mean 0 and variance σ^2, both for the data obtained at different time points for the same individual and for data obtained from different individuals. The independence assumption can be relaxed by allowing the residuals to have a random-effects structure (i.e., corr(e_{it}, e_{is}) = ρ for all t and s), which for the case of $L = 1$ is a model often used in the econometric literature (Anderson & Hsiao, 1982). Furthermore, Muñoz, Rosner, and Carey (1986) have proposed regression methods to allow the random-effects structure to be different for different types of individuals (e.g., different gender). Finally, we make the assumption of fixed effects, that is, the same relationship between outcome and exposure is assumed to exist for each individual. This can of course be relaxed by introducing the appropriate interaction terms to modify the regression coefficients for a particular exposure variable in different subgroups.

The interpretation of the regression coefficients of the model is given in the following example. Suppose, for the sake of concreteness, that y_{it} represents FEV (forced expiratory volume in one second) at time t, that x_{ijt} is a binary time-dependent covariate representing current cigarette smoking, and that we are using a first-order model ($L = 1$), that is, that we are conditioning on outcome only at the previous time point. The coefficient β_j represents the expected difference in outcome at time t between a current and a noncurrent smoker starting with the same initial level at time $t - 1$ and the same values for the other fixed and time-dependent covariates at time t. A similar interpretation holds for the regression coefficients for fixed covariates β_k^*. Furthermore, in an hypothesis-testing context, where one wishes to test $H_0: \beta = 0$ vs. $H_1: \beta \neq 0$, given a baseline difference between smokers and nonsmokers of β_0, the null hypothesis will correspond to the case of the baseline difference being transient, that is, the expected difference between smokers and nonsmokers will converge to zero over time; conversely, if $\beta = \beta_0(1 - \gamma) \neq 0$, then the expected long-term difference is constant (β_0) (i.e., the expected rate of change in smokers and nonsmokers is the same), whereas if $\beta \neq \beta_0(1 - \gamma) \neq 0$, then the expected long-term difference $\neq \beta_0$, that is, the rate of change in the two groups, would be different over the long term (Figure 5-1).

Another way of looking at this model is in cross-sectional terms, as shown in equation (2) for the case of a single time-dependent covariate x_{it} and a first-order model.

$$y_{it} = \gamma^t \alpha_0 + \frac{\alpha(1 - \gamma^t)}{1 - \gamma} + (\gamma^t \beta_0) x_{i0} + (\gamma^{t-1} \beta) x_{i1}$$

$$+ \cdots + (\gamma \beta) x_{i,t-1} + \beta x_{it} + \varepsilon_{it} \qquad 1 \leqslant t \leqslant T$$

$$y_{i0} = \alpha_0 + \beta_0 x_{i0} + \varepsilon_{i0} \tag{2}$$

$$\text{var}(\varepsilon_{it}) = \frac{\sigma^2}{1 - \gamma^2} \qquad \text{corr}(\varepsilon_{it_1}, \varepsilon_{it_2}) = \gamma^{|t_1 - t_2|}$$

Note that expected outcome at time t is modeled as a weighted linear function of exposure at all previous time points with weights diminishing for levels of exposure at times that are further removed from time t. Furthermore, the residuals at two time points t_1, t_2 have correlation $\gamma^{|t_1 - t_2|}$. This is in contrast to

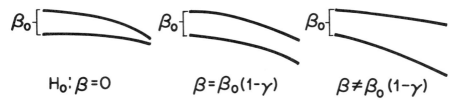

$$H_0: \beta = 0 \qquad \beta = \beta_0(1-\gamma) \qquad \beta \neq \beta_0(1-\gamma)$$

Figure 5–1. Expected pattern of change over time in smokers and nonsmokers according to the value of β and γ for a given baseline difference of β_0.

the standard first-order autoregressive model as shown in equation (3).

$$y_{it} = \alpha_1 + \beta_1 x_{it} + \varepsilon_{it}^*$$

$$\varepsilon_{it}^* \sim N(0, \theta^2) \qquad \mathrm{corr}(\varepsilon_{it_1}^*, \varepsilon_{it_2}^*) = \gamma^{|t_1 - t_2|} \tag{3}$$

Under this model, outcome at time t is modeled as a linear function of exposure only at time t. In some cases it may be more realistic to model current outcome as a function of covariate levels at many previous time points, such as in the relationship of FEV to cigarette smoking habit, but this is of course data-set specific. This distinction has also been noted previously in the econometric literature (Anderson & Hsiao, 1982). In particular, the modified autoregressive model is referred to in Anderson and Hsiao as the "state-dependence model," whereas the standard autoregressive model is referred to as the "serial correlation model." These authors pointed out that the key distinction between these two models is whether there is a dynamic response to changes in covariates. Under a *serial correlation model*, if x is increased in period t and then returned to its former level (e.g., if a nonsmoking child takes up smoking at time t and subsequently discontinues this habit), the distribution of y at time $t + 1$ is not affected. Conversely, in the *state-dependence model*, a change in x at time t will affect the distribution of y at subsequent time periods even if x is returned to its previous level. Thus, under the modified autoregressive model, if a child takes up smoking at age 12 for a five-year period and then quits, this smoking experience will have a long-term effect on pulmonary function, whereas under the standard autoregressive model it will not.

The standard autoregressive model in (3) can also be expressed in conditional form as shown in equation (4).

$$y_{it} = \alpha_1(1 - \gamma) + \gamma y_{i,t-1} + \beta_1 x_{it} - \beta_1 \gamma x_{i,t-1} + e_{it} \tag{4}$$

Note that when expressed in conditional form, the standard autoregressive model can be viewed as a special case of the previously described model, where the regression coefficient for $x_{i,t-1}$ is the negative of the product of the regression coefficients of x_{it} and $y_{i,t-1}$. Finally, in the case of a fixed covariate z_i, the models are parameterized differently but are actually equivalent.

We have applied the modified autoregressive model in equation (1) to a set of pulmonary function data collected over seven years in 1042 children/young adults ages 4 through 23 in the East Boston Childhood Respiratory Disease Study (CRD study) (Tager, Weiss, Rosner, & Speizer, 1979). Data were available in years 1, 4, 5, 6, and 7. Note that for the case of a first-degree model (i.e., $L = 1$), the units of analysis consist of all available equidistant pairs of visits for individual children. In the most straightforward implementation of this model, we use linear regression analysis and require pairs of visits that are equally spaced in time one year apart. Table 5-2 shows the pairs provided for the fitting of the model by an individual with data in years 1, 4, 5, and 6 for the case of $L = J = K = 1$ in equation (1). Thus a person with complete data in years 1, 4, 5, and 6 and missing data in year 7 would contribute two observations to the analysis consisting of the 4–5 and 5–6 pairs. The 1–4 pair cannot be used at this stage of the analysis because the number of years between the two visits is different from one. An extension of these methods to handle unequidistant visits is proposed below. For a second-order model, the observations would correspond to triplets of visits, and so on.

The first task in fitting such models is to decide on the appropriate order of the model. For this purpose, both a first- and a second-order model were fit to the data in the absence of covariates, as shown in Table 5-3. We note that 1543 pairs of visits and 869 triplets of visits were available for the first- and second-order analyses, respectively. Note that in the second-order model the coefficient for γ_2 is not statistically significant. Thus we will use a first-order model in our subsequent analyses. The covariates we considered in our analyses to predict current level of FEV were previous FEV; the time-dependent covariates of height, growth in height, age, and smoking; and the fixed covariate sex. The results are shown in Table 5-4. These are based on 1543 pairs of observations obtained from 674 individuals seen during years 4 through 7 of the study. The dependent variable in this analysis is current level of FEV. Highly significant positive effects of previous FEV, height, growth, and sex are noted in predicting current level of FEV. After controlling for height, age is not statistically significant. Finally, after controlling for all the previous covariates, current cigarette smoking at time $t - 1$ has a significant negative association with level of FEV at time t even after previous level of FEV at time $t - 1$ has been adjusted for.

Table 5–2. Contribution to the analysis for a hypothetical person[a] using a first-order regression model

Dependent variable	Independent variables (one time dependent, one fixed)
y_{i5}	y_{i4}, x_{i5}, z_i
y_{i6}	y_{i5}, x_{i6}, z_i

[a]For this hypothetical person, complete data are available in years 1, 4, 5, and 6; data are missing in year 7.

Table 5-3. Parameter estimates for a first- and second-order model, no covariates[a]

L	Number of persons	Number of observations	Model parameters	Parameter estimate	se[b]	p value
1	674	1543	α	0.855		
			γ_1	0.922	0.008	<0.001
2	474	869	α	0.857		
			γ_1	0.859	0.038	<0.001
			γ_2	0.058	0.037	NS

[a]The two models considered are of the form

$$\ln \text{FEV}_{it} = \alpha + \sum_{l=1}^{L} \gamma_l (\ln \text{FEV}_{i,t-l} - c_l) + e_{it}$$

for $L = 1, 2$, respectively, where c_l are centering constants, $c_1 = 0.75$, $c_2 = 0.65$, chosen to be close to the median $\ln(\text{FEV})$ in years 5 and 4, respectively, thereby simplifying the interpretation of the constant term (α).
[b]Standard error.

One disadvantage of the foregoing methodology is that one must restrict the analysis to pairs of visits that are an equal number of years apart. This is a severe limitation when one has examinations that are unequally spaced. In the context of this study, all information from years 1 through 4 would be lost. Furthermore, even if all examinations are planned to be equally spaced, any missing examination means that all pairs of visits, including that visit, will be lost. Thus if year 5 data were missing while year 4 and 6 data were available, all person-time from years 4 through 6 would not be utilized with the linear regression approach. To address this issue we have considered an extension of the discussed methodology in the case of a first-order model (Rosner & Muñoz, 1988). We first consider the conditional distribution of y_{it} given $y_{i,t-s}$ in the case

Table 5-4. Relationships between changes in FEV over time and other covariates based on 1543 pairs of observations obtained from 674 individuals (East Boston Childhood Respiratory Disease Study)

Variable	Regression coefficient	se[a]	p value (two-tailed)
Constant	0.7488		
$\ln(\text{FEV}_{t-1}) - 0.75$	0.7712	0.0158	<0.001
$\ln(\text{height}_{t-1}{}^{b}) - 0.33$	0.7872	0.0546	<0.001
$\ln(\text{height}_t / \text{height}_{t-1})$	1.5781	0.0953	<0.001
Sex[c]	0.0100	0.0044	0.025
$\text{Age}_t - 15.0$	−0.0006	0.0017	0.710
Current smoking$_{t-1}$[d]	−0.0503	0.0116	<0.001

[a]Standard error.
[b]Height is measured in inches.
[c]Sex is coded as 1 if male and 0 if female.
[d]Current smoking is coded as 1 if yes and 0 if no.

of one fixed covariate z_i. This is obtained by recursively applying the conditional distribution of y_{it} given $y_{i,t-1}$. The result is shown in equation (5).

$$y_{it} = \gamma^s y_{i,t-s} + \frac{(1 - \gamma^s)}{1 - \gamma}(\alpha + \beta^* z_i) + e_{it}^*$$

$$e_{it}^* \sim N\left[0, \sigma^2\left(\frac{1 - \gamma^{2s}}{1 - \gamma^2}\right)\right] \tag{5}$$

We note that for different values of s, this is a weighted nonlinear regression model with constant term α and regression parameters γ and β^*. If $s = 1$, this model reduces to the linear regression model mentioned previously. Similarly, in the case of a single time-dependent covariate x_{it}, using similar recursive methods we have the conditional distribution of y_{it} given $y_{i,t-s}$ and the x's as shown in equation (6).

$$y_{it} = \gamma^s y_{i,t-s} + \frac{(1 - \gamma^s)}{1 - \gamma}\alpha + \beta \sum_{j=0}^{s-1} \gamma^j x_{i,t-j} + e_{it}^*$$

$$e_{it}^* \sim N\left[0, \sigma^2\left(\frac{1 - \gamma^{2s}}{1 - \gamma^2}\right)\right] \tag{6}$$

This model is similar to that for a fixed covariate except that the values of x between time $t - s$ and time t are not known. To address this problem we use linear interpolation to approximate the missing values

$$\hat{x}_{i,t-j} = \frac{jx_{i,t-s} + (s - j)x_{it}}{s} \tag{7}$$

Under this assumption the summation reduces to a relatively simple function of x_{it} and $x_{i,t-s}$, as shown in Table 5-5. The exact nature of the function depends on whether the time-dependent covariate is of the form x_{it} (such as for current height), $x_{i,t-1}$ (such as for previous smoking status), or $x_{it} - x_{i,t-1}$ (such as for change in body mass index). By using the appropriate expressions from Table 5-5, one can now fit first-order or Markov models, even in the presence of missing or unequidistant time points, by forming all pairs of consecutive examinations regardless of the time s between exams. It follows that the estimation and hypothesis-testing procedures for the model reduce to those of a weighted nonlinear regression problem. Several standard statistical packages can be used to fit weighted nonlinear regression models, such as PROC NLIN of SAS, on providing the derivatives of the conditional mean of y_{it} given $y_{i,t-s}$ with respect to the regression parameters and by using the appropriate weight function. The code for such a program based on the above FEV data is less than one page long and is provided as an example in the appendix.

Note that this methodology allows one to use all available person-time rather than simply equidistant pairs and is equally applicable to a design with planned unequidistant time points as well as for missing or untimely examinations in the context of a design with planned equidistant time points. Furthermore, the unit of time used in such analyses is arbitrary, since the

Table 5–5. Contribution to nonlinear regression model for various types of covariates

Equidistant time points	Variable	Interpolation	Unequidistant time points for pairs of visits s units of time apart
z	Sex	Not needed	$zA(s)^{a}$
x_t	Current height	Linear	$x_t A(s) + \left(\dfrac{x_t - x_{t-s}}{s}\right) B(s)^{b}$
x_{t-1}	Previous smoking status	Linear	$x_t A(s) + \left(\dfrac{x_t - x_{t-s}}{s}\right)[B(s) - A(s)]$
$x_t - x_{t-1}$	Change in body mass index	Linear	$\left(\dfrac{x_t - x_{t-s}}{s}\right) A(s)$

$^{a}A(s) = (1 - \gamma^s)/(1 - \gamma)$.
$^{b}B(s) = [s\gamma^s - (s-1)\gamma^{s+1} - \gamma]/(1 - \gamma)^2$.

regression coefficients obtained from using different units of time are related as shown in equation (8).

$$\beta^{(s)} = \beta^{(1)} \frac{(1 - \gamma^s)}{1 - \gamma} \tag{8}$$

where $\beta^{(s)}$ and $\beta^{(1)}$ are regression coefficients corresponding to units of time of s units and 1 unit, respectively. Therefore, inferences are the same regardless of which unit of time is used.

The principal motivation for using the nonlinear regression model based on all available person-time rather than the linear regression model based only on equidistant pairs is to improve the efficiency of estimation of the regression parameters. We performed a study to look at the bias and mean square error (MSE) of regression parameters under each model and to quantify the gain in efficiency from using the nonlinear versus the linear regression approaches.

Specifically, 100 data sets were created, each set consisting of 100 persons with four time points ("follow-up visits") per person. A comparison was made between the two methods in the case of two time-dependent covariates. Specifically, in this case, y and x were simulated to approximate the distribution of FEV (liters), height (inches), and growth (inches) among 6- to 7-year-old boys using appropriate empirically derived regression parameters based on cross-sectional and longitudinal data from the CRD study (Tager et al., 1979). Simulation was used to identify a visit as missed by using a uniform random-number generator to allow data from each of the 300 follow-up visits to be missing with probability 0.20. In this way, twenty-five "pseudo data sets" with missing values were created for each complete data set. The ordinary least squares (OLS) model for pairs of visits one year apart and the nonlinear regression (NLR) model for all available pairs were fitted for each pseudo data set. We then computed the average bias and MSE for each estimator over the twenty-five pseudo data sets. As a summary measure over the 100 complete data sets, the percent bias for each estimator, as well as the relative efficiency of the two estimators, was obtained as follows:

$$\text{PCT BIAS}_{\text{OLS}} = 100\% \times \frac{\left(\sum\limits_{p=1}^{100} \text{bias}_{p,\text{OLS}} \Big/ 100\right)}{\beta}$$

$$\text{PCT BIAS}_{\text{NLR}} = 100\% \times \frac{\left(\sum\limits_{p=1}^{100} \text{bias}_{p,\text{NLR}} \Big/ 100\right)}{\beta} \tag{9}$$

$$\text{EFF} = \exp\left[\sum\limits_{p=1}^{100} \frac{\ln(\text{MSE}_{p,\text{OLS}}/\text{MSE}_{p,\text{NLR}})}{100}\right]$$

The results are presented in Table 5-6.

No significant or meaningful biases are present for either estimator for any of the parameters. The mean square errors are all significantly larger for the ordinary least-squares estimators versus the nonlinear regression estimators with efficiency ranging from 1.27 to 1.76. We performed similar simulations for different numbers of visits (eight), percent missed visits (5%, 10%), and also for fixed covariates and obtained comparable results. In summary, we found that in all the simulations, use of nonlinear regression based on all available person-time offers substantial gains in efficiency (in some cases over 100%) versus ordinary least squares using only equidistant pairs. The gains in efficiency is larger with an increasing number of visits, and particularly as the percentage of missed visits increases from 5 to 20 percent.

The nonlinear regression model has been applied to the previously mentioned pulmonary data set for the comparable year 4–7 period over which the linear regressions were run and also over the entire year 1–7 period. The results are given in Table 5-7. We note that for all models, the effects of previous FEV,

Table 5-6. Bias and efficiency for parameter estimates under linear and nonlinear regression models from study involving 100 simulated data sets with four visits and 20 percent of follow-up visits missing

Parameter	Percent bias[a]		EFF[c] p
	OLS[b] p	NLR[b] p	
α	−1.0 NS	−1.1 NS	1.61 <0.001
γ (previous FEV[b])	−0.0 NS	0.2 NS	1.56 <0.001
β_1 (height)	−0.7 NS	−1.0 NS	1.76 <0.001
β_2 (growth)	0.2 NS	0.7 NS	1.27 <0.001

[a]Percent bias = $100\% \times$ bias/true coefficient.
[b]OLS, ordinary least squares; NLR, nonlinear regression; FEV, forced expiratory volume.
[c]EFF = $\exp[\Sigma \ln(\text{MSE}_{\text{OLS}}/\text{MSE}_{\text{NLR}})/100]$.

Table 5-7. Relationships between changes in forced expiratory volume (FEV in litres) over time and other covariates based on linear and nonlinear regression analysis

Variable	Year 4–7 linear regression			Year 4–7 nonlinear regression			Year 1–7 nonlinear regression		
	Regression coefficient	se[a]	p[b]	Regression coefficient	se	p	Regression coefficient	se	p
Constant	−2.9688			−2.8102			−2.2520		
$\ln(FEV_{t-1})$	0.7712	0.0158	<.001	0.7797	0.0147	<.001	0.8048	0.0116	<.001
$\ln(ht_{t-1}{}^{c})$	0.7872	0.0546	<.001	0.7445	0.0504	<.001	0.5948	0.0390	<.001
$\ln(growth^{d})$	1.5781	0.0953	<.001	1.6105	0.0925	<.001	1.8352	0.0707	<.001
Sex[e]	0.0100	0.0044	.025	0.0111	0.0041	.007	0.0071	0.0030	.019
Age_t	−0.0006	0.0017	NS	−0.0002	0.0015	NS	0.0022	0.0010	.040
$Smoking_{t-1}{}^{f}$	−0.0503	0.0116	<.001	−0.0546	0.0097	<.001	−0.0337	0.0075	<.001
Number of persons	674			870			1042		
Number of pairs	1543			1675			2131		
Person-years	1543			1812			3365		

[a]Standard error.
[b]p-value (two-tailed).
[c]Height (in.).
[d]Growth = height$_t$/height$_{t-1}$.
[e]Sex = 1 if male and 0 if female.
[f]Smoking$_{t-1}$ = current smoking at time $t-1$ = 1 if yes and 0 if no.

height, and growth are highly significant predictors of current FEV ($p < 0.001$); sex is an additional significant predictor. The effect of age is inconsistent, being nonsignificant in the year 4–7 analyses but positively related to current level of FEV in the year 1–7 analyses. This may be due to the markedly younger age distribution of children seen in year 1. Finally, current smoking is an additional significant predictor ($p < 0.001$) of FEV after the other variables have been controlled for.

We note that there is very close correspondence between the regression coefficients obtained by linear and nonlinear regression over the period year 4–7. Conversely, the standard errors of the regression coefficients are consistently smaller when the nonlinear regression model based on all available person-time is used. This is in agreement with the simulation study results discussed previously. Furthermore, the standard errors of the coefficients based on experience from year 1–7 are consistently lower than the year 4–7 coefficients, reflecting the inclusion of a much larger amount of person-time in the analysis. We note that the magnitude of the coefficients for the year 1–7 analyses are slightly different from those of the year 4–7 analyses for all variables except previous FEV. This is likely to be a consequence of the markedly younger age distribution seen at year 1 of the study and the possibility of interaction effects of age and the other covariates. We should emphasize that only the nonlinear regression model in equation (5) and not the linear regression model in equation (1) can make use of the year 1–4 person-time in the analysis. Therefore it is not possible to compare directly the linear and nonlinear regression models based on year 1–7 data.

We have assumed in Table 5-7 that all covariates change linearly between successive examinations. This assumption appears reasonable for continuous covariates, but may not be reasonable for discrete covariates. Another possible assumption for binary covariates is that if a change of status is reported between successive exams (say at times $t - s$ and t), the change occurred at the latter exam (time t). For example, if we make this assumption for previous smoking status, then the contribution to the nonlinear regression model would take the form $x_{t-s}A(s)$ rather than the corresponding expression in Table 5-5. We have rerun the analyses under this "conservative" assumption for previous smoking status and have compared the results with the "linear" assumption results reported in Table 5-7 for the year 1–7 data. The results are presented in Table 5-8.

The results are similar under either analysis. Thus the linear assumption seems reasonable in this example and we will continue to use it in the remainder of this chapter.

We can use the coefficients in the model for the year 1–7 data in Table 5-7 to quantify the effect of personal smoking on a child's respiratory function over arbitrary periods of time. For illustration, consider two children with identical age, sex, height, and FEV at some time t_0 who have never smoked. We assume that at t_0 one of the children becomes a smoker and subsequently does not quit, while the other child remains a nonsmoker. We also assume that both children show the same growth in height after t_0. Using equation (1) and the model based

Table 5–8.   Relationships between changes in forced expiratory volume (FEV in liters) over time and other covariates based on nonlinear regression analysis (comparison of conservative and linear method)

Variable	Year 1–7 conservative method			Year 1–7 linear method		
	Regression coefficient	se[a]	p[b]	Regression coefficient	se	p
Constant	−2.2480	0.1471		−2.2520	0.1469	
$\ln(FEV_{t-1})$	0.8056	0.0116	<.001	0.8048	0.0116	<.001
$\ln(ht_{t-1}{}^{c})$	0.5943	0.0390	<.001	0.5948	0.0390	<.001
$\ln(growth^{d})$	1.8426	0.0708	<.001	1.8352	0.0707	<.001
Sex[e]	0.0070	0.0030	.021	0.0071	0.0030	.019
Age_{t}	0.0019	0.0010	NS	0.0022	0.0010	.040
$Smoking_{t-1}{}^{f}$	−0.0293	0.0073	<.001	−0.0337	0.0075	<.001
Number of persons	1042			1042		
Number of pairs	2131			2131		
Person-years	3365			3365		

[a]Standard error.
[b]p-value (two-tailed).
[c]Height (in.).
[d]Growth = $height_{t}/height_{t-1}$.
[e]Sex = 1 if male and 0 if female.
[f]$Smoking_{t-1}$ = current smoking at time $t-1 = 1$ if yes and 0 if no.

on year 1–7 data in Table 5-7, it can be shown that the expected difference in pulmonary function τ years after time t_0 between the two children is given by

$$E(y_{i,t_0+\tau}) - E(y_{i',t_0+\tau}) = \frac{\beta\Delta(1-\gamma^{\tau})}{1-\gamma} \tag{10}$$

where

$$x_{it} = x_{i't} + \Delta \quad \text{for all } t > t_0$$

and in this case $\Delta = 1$. We can apply this to the foregoing pulmonary function data by looking at the effect of smoking on growth of pulmonary function between two hypothetical 10-year-old boys who are both nonsmokers and have the mean FEV and height for 10-year-old boys in the CRD study (Rosner and Muñoz 1988) (viz., 1.89 liters and 55.3 inches), and who grow at an average rate over the ten-year period. One of the boys takes up smoking at age 10 and continues smoking until age 20, while the other boy remains a nonsmoker through age 20. The expected difference in log FEV or, equivalently, the expected ratio of pulmonary function at various ages is shown in Table 5-9 and Figure 5-2. Note that there is a 10.9-percent expected difference in FEV after five years and a 14.3-percent expected difference after ten years.

Table 5-9. Expected growth in pulmonary function (forced expiratory volume in liters) in two hypothetical 10-year-old boys, one of whom begins smoking at age 10 and continues to age 20, the other of whom remains a nonsmoker through age 20[a]

	FEV(1)				FEV(1)		
Age	Nonsmoker	Smoker	Ratio	Age	Nonsmoker	Smoker	Ratio
10	1.89	1.89	1.00	16	3.70	3.26	0.881
11	2.12	2.05	0.967	17	3.96	3.46	0.874
12	2.39	2.25	0.941	18	4.18	3.63	0.868
13	2.72	2.50	0.919	19	4.37	3.77	0.863
14	3.04	2.75	0.905	20	4.56	3.91	0.857
15	3.41	3.04	0.891				

[a]Initial FEV, height at age 10, and growth in height from age 10 to 20 for each boy are assumed to be the same as for an average boy in the East Boston Childhood Respiratory Disease Study.

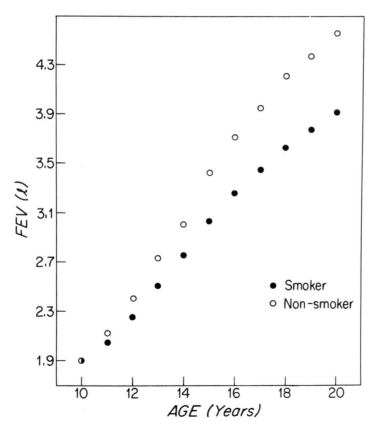

Figure 5-2. Comparison of growth of forced expiratory flow (FEV) between smoking and nonsmoking boys, ages 10–20, East Boston Childhood Respiratory Disease Study.

DISCUSSION

In summary, we have presented regression models for the analysis of longitudinal data and an application of these models in the context of a data set involving risk factors for predicting growth in pulmonary function in children. One key feature of these models is that they allow one to look at effects of changes in risk factors on changes in outcome over short periods of time, as opposed to relating slopes over long periods of time where cause-and-effect relationships and assumptions of linearity become more uncertain. Another key feature of the nonlinear regression model is that it allows for a variable length of time between examinations and thus represents an improvement over the linear regression model, which required equidistant intervals between successive exams and therefore resulted in a substantial amount of information not being used. The nonlinear regression model allows use of missing visits or of visits that were designed to be unequally spaced, or both, as was the case in the CRD study discussed in this chapter. The simulation study described here verified that no meaningful biases are introduced and that considerable gains in efficiency (in some cases over 100%) are achieved from using the nonlinear regression model based on all available person-time rather than the linear regression model based only on equidistant pairs. Furthermore, the nonlinear regression model can be fit using standard statistical packages such as PROC NLIN of SAS.

Several assumptions are made to enable the fitting of this model. Specifically, we assume that the residuals for a particular individual are independent after conditioning on outcome at time $t - 1$ and other relevant covariates. This assumption may not be warranted in some applications, and it may be necessary either to (1) consider a more general covariance structure for the residuals in the model or (2) condition on outcome at time $t - 1$, $t - 2, \ldots, t - L$ for some $L > 1$, in order to make the independence assumption valid. Finally, as in any Regression model, it is important to include the relevant covariates. In particular, in the context of the proposed autoregressive models, it is imortant to control for growth, which in our application is represented by the variable age.

Appendix
SAS Code Using PROC NLIN for the Models in Table 5-7

* LCURRFEV: natural log of current fev in liters;
* LPREVFEV: natural log of previous fev in liters;
* LNPREVHT: natural log of previous height in inches;
* LNCURRHT: natural log of current height in inches;
* SEX: 1 = male, 0 = female;
* CURRAGE: current age in years;

* PREVSMK: 1 = smoker at previous visit; 0 = nonsmoker at
previous visit;
* CURRSMK: 1 = smoker at current visit; 0 = nonsmoker at
current visit;
* S: years between previous and current visit;

```
PROC NLIN METHOD = GAUSS;
  PARMS ALPHA = 0.0
    GAMMA = 0.5
    BETAHT = 0.0
    BETAGROW = 0.0
    BETASEX = 0.0
    BETAAGE = 0.0
    BETASMK = 0.0;

BOUNDS - 1 < GAMMA < 1;

GTOS = GAMMA**S;
A = (1 - GTOS)/(1 - GAMMA);
B = (S*GTOS - (S - 1)*GTOS*
  GAMMA - GAMMA)/((1 - GAMMA)**2);
APRIME = - B/GAMMA;
BPRIME = (S*S*(GAMMA**(S - 1)) - (S*S - 1)*GTOS - 1 + 2*B*(
(1-GAMMA)) / ((1 - GAMMA)**2);

MODEL LCURRFEV = ALPHA*A
              + GTOS*LPREVFEV
              + BETAHT*(A*LNCURRHT + (B - A) *
                 (LNCURRHT - LNPREVHT)/S)
              + BETAGROW*A*
                (LNCURRHT - LNPREVHT)/S
              + BETASEX*A*SEX
              + BETAAGE*(A*CURRAGE + B)
              + BETASMK*(A*CURRSMK + (B - A)*
                (CURRSMK - PREVSMK)/S);

DER.ALPHA = A;
DER.GAMMA = ALPHA*APRIME
           + S*(GAMMA**(S - 1))*LPREVFEV
           + BETAHT*(APRIME*LNCURRHT
           + (BPRIME - APRIME)*
             (LNCURRHT - LNPREVHT)/S)
           + BETAGROW*APRIME*
             (LNCURRHT - LNPREVHT)/S
           + BETASEX*APRIME*SEX
           + BETAAGE*(APRIME*CURRAGE + BPRIME)
           + BETASMK*(APRIME*CURRSMK
           + (BPRIME - APRIME)*
             (CURRSMK - PREVSMK)/S);
```

```
DER. BETAHT     = A*LNCURRHT + (B − A)*
                  (LNCURRHT − LNPREVHT)/S;
DER. BETAGROW = A*(LNCURRHT − LNPREVHT)/S;
DER. BETASEX    = A*SEX;
DER. BETAAGE    = A*CURRAGE + B;
DER. BETASMK    = A*CURRSMK + (B − A)*
                  (CURRSMK − PREVSMK)/S;

__WEIGHT__      = (1 − GAMMA*GAMMA)/(1 − GTOS*GTOS);
```

REFERENCES

Anderson TW, Hsiao C (1982). "Formulation and estimation of dynamic models using panel data." *Journal of Econometrics* 18:47–82.

Berson EL, Sandberg MA, Rosner B, Birch DG, Hanson AH (1985). "Natural course of retinitis pigmentosa over a three-year interval." *American Journal of Ophthalmology* 99:240–251.

Muñoz A, Rosner B, Carey V (1986). "Regression analysis in the presence of heterogeneous intraclass correlation." *Biometrics* 42(3):653–658.

Rosner B, Muñoz A (1988). "Autoregressive modelling for the analysis of longitudinal data with unequally spaced examinations." *Statistics in Medicine*, 7:59–710.

Rosner B, Muñoz A, Tager I, Speizer FE, Weiss ST (1985). "Use of a generalized autoregressive model for the analysis of longitudinal data." *Statistics in Medicine* 4(4):457–467.

Tager IB, Weiss ST, Rosner B, Speizer FE (1979). Effect of parental cigarette smoking on pulmonary function in children." *American Journal of Epidemiology* 110:15–26.

6

Linear Structural Equation Modeling with Nonnormal Continuous Variables

Application: Relations Among Social Support, Drug Use, and Health in Young Adults

PETER M. BENTLER AND MICHAEL D. NEWCOMB

This chapter is a nontechnical introduction to some recent developments in linear structural equation modeling that are relevant to the study of human health-related issues. Linear structural models and the associated statistical methodology provide an extremely general and widely applicable set of procedures for representing, and evaluating, theoretical questions about how various sets of variables may influence each other. Structural modeling has its strongest domain of application in the analysis of quantitative variables obtained in nonexperimental research contexts where statistical and design controls must be used to substitute for experimental control. Statistical controls may involve such considerations as the postulation of latent variables to explain the interrelations among various measured variables and to control for the inevitable errors of measurement in variables, and the evaluation of effects of variables in the context of controls for true initial level of competing or potentially confounding variables. Design controls may involve the specification of conditions of measurement, sampling of a relevant population, and use of a longitudinal or panel research design to rule out various competing explanations of how variables affect each other. We cannot do much beyond provide the briefest glimpse of the relevant technical literature, since we use a good part of this chapter to illustrate the method with a report of a new study dealing with several topics of substantive interest to health researchers. Other sources, such as Bentler (1986a) or Bentler and Chou (1987), should be used for a broader introduction to the field.

The empirical section of this chapter will deal with the interrelations of social support, drug use, and health in a sample of 654 normal young men and women. Data were obtained in late adolescence on a large number of variables including the ten health-related variables to be studied here, and again four years later in young adulthood on essentially the same variables. Questions such as whether social support in adolescence has a positive effect on health status, or whether early drug use leads to poorer health, were evaluated. Although the study was intended primarily to determine the consequences, if any, of adolescent drug use, the importance of social support to health mandated that this variable be included in the design. The literature indicates that social support has a positive effect on mental and physical health, including decreased morbidity and mortality (see, e.g., Berkman, 1985; Berkman & Breslow, 1983; Kessler & McLeod, 1985; Newcomb & Bentler, 1988a; Reed, McGee, Yano, & Feinleib, 1983).

The proposal that social support and health be studied with structural modeling is not new. This methodology is one of the major approaches suggested by Dooley (1985) in his review of research methods that are appropriate to estimate the effect of social support on health. As we shall see, however, Dooley's conclusion that structural modeling is limited in application due to its inherent requirement for multivariate normal data is overly pessimistic and out of date.

STRUCTURAL MODELS

Recent years have seen the introduction of methods for the analysis of correlational data (as well as experimental data) that allow substantially stronger causal conclusions than methods historically considered appropriate for nonexperimental research. These newer methods are hypothesis-testing multivariate analysis procedures known by many names, such as structural equation models, covariance structure analysis, and linear structural relations models, and have become known colloquially as *causal modeling* methods because their broadest intent is to permit the testing of causal theories about data. Of course, multivariate structural methods are strictly neutral about interpretations regarding causality, but the methods permit drawing conclusions about whether a causal theory—posited by the substantive researcher, not the methodologist—may be considered plausible in the context of a given set of data. If a causal theory, as translated into a path diagram that specifies the relations among variables in the theory, and into equations and variance–covariance parameters that mirror the diagram, is consistent with a set of data, the theory is confirmed to the extent that the proposed model is not rejected by the data. On the other hand, if the data are not consistent with implications drawn about the data from the theory, one may conclude either that the theory is incorrect or that the data were not appropriate to test the theory. Since a test of a model against data should, in principle, be carried out only when the data are presumed to mirror adequately the conditions required by the theory (e.g., sample, measuring instruments, and procedures), the usual conclusion then would be that the theory has a flaw.

Although methods for multivariate analysis have been around for decades, they have been primarily for the exploration of data rather than for testing of causal theories. For example, factor analysis is usually considered a method for "finding" how many factors explain the correlations among variables. In contrast, the structural modeling approach to factor analysis would be used when the investigator has a very explicit hypothesis not only about how many factors might exist, but also about which variables might be good indicators of a given factor and, equally important, about which variables should not be indicators of a factor. Thus a critical part of structural modeling in the factor analytic context is that many factor loadings are, a priori, hypothesized to be zero, and that the number of factors is also hypothesized to be a given number. The task is to test whether such a theory might be correct. A chi-square statistic is typically used for this purpose. In large samples, goodness-of-fit indices that range from 0 to 1 also can be used to evaluate a model (Bentler & Bonett, 1980; Bentler, 1990). The second typical component of such structural models is that these factors, typically called *latent variables* or *latent constructs*, not only may be arbitrarily correlated among themselves but may be hypothesized to affect each other in a particular way. A given factor may be regressed on, or in a multiple correlation sense be predicted by, several other factors; there may be several such simultaneous regressions in which a given factor may be not only the cause of another factor but also the consequence of a different factor. In fact, the most widely known method of structural modeling, often associated with the name of the computer program LISREL (Jöreskog & Sörbom, 1983), represents the wedding of psychometric factor analytic (FA) models with econometric simultaneous equation models (SEM) just described. Developed by Ward Keesling, David Wiley, and Karl Jöreskog (Jöreskog, 1977; Wiley, 1973), this approach was called the *FASEM* approach in a recent review article (Bentler, 1986a). The FASEM equations are used to develop the covariance implications of the model. In practice it is the parameters of the resulting covariance structure that are estimated, based on a sample covariance matrix.

The distinction between latent and manifest variables is a key component of the FASEM approach to general structural models. Another approach makes no such distinction. Rather a generic linear structural matrix equation is used to relate variables of all kinds, whether measured or unmeasured, first-order or higher order common factors, errors in equations or errors in variables, and so on. The covariance matrix (Bentler & Weeks, 1980, 1982, 1985) and higher order multivariate product-moment matrices (Bentler, 1983) of the "independent" (nondependent) variables complete the parameterization. The covariance and product-moment structure of the measured variables expressed as a function of the parameter matrices completes the development. Some of the relevant equations of this approach are summarized in Appendix A. A related matrix model was given by McArdle and McDonald (1984). The Bentler–Weeks approach is used in the computer programs EQS and EQS/PC (Bentler, 1989). As will be seen in the example, while EQS makes use of the generic approach to models, it does not confront the user with any of the matrix algebra that forms a basis of the computations.

The basic procedures involved in structural modeling, based on the generic Bentler–Weeks approach, are relatively simple:

1. Draw a path diagram that includes all the variables involved in a causal system. Use two-way arrows to represent correlations or covariances between independent variables (those variables that are not explained by, or regressed on, other variables). Use one-way arrows to represent the

influences of one variable on another, with the direction indicating the direction of causation. (Figure 6-1 is an example.)

2. Transcribe the diagram into a series of multiple-regression type of equations. There will be as many equations as there are dependent variables to be explained.

3. The parameters of the model will be the regression coefficients and the variances and covariances (correlations) of the independent variables. Use a computer program such as EQS to estimate the parameters of the model against an appropriate set of data.

4. Evaluate the necessity of the parameters and the adequacy of the model by statistical and nonstatistical means.

5. If possible, or necessary, compare and contrast alternative models for the same set of data and for new data.

The data to be analyzed consist of derived moment statistics for the p variables, in particular, the $p(p + 1)/2$ different variances and covariances of the measured variables (in most models, the first moments are uninteresting means, and higher order moments are currently generally ignored). A model is created, in both diagrammatic and symbolic form. It is hypothesized that this model provides an explanation for the process that generated the data on the observed variables. If this hypothesis is true, then the model should be able to reproduce the data. In particular, in the population, if one knows the parameters θ of the model (the regression coefficients and variances and covariances of the independent variables) one would be able to plug these into a series of equations and generate precisely the covariance matrix of the observed variables. The Bentler–Weeks (1980) or Jöreskog–Keesling–Wiley model (Jöreskog & Sörbom, 1983; Wiley, 1973) could be used in this process. Note that it is the summary-moment parameters, the population variances and covariances σ_{ij}, that would be explained perfectly, since $\sigma_{ij} = \sigma_{ij}(\theta)$ is a function of the vector of parameters θ The subjects' scores on observed variables would, however, not be precisely knowable—even in the population—because of the random nature of the variables. On the other hand, if one has an incorrect model, then plugging its parameters into generating equations would lead to predictions of values of the population variances and covariances of the measured variables that would be incorrect to some extent. If the model were only marginally wrong, the reproduction would be close to perfect; if it were substantially wrong, the reproduction would be very bad. However, in principle it would be easy to see whether a model were correct or incorrect by evaluating its ability to reproduce moments, especially the variances and covariances.

In a sample, the problem of evaluating a structural hypothesis is more complex. In the first place, one does not know the parameters of the model but has to estimate them. Second, even if the estimates of parameters were close to their population values, one might not expect these estimates to be able to reproduce the sample covariance matrix exactly. The sample matrix will differ from sample to sample, even though the population matrix is a fixed matrix. Thus one turns to statistical criteria that can be used simultaneously to estimate the parameters of the model and to evaluate the model probabilistically. If the hypothesized model is in fact true, one should expect to see sample covariance matrices that do not depart much from a predicted covariance matrix that is generated after optimal parameter estimation. That is, one would expect to see reproduced matrices that are close to the population matrix within the limits of sampling error. Hence they should also be close to a sample covariance matrix drawn from the population.

The sample data under consideration consist of the covariances s_{ij} between pairs of variables i, j. The problem is to obtain an estimate of parameters $\hat{\theta}$ so that the estimated covariance $\hat{\sigma}_{ij} = \hat{\sigma}_{ij}(\hat{\theta})$ is close to the data s_{ij} (the population value σ_{ij} is not known, so it cannot be used).

It will be apparent from the foregoing discussion that structural models can be discussed with only minimal attention focused on the random variables. Whereas the FASEM and generic approaches specify a linear structure relating variables, the model-free approach $\sigma_{ij} = \sigma_{ij}(\boldsymbol{\theta})$ is in principle broader because it is not limited by a linearity assumption. This approach tends to be used in the statistical literature. As developed by Browne (1974), Lee and Bentler (1980), Browne (1984), Bentler and Dijkstra (1985), Shapiro (1986), and others, the elements of a covariance matrix Σ are assumed to be generated as a function of a vector of more basic parameters θ. Thus $\Sigma = \Sigma(\theta)$. For purposes of this chapter, as discussed next, the major virtue of the model-free approach is that it allows a simple discussion of the statistical issues in structural modeling. The EQS approach, of course, assumes that the parameter vector θ contains the parameters of the Bentler–Weeks model, whereas the FASEM approach might consider the parameters to be the relevant matrices of the LISREL program.

STATISTICAL METHODS

Historically, the most popular method for estimating parameters and testing hypotheses about specific structures, within the large class of structural models, is based on the assumption that the measured variables that generate a specific covariance structure are multivariate normally distributed (see e.g., Anderson, 1984; Jöreskog, 1977). As a consequence, normal-theory maximum likelihood (ML) methods have become almost standardly applied in structural modeling, especially due to their wide availability via the LISREL program. Normal-theory generalized least-squares (GLS) approaches to structural models have also been developed (e.g., Browne, 1974; Lee & Bentler, 1980). The optimal or best GLS estimators and test possess the same large sample properties as exhibited by the ML statistics. ML and GLS methods are now available in LISREL and EQS.

The assumption that variables are multivariate normally distributed is typically either plain wrong or at least troubling in applied research, having the consequence that, while the parameter estimates are appropriate (consistent) under violation of assumptions, the statistics (e.g., the goodness-of-fit test) may not have the assumed distribution (e.g., χ^2). Consequently, recent statistical research has been directed toward developing methods that hold under more general circumstances. Two major achievements in this regard have been obtained: elliptical and distribution-free covariance structure methods. Browne (1982, 1984) produced a major breakthrough by developing asymptotically efficient estimators and tests for covariance structures for variables that may not be normally distributed. Elliptical distributions are a general class of symmetric distributions that allow heavier or lighter kurtosis than the normal distribution and include the normal as a special case (e.g., Cambanis, Huang, & Simons, 1981; Muirhead, 1982). Variables are assumed to have no skew and homogeneous kurtosis. Thus the elliptical generalization of normal-theory statistics is a major competitor to normal-theory methods such as ML or GLS. Extending the work of Muirhead and Waternaux (1980), Browne emphasized certain types of elliptical tests, namely, corrected likelihood ratio statistics, that apply when a model is invariant with respect to a constant-scale factor; Satorra and Bentler (1986) provided a test for this model characteristic. Tyler (1982, 1983) developed the same likelihood ratio statistics. Bentler (1983) emphasized elliptical GLS statistics that hold for all classes of models. Bentler and Dijkstra (1985) developed the distribution of elliptical GLS estimators when the elliptical assumption is false, and provided an efficient linearized estimator as a one-step improvement over normal-theory least-squares, GLS, or ML estimators. Bentler and Berkane (1986) provided a bound for the elliptical kurtosis parameter that describes the homogeneous kurtoses of variables, and Satorra and Bentler (1986) provided a new estimator of this parameter. Berkane and Bentler (1986, 1987a) provided a series of parameters that describe the relations of centered second to all higher order moments. Berkane and Bentler (1987b) provided a GLS-based test of the homogeneity of kurtosis assumption. As yet, little experience has been gained regarding the practical use of elliptical theory. Harlow (1985) noted that normal-theory goodness-of-fit tests sometimes work well even when data are not multivariate normal, and that, when this happens, elliptical corrections to normal tests may be overly optimistic. This appears to be due to special model conditions that enable robustness to occur. Some work on the robustness of misspecified statistics has begun to appear (e.g., Browne, 1987; Satorra & Bentler, 1986, 1990; Shapiro, 1987) and much additional work is under way (e.g., Amemiya, 1985; Mooijaart & Bentler, 1991).

Browne (1982, 1984) and Chamberlain (1982) developed an estimator and goodness-of-fit test that holds when the variables have arbitrary distributions (see also Dijkstra, 1981). This asymptotically distribution-free method is based on a minimum chi square (Berkson, 1980; Ferguson, 1958), minimum distance, or GLS rationale applied to the distribution of sample covariances (called AGLS in EQS). Although the rationale for this method has a long history in statistics, this development for the first time explicitly frees structural modeling from making strong assumptions about the distribution of variables. Bentler and Dijkstra (1985) and Shapiro (1983, 1986) provided an explication of the relevant general asymptotic theory. Bentler (1983) developed a parametric form for the optimal-weight matrix used in estimation that was applied to the exploratory factor analytic model by Mooijaart and Bentler (1985) and that is critical to recent work on robustness. Bentler and Dijkstra (1985) developed a linearized alternative to the iterated GLS estimator, and showed that it is also asymptotically efficient and can be used for appropriate model tests. It seems to work well in practice (Tanaka, 1984; Tanaka & Bentler, 1985) and is cheaper to implement than the fully iterated estimator. This distribution-free theory is also relevant to specialized models such as univariate and multivariate regression (Chamberlain, 1982; Van Praag, Dijkstra, & Van Velzen, 1985).

A summary of the GLS approach to statistical theory in structural models that includes normal theory, elliptical theory, and arbitrary distribution theory as a special case is given in Appendix B. The appendix does not provide the technical details; but rather an overview of how the problem is addressed abstractly. The EQS program uses this generic theory to provide estimators and tests under the various distributional conditions. It also provides some indices for determining whether outliers exist in the data, and provides simple methods for eliminating these outliers, as will be shown in the example.

A recent release of the EQS program also contains statistical tests (Bentler, 1986b) that are familiar in several other research contexts but are not well known in the context of covariance structure analysis. In particular, Wald and Lagrange Multiplier tests (Chou & Bentler, 1990) are provided to evaluate hypotheses on subsets of parameters. Current statistical methods for comparing competing models are based on likelihood ratio criteria, or on chi-square difference tests that operate similarly to likelihood ratio tests. In this traditional approach, two nested models are each estimated separately and a goodness-of-fit test is obtained for each model. The difference between the two statistics is then taken as a chi-square difference statistic for evaluating whether the restrictions of the more restricted model are statistically plausible. This procedure thus requires estimating both the less restricted and more restricted models, which can be expensive and time consuming. The Wald statistic provides equivalent information by use of the less restricted model alone (see, e.g., Lee, 1985a), whereas the Lagrange Multiplier statistic provides equivalent information by use of the more restricted model alone (see, e.g., Lee & Bentler, 1980). An overview of these tests is provided by Buse (1982) and Engle (1984), and their large sample equivalence in a wide variety of ways in covariance structure analysis is demonstrated by Satorra (1989).

One of the major practical problems in structural modeling is that the methods are very demanding of researchers' knowledge, especially in large samples. In such samples virtually any a priori reasonable model may be statistically inadequate, that is, not all covariation will be explainable in terms of a priori hypothesized model parameters. One helpful tool in such circumstances is to use fit indices that range in an approximate or exact 0 to 1 range to determine how good a model may be (the closer to 1.0, the better), irrespective of whether a model may be statistically inadequate (e.g., Bentler, 1990; Bentler & Bonett, 1980; Tanaka & Huba, 1985). Another approach involves using empirical procedures to improve the fit of the model to the data. LISREL's model modification indices have proven invaluable. Bentler's (1989) EQS program provides various forms of univariate and multivariate Lagrangian model modification statistics. The univariate indices are very similar to those of LISREL, but in the context of the EQS program they provide information on potentially unnecessary parameter restrictions that cannot be obtained with LISREL, due to its use of the FASEM model. For example, LISREL does not provide an index of whether a measured variable should influence a latent factor, since a matrix to describe such a structural parameter is not routinely available. The multivariate indices are obtained in a stepwise fashion, with potential restrictions to be released, or parameters freed to be estimated, added in a sequential way so as to maximize the given step's Lagrange Multiplier statistic. Thus EQS will provide information on an entire set of possible restrictions to lift, or parameters to add, when a significant Lagrange test can be developed. The process is substantially under the user's control, so that only types of parameters of interest to the researcher are considered. Taken together with the Wald test, the forward Lagrange stepwise procedure acts very much like stepwise regression in the context of multiple regression. And, just as in stepwise regression, the methods can be misused or misleading (see MacCallum, 1986), but in appropriate circumstances they can be very valuable.

A nontrivial extension of single-population structural models involves estimating such models simultaneously in several populations. In such an approach it is possible to evaluate the hypothesis that key parameters of a model may be invariant across subgroups, such as sex or ethnic groups (Jöreskog, 1971; Sörbom, 1974, 1978). LISREL and EQS permit testing such multiple group models under the assumption that variables in each group are multivariate normally distributed, using ML estimation. Bentler, Lee, and Weng (1987) and Bentler (1989) have extended Lee and Tsui's (1982) GLS theory for multiple-population models to the case of populations with nonnormal distributions as well as mean structures under nonnormality. A multiple group option involving this theory will be made available with the next release of EQS.

Two other planned improvements in EQS involve methods for the correct statistical evaluation of models beyond covariance matrices. Current methods are correctly rationalized primarily as covariance structure methods, yet there are some situations where an analysis of standardized variables (i.e., correlation structures) is appropriate. It would thus be valuable to see some of the recent statistical theory that covers this situation to be implemented in EQS (e.g., Bentler & Lee, 1983; Lee, 1985b). In addition, it would be desirable to develop routine procedures for the use of higher multivariate product-moment data (e.g., third or fourth moments associated with multivariate skewness or kurtosis) in structural modeling. The theory is already developed (Bentler, 1983), and important applications exist (Mooijaart, 1985). The applied researcher, however, currently has no access to such methods that yield new statistical information about models, such as skewness and kurtosis of latent variables, and also yield greater efficiency in estimation and testing compared with extant methods when data are nonnormal.

Methods for dealing with nonlinear relations, such as interactions among latent variables, are still further on the horizon. Although theory (Bentler, 1983) and special cases such as polynomial models (Mooijaart & Bentler, 1985b) have been developed, routine implementation is still some years away. Fortunately, some nonlinear relations can be handled by reparameterization with existing programs (Wong & Long, 1987). Structural models also may be considered for measured variables that are categorical or ordinal in nature. When there are few categories in a response, for example when the variables are binary, then linear models such as the Bentler–Weeks model may not be appropriate. If the categorical variables arise from normally distributed continuous variables that have been arbitrarily cut to create categories, one may utilize a nonlinear probit-type structure relating observed to latent variables, while also considering a linear structure to interrelate the underlying latent variables. Methods for the analysis of ordered categorical data with latent variables have been developed by Muthén (1984), Lee, Poon, and Bentler (1990), and Arminger and Küsters (see Chapter 15 in this volume). When the number of response categories on a variable is large, or when several categorical variables are summed to create a more or less continuous variable (as in the example that follows), such variables can be used as if they were continuous in structural models for continuous variables. In that case one usually also adopts a particular scoring system for the variables (e.g., the integers 1–7) that may be nonoptimal in the sense that equal distances between categories on the variable are implicitly assumed. While continuity and equidistance may then be technically incorrect assumptions, the degree of violation of these assumptions will be sufficiently minor to affect the results trivially, compared with the other many sources of model misspecification that may occur. A typical consequence will be that a few extra "junk" parameters will be needed to make the model fit the data. In general, these potential junk parameters are small in magnitude and do not appear to affect the substance of the critical model parameters. For an illustration showing how a theoretically inferior method (ignoring continuity and category distances) may work better at recovering a true model than a theoretically appropriate method (based on tetrachoric correlations), see Collins, Cliff, McCormick, and Zatkin (1986). It is also the case that the computations required for structural models with categorical variables are quite extensive and grow rapidly with the number of categories. As a consequence, such methods are not practicable for large models such as are used here.

LONGITUDINAL STUDY

Sample

As part of an eight-year study of adolescent and young adult drug use and development, 654 individuals provided questionnaire data as older adolescents and again as young adults four years later. At all stages of the study, participants were informed of a grant of confidentiality given by the U.S. Department of Justice, which legally protects their responses. Each respondent at the young adult follow-up was paid $12.50 for participation.

Seventy percent of the sample were women and 30 percent were men, a proportion consistent with the initial survey. Breakdowns by other demographic characteristics such as income, life pursuit, ethnicity, and living arrangements are also provided in Table 6-1.

An extensive series of attrition analyses, reported elsewhere (Newcomb, 1986; Newcomb & Bentler, 1988b), revealed that patterns of dropping out of the study were only slightly systematic due to drug use, personality, or gender of the respondent. Trivial amounts of variance were associated with these factors. For example, when comparing retention and dropout in the study from 1976 to 1984 on thirty-eight personality and drug-use variables at initial testing, none of the variables differentiated the two groups significantly ($p < .05$). The average absolute-point biserial correlation for these thirty-eight tests was .04, whereas the average squared correlation was .002. The largest difference accounted for

Table 6–1.   Description of sample

Variable	Number of subjects	Percent of sample
Total	654	100
Sex		
Male	192	29
Female	462	71
Age		
21	253	39
22	214	33
23	170	26
24	17	2
Ethnicity		
Black	97	15
Hispanic	64	10
White	432	66
Asian	61	9
Current life activity		
Military	17	3
Junior college	79	12
University	139	21
Part-time job	89	14
Full-time job	305	47
None	25	4
Income last year		
None	62	9
Less than $5,000	215	33
Between $5,000 and $15,000	300	46
Over $15,000	76	12
Current living arrangements		
Alone	27	4
With parent(s)	311	48
Spouse	68	10
Spouse and child(ren)	43	7
Cohabitation	58	9
Dormitory	37	6
With roommates	81	12
Other	29	4

less than 1 percent of the variance between groups and was not significant when the Bonferroni method was used to correct for capitalizing on chance. With stepwise regression used to select the best predictors, nine of thirty-eight variables yielded an R^2 of .05 in accounting for between-group variance; the addition of sex and ethnicity yielded further 1- and 3-percent increments in attrition variance (showing women, Whites, Asians, and non-Blacks were more likely to stay in the study). Thus, although the retention rate after eight years was 45 percent, not surprising considering the nature and length of the research, results should not be severely biased due to subject loss.

Method

Embedded in the questionnaires at each occasion were a series of items dealing with social support, drug use, and health. Three indicators or measured variables from each of these domains were chosen to represent the relevant constructs in a latent-variable methodology. Effects of variables on each other across time were expected to be found primarily in the regressions of latent constructs on each other, controlling for initial levels in the other constructs. On the basis of knowledge of the domain, and preliminary analyses, an additional measured variable involving relations with peers was included in the analysis, but this variable was not taken as an indicator of a latent construct of general social support.

Ten variables (called V1–V10 in adolescence and V11–V20 in young adulthood) were thus measured at each of the two occasions. Nine of these variables were identical at the two occasions, but one, involving health symptomatology, was improved and refined in the interval between the two measurement occasions (details are given below).

The twenty variables were included in a series of structural models that differed only in minor ways, as will be noted. Since some of the variables were expected to be heavily skewed and kurtotic, ML analyses were backed up by the arbitrary distribution GLS (AGLS) estimator of the EQS program.

Measures

Drug Use

Drug-use measures included frequency of use during the past six months for twenty-two different substances. Frequency responses were given on a 7-point anchored rating scale that ranged from never use (1) to use more than once per day (7). Beer, wine, and liquor frequency-of-use variables were summed to yield a measured variable (V1) of alcohol use. Marijuana and hashish use yielded a cannabis variable (V2). The fifteen hard-drug use frequencies included five stimulants (substances such as amphetamines, cocaine, and inhalants), seven sedatives (substances such as barbiturates, tranquilizers, and narcotics), and three psychedelics (LSD, other psychedelics, and PCP). The frequencies were summed to yield a hard-drug measured variable (V3). Variables V1, V2, and V3 (indicators of latent variable F2) were measured in young adulthood as V11, V12, and V13 (taken as indicators of the factor F5).

Relationships

Four scales assessed the perceived quality of socially supportive relationships with family, parents, adults, and peers. Each scale consisted of four bipolar items rated on a 5-point scale anchored at each end by opposing descriptions (Newcomb & Bentler, 1986). For instance, an item on the "Good Relationship with Parents" scale had endpoints of "Parents don't think my ideas are worth much" and "Parents usually respect my ideas." The items typically assess the amount of respect, support, and inclusion experienced in each of these types of relationships. Internal consistency of the scales was quite good. Cronbach alpha for "Good Relationship with Parents" (V4) was .82, whereas the internal consistencies for "Good Relationship with Family" (V5) was .84, and "Good Relationship with Adults" (V6) was .54. The relations with parents, family, and adult scales were used as indicators of a general factor (F1) of social support. The same variables as V4, V5, and V6 were measured subsequently as V14, V15, and V16, while F4 was the factor presumed to underlie these indicators. "Good Relationships with Peers" (V7 and V17) also had an acceptable internal consistency of .74.

Health Status

Three measures were used to reflect a construct of poor health status during adolescence. These included times felt really ill (V10 and V20, rated for the past six months on a 7-point anchored scale that ranged from none [0] to six times or more [6]); illness sensitive (V8 and V18, a sum of four bipolar rating scales that assessed perceived vulnerability or sensitivity to illness, taken from the Bentler Medical-Psychological Inventory [Newcomb, Huba, & Bentler, 1981]), and a symptom index (V9, a sum of the presence [1] or absence [0] of twenty-five physical symptoms such as frequent headaches, wheezing, allergies, tightness in chest, high blood pressure, frequent constipation, and shake or tremble).

The symptom index was expanded for the young adult follow-up (V19). Each respondent indicated how frequently he or she had experienced each of twenty-two physical symptoms on a 3-point rating scale that ranged from not at all (0) to a lot (2). These items were developed by a physician and were taken from the marijuana consequences sourcebook (Huba, Bentler, & Newcomb, 1981). Items included descriptions of respiratory symptoms (seven items such as sore throat, wheezing, coughing spells, and shortness of breath), psychosomatic symptoms (eleven items such as headaches, trouble falling asleep, and skin problems), and seizure symptoms (four items such as dizzy spells, convulsions, and passed out). Item responses were summed to yield the variable included in the analysis. Health variables V8, V9, and V10 were taken as an indicator of a poor health factor (F3), while V18, V19, and V20 indicated the corresponding young-adult factor (F6) (Newcomb & Bentler, 1987).

Table 6–2. Job setup for EQS program

```
/TITLE
  SOCIAL SUPPORT, DRUG USE, AND POOR HEALTH
/SPECIFICATIONS
  CASES = 654; VAR = 20; ME = ML,AGLS; MA = RAW; DEL = 137,359;
/LABELS
  V1=ALCOHOL5;    V2=CANNBIS5;    V3=HARDDRG5;    V4=RELPAR5;    V5=RELFAM5;
  V6=RELADU5;     V7=RELPEER5;    V8=SENSIL5;     V9=SYMPTM5;    V10=FLTSICK5;
  V11=ALCOHOL9;   V12=CANNBIS9;   V13=HARDDRG9;   V14=RELPAR9;   V15=RELFAM9;
  V16=RELADU9;    V17=RELPEER9;   V18=SENSIL9;    V19=SYMPTM9;   V20=FLTSICK9;
  F1=SOCSPRT5;    F2=GENDRUG5;    F3=POORHLT5;    F4=SOCSPRT9;   F5=GENDRUG9;
  F6=POORHLT9;
/EQUATIONS
  V1  = .9*F2                        + E1;
  V2  = 1 F2       - .2*F3           + E2;
  V3  = .9*F2                        + E3;
  V4  = .9*F1                        + E4;
  V5  = 1 F1                         + E5;
  V6  = .6*F1  -.1*F2      + .1*V7   + E6;
  V8  =         .9*F3                + E8;
  V9  =         1 F3                 + E9;
  V10 =         .4*F3                + E10;
  V11 =               1*F5  + .1*V17 + E11;
  V12 =               1 F5           + E12;
  V13 =               1.4*F5         + E13;
  V14 = .9*F4                        + E14;
```

```
                                   1 F4                              + E15;
V15  =                             .6*F4                             + E16;
V16  =                                                               + E18;
V18  =                             .7*F6                             + E19;
V19  =                             1 F6                              + E20;
V20  =                             .4*F6                             + D4;
F4   =   .8*F1                               + .1*V1                 + D5;
F5   =   .5*F2      + .1*F3                            + .1*V17       + D6;
F6   =   -.1*F1     + .8*F3                   + .1*V7                 + E17;
V17  =   .1*F1                                         + .5*V7

/VARIANCES
V7  =  8*;    E17 = 9*;
F1  =  7*;    F2  = 7*;    F3  = 5*;    D4  = 1*;    D5  = 1*;    D6  = 8*;
E1  =  8*;    E2  = 1*;    E3  = 7*;    E4  = 5*;    E5  = 10*;   E6  = 4*;
E8  = 11*;    E9  = 5*;    E10 = 2*;    E11 = 11*;   E12 = 2*;    E13 = 4*;    E14 = 5*;
E15 =  9*;    E16 = 4*;
E18 =  6*;    E20 = 2*;

/COVARIANCES
F1  TO  F3 = *;
                        D4  TO  D6  ×  D5,D4 = *;
    F1,V7 = *;      F2,V7 = *;      F3,V7 = *;
    E1,E11 = *;     E3,E13 = *;     E5,E15 = *;     D4,E17 = *;     D6,E17 = *;
    E10,E20 = *;    E4,E6 = *;      E6,E8 = *;      E6,E16 = *;     E8,E18 = *;
    E1,E18 = *;     E2,E13 = *;     E2,E17 = *;     E14,E15 = *;    E18,E19 = *;
    E3,E19 = *;     E4,E11 = *;     E4,E18 = *;
    E6,E17 = *;     E8,E11 = *;     E9,E17 = *;                     E9,E19 = *;

/TECHNICAL
ITR = 15;  AITR = 15;
/END
```

Method

The basic model involved three factors F1, F2, and F3, as generators of the measured variables V1 through V10 at initial measurement, with factors F4, F5, and F6 generating variables V11 through V20, as noted previously. Variables V1 through V20 were assumed to contain errors of measurement, which were permitted to be pairwise correlated (e.g., error terms E1, E11 were correlated, as were E2, E12, etc.). Factors F1–F3 were allowed to correlate freely at time 1, and to correlate freely with V7, the peer relations variable. In a sense, V7 was considered to have a status equivalent to F1–F3, although of course it contains error of measurement. Factors F4–F6 and V17 were freely regressed on variables F1–F3 and V7, and the residuals in those regressions D4–D6 and E17 were allowed to correlate freely.

It was expected that the postulated highly restricted measurement model might not suffice, and additional paths were planned to be added in accord with Lagrange Multiplier statistics. Wald statistics were used to drop parameters that were not significant.

In preliminary analyses, variable V3 was found to be quite nonnormal, with coefficients of marginal skew and kurtosis of 5.1 and 35.4, respectively. Mardia's (1970) normalized coefficient of multivariate kurtosis was 55.5, indicating that the assumption of multivariate normality was highly questionable. It was observed that two subjects contributed substantially to Mardia's coefficient, so they were dropped from further analyses (which were then based on 652 cases). V3 behaved better as a result, with a skew of 4.2 and kurtosis of 23.7. However, Mardia's coefficient remained at 48.4.

The final model was submitted to EQS as shown in Table 6-2, which is reproduced here to illustrate how estimation is achieved in practice. The program requires several types of information, provided in keyworded sections preceded by a slash (/). The "Specifications" section indicates that twenty variables are in the data file. Two methods of estimation, ML and AGLS, are requested, and raw data input is used. Although the ML solution will not be interpreted, its test statistic was desired. Cases 137 and 359 are to be eliminated from the computations. The labels are optional reminders of what the V's and F's represent in the program.

The heart of the model set-up is in the "Equations," Variances," and "Covariances" sections, since the parameters of any model in the Bentler–Weeks framework are the variances and covariances of independent variables and the regression coefficients. There are twenty-two equations, hence twenty-two dependent variables as listed on the left of the "=" sign. None of these variables will have variance or covariance parameters. All other variables are independent variables. Each equation can be read as an ordinary linear regression equation, with "*" indicating that a parameter is free to be estimated and the number next to "*" being the guessed start value provided for the program to aid its function minimization. Values without a star were used to identify the scale of the latent variables (every unmeasured variable, i.e., non "V" variable, has an arbitrary scale). Blank space in the "Equations" section is given to help visualize which variables are influenced by a given factor. Independent variables require variances as parameters, as listed in the "Variances" section. Pairs of labels indicate those variables involved in a covariance, with "*" again representing a free parameter in the "Covariances" section. The absence of a value tells the program to use a default start value. Finally, the "Technical" section tells the program to limit the number of iterations for each method to fifteen.

RESULTS

The basic statistical output from the program is similar in form to the input. Free parameters are now optimally estimated and standard errors (with test values or critical ratios) associated with each estimate permit evaluation of the hypothesis that the parameter may be zero in the population. Additional information is, of course, also provided; this cannot be duplicated here for lack of space.

The final model fit the data acceptably with both ML and AGLS estimation, with the chi-square statistics being 114.2 and 118.8 on 128 degrees of freedom ($p = .8$ and $p = .7$, respectively). Bentler–Bonett normed fit indices were .98 and .94, respectively, while the nonnormed indices were essentially 1.0, indicating excellent fit.

Table 6-3 presents the final parameter estimates of the model, organized into a format that may be more interpretable substantively than the input material of Table 6-2. For reasons of visual presentation associated with Figure 6-1, the equation for V17 is listed in the "Construct Equations" section, although of course V17 is a measured variable and not a latent construct. Now each estimate has an estimated standard error as well, given in parentheses below the estimate. Each of the estimates is statistically necessary by a two-tailed z-test (estimate divided by standard error). The bottom part of the table makes clear that a number of a posteriori covariances were added to the model during model modification. In addition to the cross-time covariances listed, two covariances were needed within each occasion as well. A dash indicates that the parameters had been dropped from the model due to nonsignificance by the Wald test.

The path diagram in Figure 6-1 presents the results in a much more pleasing manner. In the first place, the various unidirectional paths, representing regression coefficients, are easily seen at once. Second, the values of the coefficients are now more comparable. In fact, the numbers are the transformed results that are obtained when all variables in the linear system are standardized to unit variance (including the residuals E and D). Thus all variables have unit variance, and their covariances become correlations. The correlations are not shown in the figure solely for aesthetic reasons (they could be added). Instead, they have been provided in Table 6-4. Although a variety of issues arise in standardization (see, e.g., Kim & Ferree, 1981), interpretations of results in a standardized metric is a recommended procedure (Bielby, 1986).

A posteriori parameters added as paths are shown in Figure 6-1 as paths from F2 to V6, F3 to V2, V1 to F4, V7 to V6, V17 to V16, and V17 to V11. It will be noted that all of these paths are small in size (the largest is .17), but are

Table 6–3. Parameter estimates and standard errors

MEASUREMENT EQUATIONS

```
ALCOHOL5  = V1 =              .92*F2                                           + E1
                              (.05)
CANNBIS5  = V2 =              1.00 F2   - .14*F3                               + E2
                                          (.05)
HARDDRG5  = V3 =              .67*F2                                           + E3
                             (.05)
RELPAR5   = V4 =   .94*F1                                                      + E4
                  (.04)
RELFAM5   = V5 =   1.00 F1                                                     + E5
RELADU5   = V6 =   .26*F1    - .09*F2                            + .14*V7      + E6
                  (.03)      (.03)                                (.03)
SENSIL5   = V8 =              .93*F3                                           + E8
                             (.08)
SYMPTM5   = V9 =              1.00F3                                           + E9
FLTSICK5  = V10 =             .38*F3                                           + E10
                             (.04)
ALCOHOL9  = V11 =                            1.09*F5     + .11*V17            + E11
                                             (.10)          (.03)
CANNBIS9  = V12 =                            1.00 F5                          + E12
HARDDRG9  = V13 =                            1.34*F5                          + E13
                                             (.10)
RELPAR9   = V14 =                  .92*F4                                     + E14
                                  (.04)
RELFAM9   = V15 =                  1.00 F4                                    + E15
RELADU9   = V16 =                  .27*F4               + .12*V17             + E16
                                  (.04)                   (.03)
SENSIL9   = V18 =                                .71*F6                       + E18
                                                (.05)
SYMPTM9   = V19 =                                1.00*F6                      + E19
FLTSICK9  = V20 =                                .19*F6                       + E20
                                                (.02)
```

CONSTRUCT EQUATIONS

```
SOCSPRT9 = F4  =   .57*F1                      + .09*V1   + .09*V7    + D4
                  (.04)                         (.02)       (.04)
RELPEER9 = V17 =   .21*F1                                  + .36*V7   + E17
                  (.03)                                      (.04)
GENDRUH9 = F5  =            .49*F2   - .07*F3                         + D5
                           (.03)     (.03)
POORHLT9 = F6  =  - .17*F1           + .90*F3                         + D6
                   (.04)             (.10)
```

VARIANCES

CONSTRUCTS – TIME 1

F1 = 11.09*	V7 = 7.81*	F2 = 6.10*	F3 = 4.60*
(.80)	(.44)	(.46)	(.56)

CONSTRUCT RESIDUALS – TIME 2

D4 = 2.85*	E17 = 7.17*	D5 = .72*	D6 = 10.16*
(.86)	(.42)	(.14)	(1.71)

Table 6-3. *(Continued)*

			VARIANCES			

ERROR VARIABLES

E1 = 7.57*	E2 = .31*	E3 = 4.44*	E4 = 1.59*	E5 = 6.05*	E6 = 4.00*	
(.41)	(.23)	(.66)	(.36)	(.54)	(.22)	
--	E8 = 10.88*	E9 = 4.34*	E10 = 1.27*	E11 = 11.06*	E12 = 1.52*	
	(.63)	(.46)	(.11)	(.44)	(.18)	
E13 = 2.02*	E14 = 4.44*	E15 = 7.36*	E16 = 3.49*	--	E18 = 6.57*	
(.44)	(.76)	(.96)	(.19)		(.85)	
E19 = 3.47*	E20 = 1.08*					
(1.65)	(.09)					

COVARIANCES

	Within-time		
	Time 1		Time 2

Es	F/Vs	D/Es	Es
E4,E6 = .74* (.17)	V7,F1 = 3.17* (.36)	E17,D4 = .70* (.28)	E14,E15 = 3.08* (.79)
E6,E8 = − .52* (.20)	V7,F2 = − .29* (.24)	E17,D5 = --	E18,E19 = −3.20* (1.00)
	V7,F3 = − .98* (.26)	E17,D6 = − 2.25* (.33)	
	F1,F2 = − 1.77* (.35)	D4,D5 = --	
	F1,F3 = − 2.16* (.36)	D4,D6 = − 1.38* (.33)	
	F2,F3 = 1.17* (.35)	D5,D6 = .36* (.15)	

Cross-time

A priori	A posteriori
E1,E11 = 4.31* (.33)	E1,E18 = − .81* (.25)
E2,E12 = --	E2,E13 = − .57* (.17)
E3,E13 = .74* (.33)	E2,E17 = − .57* (.16)
E4,E14 = --	E3,E19 = .64* (.28)
E5,E15 = 2.30* (.25)	E4,E11 = .43* (.21)
E6,E16 = 1.00* (.13)	E4,E18 = .66* (.21)
E8,E18 = 4.08* (.45)	E6,E17 = .65* (.17)
E9,E19 = .99* (.43)	E8,E11 = − .61* (.31)
E10,E20 = .15* (.06)	E9,E17 = .98* (.24)

nonetheless statistically significant. These paths represent areas of incompleteness of the a priori theoretical specification. For example, the factor structure was incomplete due to lack of knowledge of two of the paths. Most of the a posteriori added correlations shown in Table 6-4 are also quite small in magnitude, except for the following: E14, E15 = .54; E18, E19 = − .67; and E2, E13 = −.72. The high correlation of these residuals suggests that a more complete model should include additional variables that can help to account for these unexpected residual associations.

The key substantive questions that generated the model lie in the cross-time paths of the inner variables in the figure. (Missing paths indicate that the

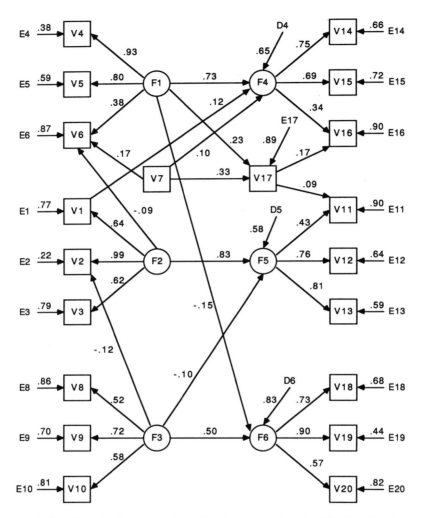

Figure 6-1. Standardized solution. Numbers associated with directional arrows are standardized coefficients. The correlations among independent variables are not shown; they are reported in Table 6-4.

coefficients were not significant and have been dropped.) Aside from the obvious stability effects of factors and variables predicting themselves across time, we note the following significant, though relatively weak, results:

1. High levels of general social support (F1) during adolescence lead to decreasing poor health (F6) (i.e., better health) four years later.
2. High amounts of general social support (F1) during adolescence lead to increasingly better peer support (V17) during young adulthood.
3. High amounts of general social support (F4) received during young

Table 6–4. Correlations for model in Figure 6-1

		Within-time correlations		
	Time 1		Time 2	
Es	F/Vs	D/Es		Es
E4, E6 = .29	V7, F1 = .34	E17, D4 = .16		E14, E15 = .54
E6, E8 = −.08	V7, F2 = −.04	E17, D5 = —		E18, E19 = −.67
	V7, F3 = −.16	E17, D6 = −.26		
	F1, F2 = −.22	D4, D5 = —		
	F1, F3 = −.30	D4, D6 = −.26		
	F2, F3 = .22	D5, D6 = .13		

Cross-time correlations	
A priori	A posteriori
E1, E11 = .47	E1, E18 = −.12
E2, E12 = —	E2, E13 = −.72
E3, E13 = .25	E2, E17 = −.38
E4, E14 = —	E3, E19 = .16
E5, E15 = .34	E4, E11 = .10
E6, E16 = .27	E4, E18 = .20
E8, E18 = .48	E6, E17 = .12
E9, E19 = .26	E8, E11 = −.06
E10, E20 = .13	E9, E17 = .18

adulthood are a consequence of higher levels of peer support (V7) and alcohol use (V1) during adolescence.

4. Poor health (F3) during adolescence leads to decreased levels of drug use (F5) during young adulthood.

No other effects could be demonstrated.

DISCUSSION

Linear structural modeling has in recent years grown in statistical sophistication as well as in practicality of application, as the review materials at the beginning of this chapter and the illustration were meant to convey. Of course, many technical and applied problems remain to be addressed in the field, but a useful technology for the study of longitudinal data has certainly been developed.

Although the AGLS (called ADF, asymptotically distribution free, by Browne, 1984) method has robustness properties to recommend it, two of its major limitations should be understood. First, it requires very large sample sizes for the estimated weight matrix, based on fourth-moment data, to become stable. One may suspect that the asymptotic statistics that justify its probability statements are not as readily applicable to small-sample data as are methods based only on covariance data. Second, this method becomes impractical as the number of variables exceeds about twenty or so, since the size of the weight matrix expands quadratically with the number of variables. Consequently the method can become quite expensive to implement. Costs can be kept down by using the linearized estimator also available in the program (not illustrated above), but the computer storage requirements cannot be overcome this way. Actually, the size limitation served to minimize the number of variables that we studied in our model. Elliptical methods, not demonstrated here, do not share this drawback since they are computationally almost as easy to apply as normal-theory methods.

Normal-theory maximum likelihood methods are in principle incorrect to apply when data are severely nonnormal. Although ML estimates of parameters are no doubt trustworthy due to the consistency of the estimator, the standard errors and goodness-of-fit chi-square statistics may well be questionable. However, as in the example, there appear to be some situations when the chi-square value is actually surprisingly similar to that of AGLS. In fact, all statistical conclusions on key parameters were the same whether considered from ML or AGLS perspectives. Thus the AGLS construct equations in the middle of Table 6-3 are virtually identical in the ML solution: $F4 = .55*$ $F1 + .07* V1 + .09* V7 + D4$; $V17 = .17* F1 + .39* V7 + E17$; $F5 = .50*$ $F2 - .07* F3 + D5$; and $F6 = -.15*F1 + .80*F3 + D6$. The median difference in parameter estimates is .02, and only one estimate is substantially off (.9 vs. .8). The standard error estimates differed by .01 at most. Research is currently addressed toward gaining greater understanding of these phenomena.

Statistical goodness-of-fit tests are quite unforgiving about lack of a priori theoretical knowledge of influences that might exist among a set of variables. Virtually any a priori model for a large number of variables, especially when based on data arising from a sizable sample, inevitably tends to be rejected statistically because the model covariance matrix reproduced from the estimated parameters is not sufficiently close to the sample covariance matrix. While the discrepancies between data and model may be small, the power of the method to detect model misspecification is often extremely high. (When testing someone else's theory, this is desirable; but when evaluating one's own theory, one would like to have a more forgiving procedure!) As a consequence, empirical model modification, based on Lagrange Multiplier statistics or similar indices, is frequently made. This was done in the present illustration as well. The purely a priori model yielded a χ^2 of 278.4 and 307.3 for ML and AGLS methods, respectively, too high for an acceptable model with 143 degrees of freedom ($p < .001$). While the Bentler–Bonett normed (.94, .85) and nonnormed (.96, .89) fit indices for ML and AGLS solutions indicated that the degree of model fit was already quite high, and that any potential model modifications would yield relatively minor increases in fit, statistical fit at the .05 level or beyond required adding a posteriori parameters as described previously. The effect of these a posteriori parameters on key substantive conclusions was relatively minor, typically having the effect that a marginally significant effect might become nonsignificant, or the reverse. Thus the AGLS estimates of the construct equations of the a priori model were as follows: $F4 = .59*F1 + .06*V7 + D4$; $V17 = .18*F1 + .31*V7 + E17$; $F5 = .50*F2 + .00*F3 + D5$; and $F6 = -.11*F1 + .86*F3 + D6$. These estimates are quite close to the final results shown in the middle of Table 6-3, the median being .035 different. The two least significant effects in Table 6-3, as judged by z-test ($F4 \leftarrow V7$ and $F5 \leftarrow F3$), were nonsignificant in the a priori model. While the resulting model cannot be rejected statistically, it must be remembered that the statistics cannot be presumed to be precisely distributed as under the null hypothesis due to the empirical nature of model modification, which lends itself to capitalizing on chance. Thus a certain amount of caution, especially regarding small effects in models, is appropriate. Certainly one cannot claim to have "discovered" the "true" process that generated the data with this methodology (Cliff, 1983; MacCallum, 1986).

Finally, the empirical results observed in the study of social support, drug use, and health are quite positive in nature. Social support was seen in this sample of essentially normal youth to have the beneficial effect on health that has been observed in older subjects, in whom one would expect to see substantially greater variance in both health and social support. Thus the phenomenon, while no doubt attenuated here, remained verifiable in a causal modeling context covering a four-year time span. Happily, no negative effects on health were observed for drug use. Although early poor health was found to inhibit subsequent drug use, this effect was quite small and seems to have no policy implications. Whereas social variables such as peer pressure have been found to have a strong impact on drug use, social support has no direct impact one way or the other. Future research could be directed at evaluating whether specific health problems, ideally verified by medical measurements, relate to social support and drug use in a similar fashion as the global self-report indices used in the current study.

GUIDE TO THE LITERATURE

A nontechnical overview of developments in structural modeling across several decades can be found in the review article by Bentler (1986a). A practical introduction to the field that is accessible to anyone familiar with multiple regression can be found in Bentler (1989). Chapter 2, in particular, shows how several models are conceptualized and set up for computer analysis, and Chapter 5 provides details on several examples. Introductory textbooks on the topic include those by Everitt (1984); James, Mulaik, and Brett (1982); Loehlin (1987); Long (1983), and Saris and Stronkhorst (1984). Browne (1982) and Bentler (1983) have provided treatment of more technical topics as well. The February, 1987, issue of *Child Development* contains a special section on structural equation modeling with articles addressing general issues, a variety of applications, and some technical issues. The Summer 1987 issue of the *Journal of Educational Statistics* provides critical discussions of limitations of the method.

The statistical theory, considered from relatively general mathematical. perspectives, can be found in such sources as Browne (1984), Bentler and

Dijkstra (1985), Satorra (1989), and Shapiro (1986). Measurement error models are reviewed in Fuller (1987).

Appendix A
Bentler–Weeks Model

Every variable in a linear system is considered to be an "independent" or a "dependent" variable. Dependent variables, placed into a vector η, can be expressed as a structural regression function of other variables. Independent variables, placed into a vector ξ, are never structurally regressed on other variables. The variables are linearly related via the matrix equation

$$\eta = \beta\eta + \gamma\xi \tag{A1}$$

where β contains the coefficients for the regression of η variables on each other and γ contains the coefficients for the regression of η variables on ξ variables. Assuming that all variables are in deviation from mean form, for simplicity (see Bentler, 1983, otherwise),

$$\Phi = E(\xi\xi') \tag{A2}$$

represents the covariance matrix of the independent variables. The parameters of the model are the unknown and known elements of the matrices β, γ, and Φ.

A supermatrix variant of (A1) is easier to manipulate further. Let $v = (\eta', \xi')'$, B be a partitioned matrix containing rows $(\beta, 0)$ and $(0, 0)$, and $\Gamma' = (\gamma', I)$. Then

$$v = Bv + \Gamma\xi \tag{A3}$$

is equivalent to (A1). It follows that all variables can be expressed as

$$v = (I - B)^{-1}\Gamma\xi \tag{A4}$$

namely, a linear combination of independent variables. Now, letting z be the vector of measured variables that are a subset of all variables v, they can be expressed as

$$z = Gv \tag{A5}$$

where G is a known matrix of zeros and ones. Thus

$$z = G(I - B)^{-1}\Gamma\xi \tag{A6}$$

and the covariance matrix Σ of z is obtained as $\Sigma = E(zz')$, or

$$\Sigma = G(I - B)^{-1}\Gamma\Phi\Gamma'(I - B)^{-1'}G' \tag{A7}$$

Thus if θ is the vector of parameters in β, γ, and Φ, $\Sigma = \Sigma(\theta)$ in model-free form is specialized to linear structures via (A7) with the Bentler–Weeks approach.

Appendix B
Estimation and Testing via Generalized Least Squares (GLS)

Let σ be the $p^* = p(p + 1)/2$ vector of nonduplicated elements in the $p \times p$ matrix Σ. Thus $\sigma = \sigma(\theta)$. Let s be the corresponding vector of nonduplicated elements in the sample covariance matrix S obtained from a sample of size n, and let W be a weight matrix of appropriate order. Then

$$Q = [s - \sigma(\theta)]'W[s - \sigma(\theta)] \tag{B1}$$

is a GLS function to be minimized with respect to choice of estimator $\hat{\theta}$. Under appropriately optimal weight matrices, $n\hat{Q} = nQ(\hat{\theta})$ is a large sample chi-square variate with $p^* - q$ degrees of freedom, where q is the effective number of free parameters estimated.

Optimal weight matrices under minimum chi-square estimation are those that converge in probability to the inverse of the covariance matrix V of the data vector s. The matrix $W = V^{-1}$ that holds under arbitrary distribution of variables can be obtained from the elements

$$\sigma_{ijkl} - \sigma_{ij}\sigma_{kl} \tag{B2}$$

where σ_{ijkl} is a centered multivariate fourth-order product moment of variables $i, j, k,$ and l, and σ_{ij} and σ_{kl} are covariances among pairs of variables. In practice, σ_{ijkl} is estimated by

$$s_{ijkl} = n^{-1}\Sigma_1^n(z_{it} - \bar{z}_i)(z_{jt} - \bar{z}_j)(z_{kt} - \bar{z}_k)(z_{lt} - \bar{z}_l) \tag{B3}$$

and σ_{ij} by the sample covariance s_{ij}. The arbitrary distribution GLS function (B1) may be called AGLS.

When the variables have an elliptical distribution, the optimal weight matrix can be computed more simply because

$$\sigma_{ijkl} = (\kappa + 1)(\sigma_{ij}\sigma_{kl} + \sigma_{ik}\sigma_{jl} + \sigma_{il}\sigma_{jk}) \tag{B4}$$

where κ is the kurtosis parameter of the distribution. Given an estimate of κ, such as

$$\hat{\kappa} = n^{-1}\frac{\Sigma_1^n[(z_t - \bar{z})'S^{-1}(z_t - \bar{z})]^2}{[p(p + 2)]} - 1 \tag{B5}$$

the fourth-moment computations (B3) are no longer needed, since via (B4) the fourth moments are an explicit function of covariances only. Under multivariate normal distributions, $\kappa = 0$, so that the optimal weight matrix is still more simple to compute.

Another perspective on GLS estimation can be obtained by noting that the function (B1) itself simplifies under elliptical distributions. If (B4) is true and a consistent estimator of the optimal weight matrix V^{-1} is used, (B1) specializes to

$$Q_E = 2^{-1}(\kappa + 1)^{-1}\text{tr}[(S - \Sigma)W_2]^2 - \delta[\text{tr}(S - \Sigma)W_2]^2 \qquad \text{(B6)}$$

where W_2 is any consistent estimator of Σ^{-1} and

$$\delta = \kappa/[4(\kappa + 1)^2 + 2p\kappa(\kappa + 1)].$$

The elliptical distribution GLS function may be called EGLS. The normal-theory GLS function is obtained from (B6) by setting $\kappa = 0$. The normal-theory maximum-likelihood estimator can be obtained with $\kappa = 0$ by iteratively updating the weight matrix W_2 by $\hat{\Sigma}^{-1}$ at the current iteration. EQS calls such functions reweighted least-squares functions, for example, ERLS or RLS.

Distributional misspecification occurs when a nonoptimal function (B6) (with $\kappa \neq 0$ or $\kappa = 0$) is minimized and the variables do not in fact have the assumed distribution. The resulting statistic, say $n\hat{Q}_E$, is then not distributed as χ^2, and standard errors computed from the Hessian or information matrix associated with (B6) will be incorrect. The robustness of these statistics to misspecification is currently under investigation (e.g., Amemiya, 1985; Browne, 1987; Satorra & Bentler, 1986, 1990). In addition, new estimators that are more general than ellipticial theory but are not more expensive to compute are being developed (Kano, Berkane, & Bentler, 1990).

REFERENCES

Amemiya Y (1985). *On the Goodness-of-fit Test for Linear Statistical Relationships.* Technical Report, no. 10, Stanford University, Stanford, Calif.

Anderson TW (1984). "Estimating linear statistical relationships." *Annals of Statistics* 12:1–45.

Bentler PM (1983). "Some contributions to efficient statistics in structural models: Specification and estimation of moment structures." *Psychometrika* 48:493–517.

Bentler PM (1986a). "Structural modeling and psychometrika: An historical perspective on growth and achievements." *Psychometrika* 51:35–51.

Bentler PM (1986b). *Lagrange Multiplier and Wald Tests for EQS and EQS/PC.* Los Angeles, BMDP Statistical Software.

Bentler PM (1989). *EQS Structural Equations Program Manual.* Los Angeles, BMDP Statistical Software.

Bentler PM (1990). "Comparative fit indexes in structural models." *Psychological Bulletin* 107:238–246.

Bentler PM, Berkane M (1986). "The greatest lower bound to the elliptical theory kurtosis parameter." *Biometrika* 73:240–241.

Bentler PM, Bonett (1980). "Significance tests and goodness of fit in the analysis of covariance structures." *Psychological Bulletin* 88:588–606.

Bentler PM, Chou CP (1987). "Practical issues in structural modeling." In Long JS (ed), *Common Problems in Quantitative Social Research* Beverly Hills, Calif., Sage.

Bentler PM, Dijkstra T (1985). "Efficient estimation via linearization in structural models." In Krishnaiah PR (ed), *Multivariate Analysis VI*. Amsterdam, North-Holland, pp 9–42.

Bentler PM, Lee S-Y (1983). "Covariance structures under polynomial constraints: Applications to correlation and alpha-type structural models." *Journal of Educational Statistics* 8:207–222, 315–317.

Bentler PM, Lee S-Y, Weng J (1987). "Multiple population covariance structure analysis under arbitrary distribution theory." *Communications in Statistics-Theory* 16:1951–1964.

Bentler PM, Weeks DG (1980). "Linear structural equations with latent variables." *Psychometrika* 45:289–308.

Bentler PM, Weeks DG (1982). "Multivariate analysis with latent variables." In Krishnaiah PR, Kanal L (eds), *Handbook of Statistics*. Amsterdam, North-Holland, pp 747–771.

Bentler PM, Weeks DG (1985). "Some comments on structural equation models." *British Journal of Mathematical and Statistical Psychology* 38:120–121.

Berkane M, Bentler PM (1986). "Moments of elliptically distributed random variates." *Statistics & Probability Letters* 4:333–335.

Berkane M, Bentler PM (1987a). "Characterizing parameters of multivariate elliptical distributions." *Communications in Statistics-Simulation* 16:193–198.

Berkane M, Bentler PM (1987b). "Distribution of kurtoses, with estimators and tests for homogeneity of kurtosis." *Statistics & Probability Letters* 5:201–207.

Berkman LF (1985). "The relationship of social networks and social support to morbidity and mortality." In Cohen S, Syme SL (eds), *Social Support and Health*. Orlando, Fla., Academic Press, pp 241–262.

Berkman L, Breslow L (1983). *Health and Ways of Living: Findings from the Alameda County Study*. New York, Oxford University Press.

Berkson J (1980). "Minimum chi-square, not maximum likelihood!." *Annals of Statistics* 8:457–487.

Bielby WT (1986). "Arbitrary matrices in multiple-indicator models of latent variables." *Sociological Methods & Research* 15:3–23, 62–63.

Browne MW (1974). "Generalized least squares estimators in the analysis of covariance structures." *South African Statistical Journal* 8:1–24.

Browne MW (1982). "Covariance structures." In Hawkins DM (ed), *Topics in Applied Multivariate Analysis*. London, Cambridge University Press, pp 72–141.

Browne MW (1984). "Asymptotically distribution free methods for the analysis of covariance structures." *British Journal of Mathematical and Statistical Psychology* 37:62–83.

Browne MW (1987). "Robustness of statistical inference in factor analysis and related models." *Biometrika* 74:375–384.

Buse A (1982). "The likelihood ratio, Wald, and Lagrange multiplier tests: An expository note." *American Statistician* 36:153–157.

Cambanis S, Huang S, Simons G (1981). "On the theory of elliptically contoured distributions." *Journal of Multivariate Analysis* 11:368–385.

Chamberlain G (1982). "Multivariate regression models for panel data." *Journal of Econometrics* 18:5–46.

Chou C-P, Bentler PM (1990). "Model modification in covariance structure modeling: A comparison among likelihood ratio, Lagrange Multiplier, and Wald tests." *Multivariate Behavioral Research* 25:115–136.

Cliff N (1983). "Some cautions concerning the application of causal modeling methods." *Multivariate Behavioral Research* 18:115–128.

Collins LM, Cliff N, McCormick DS, Zatkin JL (1986). "Factor recovery in binary data sets: A simulation." *Multivariate Behavioral Research* 21:377–391.

Dijkstra TK (1981). "Latent variables in linear statistic models." Ph.D. diss., Groningen University, Groningen, Netherlands.

Dooley D (1985). "Causal inference in the study of social support." In Cohen S, Syme L (eds), *Social Support and Health*, Orlando, Fla., Academic Press, pp 109—125.

Engle RF (1984). "Wald, likelihood ratio, and Lagrange multiplier tests in econometrics." In Griliches Z, Intriligator M (eds), *Handbook of Econometrics, Vol. 2*. Amsterdam, North-Holland, pp 776–826.

Everitt BS (1984). *An Introduction to Latent Variable Models*. London, Chapman and Hall.

Ferguson T (1958). "A method of generating best asymptotically normal estimates with application to the estimation of bacterial densities." *Annals of Mathematical Statistics* 29:1046–1062.

Fuller WA (1987). *Measurement Error Model*. New York, Wiley.

Harlow LL (1985). *Behavior of Some Elliptical Theory Estimators with Nonnormal Data in a Covariance Structures Framework: A Monte Carlo Study*. Ph.D diss., University of California, Los Angeles.

Huba GJ, Bentler PM, Newcomb MD (Eds.) (1981). *Assessing Marijuana Consequences: Selected Questionnaire Items*. Rockville, Md, National Institute on Drug Abuse.

James LR, Mulaik SA, Brett JM (1982). *Causal Analysis: Assumptions, Models, and Data*. Beverly Hills, Calif., Sage.

Jöreskog KG (1971). "Simultaneous factor analysis in several populations." *Psychometrika* 36:409–426.

Jöreskog KG (1977). "Structural equation models in the social sciences: Specification, estimation and testing." In Krishnaiah PR (ed.), *Applications of Statistics*. Amsterdam, North-Holland, pp 265–287.

Jöreskog KG, Sörbom D (1983). *LISREL User's Guide*. Chicago, International Educational Services.

Kano Y, Berkane M, Bentler PM (1990). "Covariance structure analysis with heterogeneous kurtosis parameters." *Biometrika* 77:575–585.

Kessler RC, McLeod JD (1985). "Social support and mental health in community samples." In Cohen S, Syme SL (eds.), *Social Support and Health*, Orlando, Fla., Academic Press, pp 219–240.

Kim JO, Ferree GD (1981). "Standardization in causal analysis." *Sociological Methods & Research* 10:187–210.

Lee S-Y (1985a). "On testing functional constraints in structural equation models." *Biometrika* 72:125–131.

Lee S-Y (1985b). "Analysis of covariance and correlation structures." *Computational Statistics & Data Analysis* 2:279–295.

Lee S-Y, Bentler PM (1980). "Some asymptotic properties of constrained generalized least squares estimation in covariance structure models." *South African Statistical Journal* 14:121–136.

Lee S-Y, Poon W-Y, Bentler PM (1990). "A three-stage estimation procedure for structural equation models with polytomous variables." *Psychometrika* 55:45–51.

Lee S-Y, Tsui KL (1982). "Covariance structure analysis in several populations." *Psychometrika* 47:297–308.

Liker J, Augustyniak S. Duncan GJ (1985). "Panel data and models of change: A comparison of first difference and conventional two-wave models." *Social Science Research* 14:80–101.

Loehlin JC (1987). *Latent Variable Models: An Introduction to Factor, Path, and Structural Analysis.* Hillsdale, N.J., Erlbaum.

Long JS (1983). *Covariance Structure Models: An Introduction to LISREL.* Beverly Hills, Calif., Sage.

McArdle JJ, McDonald RP (1984). "Some algebraic properties of the reticular action model for moment structures." *British Journal of Mathematical and Statistical Psychology* 37:234–251.

MacCallum R (1986). "Specification searches in covariance structure modeling." *Psychological Bulletin* 100:107–120.

Mardia KV (1970). "Measures of multivariate skewness and kurtosis." *Biometrika* 57:519–530.

Mooijaart A (1985). "Factor analysis for non-normal variables." *Psychometrika* 50:323–342.

Mooijaart A, Bentler PM (1985). "The weight matrix in asymptotic distribution-free methods." *British Journal of Mathematical and Statistical Psychology* 38:190–196.

Mooijaart A, Bentler PM (1986). "Random polynomial factor analysis." In Diday et al. (eds.), *Data Analysis and Informatics.* Amsterdam, Elsevier Science, pp 241–250.

Mooijaart A, Bentler PM (1991). "Robustness of normal theory statistics in structural equation models." *Statistica Neerlandica.*

Muirhead RJ (1982). "Aspects of Multivariate Statistical *Theory.*" New York, Wiley.

Muirhead RJ, Waternaux C (1980). "Asymptotic distributions in canonical correlation analysis and other multivariate procedures for nonnormal populations." *Biometrika* 67:31–43.

Muthén B (1984). "A general structural equation model with dichotomous, ordered categorical, and continuous latent variable indicators." *Psychometrika* 49:115–132.

Newcomb MD (1986). "Nuclear attitudes and reactions: Associations with depression, drug use, and quality of life." *Journal of Personality and Social Psychology* 50:906–920.

Newcomb MD, Bentler PM (1986). "Loneliness and social support: A confirmatory hierarchical analysis." *Personality and Social Psychology Bulletin* 12:520–535.

Newcomb MD, Bentler PM (1987). "Self-report methods of assessing health status and health service utilization: A hierarchical confirmatory analysis." *Multivariate Behavioral Research* 22:415–436.

Newcomb MD, Bentler PM (1988a). "Impact of adolescent drug use and social support on problems of young adults: A longitudinal study." *Journal of Abnormal Psychology* 97: 64–75.

Newcomb MD, Bentler PM (1988b). *Consequences of Adolescent Drug Use: Impact on the Lives of Young Adults.* Beverly Hills, Calif., Sage.

Newcomb MD, Huba GJ, Bentler PM (1981). "A multidimensional assessment of stressful life events among adolescents: Derivation and correlates." *Journal of Health and Social Behavior* 22:400–415.

Permutt T, Hebel JR (1989). "Simultaneous-equation estimation in a clinical trial of the effect of smoking on birth weight." *Biometrics* 45:619–622.

Reed D, McGee D, Yano K, Feinleib M (1983). "Social networks and coronary heart disease among Japanese men in Hawaii." *American Journal of Epidemiology* 117:384–396.

Saris WE, Stronkhorst LH (1984). *Causal Modelling in Nonexperimental Research.* Amsterdam, Sociometric Research Foundation.

Satorra A (1989). Alternative test criteria in covariance structure analysis: A unified approach." *Psycgometrica* 54:131–151.

Satorra A, Bentler PM (1990). "Model conditions for asymptotic robustness in the analysis of linear relations." *Computational Statistics and Data Analysis* 10: 235–249.

Shapiro A (1983). "Asymptotic distribution theory in the analysis of covariance structures." *South African Statistical Journal* 17:33–81.

Shapiro A (1986). "Asymptotic theory of overparameterized structural models." *Journal of the American Statistical Association* 81:142–149.

Shapiro A (1987). "Robustness properties of the MDF analysis of moment structures." *South African Statistical Journal* 21:39–62.

Sörbom D (1974). "A general method for studying differences in factor means and factor structure between groups." *British Journal of Mathematical and Statistical Psychology* 27:229–239.

Sörbom D (1978). "An alternative to the methodology for analysis of covariance." *Psychometrika* 43:381–396.

Tanaka JS (1984). *Some Results on the Estimation of Covariance Structure Models.* PhD diss., University of California, Los Angeles.

Tanaka JS, Bentler PM (1985). "Quasi-likelihood estimation in asymptotically efficient covariance structure models." *1984 Proceedings of the American Statistical Association, Social Statistics Section,* pp 658–662.

Tanaka JS, Huba GJ (1985). "A fit index for covariance structure models under arbitrary GLS estimation." *British Journal of Mathematical and Statistical Psychology* 38:197–201.

Tyler DE (1982). "Radial estimates and the test for sphericity." *Biometrika* 69:429–436.

Tyler DE (1983). "Robustness and efficiency properties of scatter matrices." *Biometrika* 70:411–420.

Van Praag BMS, Dijkstra TK, Van Velzen J (1985). "Least squares theory based on general distributional assumptions with an application to the incomplete observations problem." *Psychometrika* 50:25–36.

Wiley DE (1973). "The identification problem for structural equation models with unmeasured variables." In Goldberger AS, Duncan OD (eds), *Structural Equation Models in the Social Sciences.* New York, Seminar, pp 69–83.

Wong SK, Long JS (1987). *Parameterizing Nonlinear Constraints in Models with Latent Variables.* Technical Report, Washington State University, Pullman.

II

Models for Categorical Data

7

Use of the Logistic and Related Models in Longitudinal Studies of Chronic Disease Risk
Application: Coronary Heart Disease Mortality in Framingham

NORMAN BRESLOW

Linear models, including multiple linear regression and the analysis of variance and covariance, form the conceptual foundation for the most powerful and widely used statistical methods of analysis of both experimental and observational data. Such models are typically written in the form $y = x^t\beta + \varepsilon$ where y is a continuous outcome measure, x is a K vector of explanatory variables, β is a K vector of regression coefficients, and ε is a random-error term with mean 0 that represents the unexplained variability in the response (t denotes transpose). Usually x contains a component x_0 that takes the value 1 for each subject; its coefficient β_0, known as the "grand mean," is given special treatment.

Many outcomes of interest in laboratory, clinical, and epidemiologic studies are not continuous but instead are binary variables such as whether or not a cell is transformed by a putative mutagen, whether or not a cancer patient survives five years from time of diagnosis, or whether or not an adult male develops coronary heart disease (CHD) during a defined study period. A challenging statistical problem has been the development of linear model techniques for use with such discrete outcomes. The earliest efforts were directed to the analysis of grouped data, where in the ith of I cells there are d_i responders out of n_i subjects with regression variables x_i. However, use of the observed proportion $y_i = d_i/n_i$ as the outcome measure distorts the basic linear model. The expected outcome $E(y_i) = p_i$ (the probability of response) is constrained to the interval $0 \leqslant p_i \leqslant 1$, whereas the "linear predictor" $x_i^t\beta$ is unbounded. Also, the variance $\text{var}(y_i) = p_i(1 - p_i)/n_i$ depends on the unknown mean. This conflicts with the standard linear model, for which the error variances $\sigma_i^2 = \text{var}(\varepsilon_i)$ are assumed to be constant (σ^2) or else are multiples $\sigma_1^2 = w_i^{-1}\sigma^2$ involving known "prior weights" w_i.

A better approximation to the linear model is obtained with transformed outcome measures of the form $y_i = F^{-1}(d_i/n_i)$, where F is a cumulative distribution function. The logit (inverse logistic) and probit (inverse normal) transforms have a long history of use in bioassay (Berkson, 1944; Finney, 1952). The arcsin transform (Gabriel, 1963) stabilizes the variance of the observed proportion for large n_i. The complementary log-log (inverse extreme value) transform arises naturally from survival analysis considerations (Kalbfleisch & Prentice, 1980, Section 4.6).

Linear models can be fitted easily to transformed proportions using weighted least-squares methodology that accounts for the mean-variance relationship (Grizzle, Starmer, & Koch, 1969; Chapter 9 in this volume). This approach is commonly taken with grouped data where the numbers in each cell are reasonably large. When there are a large number of explanatory variables to consider simultaneously, however, and especially when many of them are continuous, least-squares methods tend to break down. Indeed, Truett, Cornfield, and Kannel (1967) began their landmark paper on the logistic analysis of the Framingham data with the following observation:

> It is the function of longitudinal studies, like that of coronary heart disease in Framingham, to investigate the effects of a large variety of variables, both singly and jointly on the effects of disease. The traditional approach of the epidemiologist, multiple cross-classification, quickly becomes impracticable as the number of variables to be investigated increases. Thus if 10 variables are under consideration, and each is to be studied at only 3 levels...there would be 59,049 cells in the multiple cross-classification. p. 511)

The Framingham study stimulated the development of the logistic model for the analysis of binary outcomes, just as the National Halothane Study stimulated the development of the log-linear model for the analysis of high dimensional contingency tables (Bishop, Fienberg, & Holland, 1975). This review explores its connections with modern methods of survival analysis (Cox & Oakes, 1984; Kalbfleisch & Prentice, 1980) and the theory of generalized linear models (McCullagh & Nelder, 1983), illustrating the methods where possible by application to bona fide epidemiologic data.

FITTING THE LOGISTIC MODEL*

Today the standard method for the regression analysis of binary outcomes involves fitting the logistic response function to the observed data (d_i, n_i, x_i) by maximum likelihood, assuming that the d_i are binomially distributed. The probability of response p_i for an individual with explanatory variables x_i is assumed to satisfy

$$p_i = \frac{\exp(x_i^t \beta)}{1 + \exp(x_i^t \beta)}, \qquad (1)$$

or equivalently

$$\text{logit } p_i = \log\left(\frac{p_i}{1 - p_i}\right) = x_i^t \beta$$

---

*This section reviews as briefly as possible the standard approach to likelihood analysis for the logistic model. It may be skipped or skimmed by those already familiar with this subject.

where here and elsewhere "exp" denotes exponentiation to a power of e. One reason for the widespread use of the logistic transform is its connection to normal-theory linear discriminant analysis, as demonstrated by Cornfield's (1962) analysis of the Framingham data. Suppose the distributions of covariables x among responders and nonresponders are multivariate normal with means μ_1 and μ_0 and common covariance matrix Σ, and that π_1 and $\pi_0 = 1 - \pi_1$ denote prior probabilities of response. Then the posterior response probabilities after observation of x are given by (1) with $\beta = \Sigma^{-1}(\mu_1 - \mu_0)$ (the coefficients of the linear discriminant) and $\beta_0 = \ln(\pi_1/\pi_0) - 1/2\beta^t(\mu_1 - \mu_0)$. Cornfield fit the model by substituting sample means and the (pooled) covariance matrix for the μ's and Σ.

An alternative derivation of the logistic equation arises from consideration of the tolerance distribution of a latent continuous variable E that has a linear regression on x. The event $[y = 1]$ corresponds to $[E \geqslant C]$, where C is a critical constant. If one assumes that $E = x^t\beta + \varepsilon$, where ε has the logistic distribution, equation (1) follows with $\beta_0 = -C$. (See the introductory chapter to this volume for details.) It should be stressed, however, that the machinery of latent variables and tolerance distributions is not necessary for this development; (1) may be regarded as a simple and convenient description of the dependence of the response probabilities on x that has desirable statistical properties (Cox, 1970) quite apart from its connections to normal-theory discriminant analysis or logistic tolerance distributions. Several of these properties are mentioned here.

Maximum Likelihood Estimation

Cox (1958, 1966) and Walker and Duncan (1967), the latter two also motivated by Framingham, advocated robust likelihood methods of estimation that use (1) directly, without assumptions concerning the marginal distribution of x. One finds the parameter estimates $\hat{\beta}$ that maximize the probability of occurrence of the observed data, or what is the same thing, that maximize the log likelihood function

$$L(\beta) = \sum_i [d_i \log p_i + (n_i - d_i)\log(1 - p_i)]$$

It is equally applicable to grouped-data problems with large n_i and to continuous-data problems where all n_i equal one. Maximum likelihood estimates are known to be efficient in large samples and their use gains one access to an enormous body of statistical methodology, for example likelihood ratio and score tests and likelihood confidence intervals (Cox & Hinkley, 1974).

Walker and Duncan were concerned primarily with numerical techniques for finding $\hat{\beta}$. Cox noted that the "score" equations solved by $\hat{\beta}$ involved equating linear combinations of observed and expected values:

$$U(\beta) = \frac{\partial L}{\partial \beta} = X^t(d - np) = 0 \tag{2}$$

Here X denotes the $I \times K$ matrix with rows x_i, $d = (d_1, \ldots, d_I)^t$ is a vector with numbers of responders in each cell ($d_i = 0$ or 1 for continuous data), and

$np = (n_1 p_1, \ldots, n_I p_I)^t$ is its expectation. Since these resemble the normal equations of linear regression analysis, namely $X^t(y - X\beta) = 0$ where y denotes the observations and $X\beta$ the expectations, the logit model is justifiably viewed as the "normal theory" of binary regression.

The maximum likelihood estimate $\hat{\beta}$ has an approximate normal distribution with mean β and covariance matrix Σ equal to the inverse of the (Fisher) information matrix: $\Sigma = \mathscr{I}^{-1}$. In logistic regression $\mathscr{I}$ takes the simple form $X^t V X$, where V is diagonal with variances $v_i = \text{var } d_i = n_i p_i(1 - p_i)$ on the diagonal. Using Fisher scoring to solve (2), the change in $\hat{\beta}$ from one iteration to the next is given by

$$\Delta\hat{\beta} = (X^t V X)^{-1} X^t(d - np) \tag{3}$$

where p and V are evaluated using the current values of $\hat{\beta}$. This may be viewed as iterated least-squares regression where "dependent" variables $y_i = (d_i - n_i p_i)/v_i$ are regressed on the independent variables x_i using weights v_i. Equation (3) lies at the heart of the theory of generalized linear models, of which the logit model is a paradigm, and of the computer program GLIM that was developed to fit them (Baker & Nelder, 1978; McCullagh & Nelder, 1983).

The Deviance

When data are grouped, a global assessment of the goodness-of-fit of model to data is given by the deviance

$$\text{dev} = 2[L^* - L(\hat{\beta})] = 2\sum_i \left[d_i \log\left(\frac{d_i}{n_i p_i}\right) + (n_i - d_i) \log\frac{(n_i - d_i)}{[n_i(1 - \hat{p}_i)]} \right] \tag{4}$$

Here the $\hat{p}_i = 1/\{1 + \exp(-x_i^t\hat{\beta})\}$ are fitted probabilities of response and L^* is the absolute maximum likelihood that arises by attaching a separate parameter to each data point. When I is small and the n_i are reasonably large, the deviance may be referred to tables of chi square (with $I - K$ degrees of freedom) for a rough indication of fit. However, this method breaks down if the data are sparse. A later section of this chapter ("Goodness of Fit...") considers more powerful methods for assessing fit that apply to both grouped and ungrouped data.

Testing Regression Variables for Significance

Regression models are usually developed in a hierarchical fashion with (sets of) variables being added to the model equation depending on their ability to further contribute to the prediction or explanation of response. Suppose that K_1 variables x_1 with coefficients β_1 are already in the model and one desires to test whether K_2 additional variables x_2 with coefficients β_2 should be included. Three general procedures exist for testing the composite hypothesis $\beta_2 = 0$ (Rao, 1965). Denoting by $\hat{\beta} = (\hat{\beta}_1, \hat{\beta}_2)$ the maximum likelihood estimate under the full model and by $\tilde{\beta} = (\tilde{\beta}_1, 0)$ the estimate under the constrained model, these are: (1) the (log) likelihood ratio or deviance test $2\{L(\hat{\beta}) - L(\tilde{\beta})\}$; (2) the score test $U(\tilde{\beta})^t \mathscr{I}^{-1}(\tilde{\beta})U(\tilde{\beta})$ (see equation (2)); and (3) the Wald test $\hat{\beta}_2^t \Sigma_{22}^{-1} \hat{\beta}_2$, where Σ_{22}

denotes the covariance matrix of β_2. The likelihood ratio test compares maximized likelihoods under full and restricted models; the score statistic tests whether the first derivative (score) of the log-likelihood function evaluated under the restricted model departs significantly from zero; and Wald's statistic tests directly, whether the β_2 parameters are equal to zero. The score test is particularly valuable for use in variable selection algorithms, since it does not require fitting the full model. Wald's test may give aberrant results when $|\hat{\beta}_2|$ is large or the range of parameter values is restricted (Hauck & Donner, 1977; Vaeth, 1985), but it is usually adequate for the standard logit model.

Each of these tests may be inverted to yield confidence intervals for individual regression coefficients, for sets of coefficients, or for prediction functions based on the coefficients. For example (Hauck, 1983), a simultaneous $100(1 - \alpha)$-percent confidence set based on Wald's test for the fitted probabilities of response $p(x)$ is given by the intervals $[p_L(x), p_U(x)] = (1/\{1 + \exp[-\lambda_L(x)]\}, 1/\{1 + \exp[-\lambda_U(x)]\})$, where

$$[\lambda_L(x), \lambda_U(x)] = x^t\hat{\beta} \pm \chi_{K,\alpha}(x^t \mathscr{I}^{-1}x)^{1/2} \tag{5}$$

and $\chi^2_{K,\alpha}$ is the corresponding percentile of the chi-square distribution with K degrees of freedom. The interval (5) is simultaneous in the sense that it covers the true value of the linear predictor $x^t\beta$ for all x, rather than at a single value, with approximate probability $1 - \alpha$.

Example

Table 7-1 presents grouped data on 1329 subjects classified by serum cholesterol level and blood pressure, the binary outcome being whether or not they developed CHD during a defined study period (Cornfield, 1962; Ku & Kullback, 1974). Three indicator variables x_1, x_2, and x_3 were defined to represent the level of serum cholesterol (SC), $< 200 \, mg/100 \, cc$ being treated as a reference level, and likewise three more indicator variables, x_4, x_5, x_6, defined the level of blood pressure (BP), with $< 127 \, mm \, Hg$ as reference. Thus the full model becomes

$$\text{pr(CHD)} = \frac{\exp(\beta_0 + \beta_1 x_1 + \beta_2 x_2 + \beta_3 x_3 + \beta_4 x_4 + \beta_5 x_5 + \beta_6 x_6)}{1 + \exp(\beta_0 + \beta_1 x_1 + \beta_2 x_2 + \beta_3 x_3 + \beta_4 x_4 + \beta_5 x_5 + \beta_6 x_6)}$$

where $x_1 = 1$, if $200 \leqslant SC \leqslant 219$; 0, otherwise
$x_2 = 1$, if $220 \leqslant SC \leqslant 259$; 0, otherwise
$x_3 = 1$, if $260 \leqslant SC$; 0, otherwise
$x_4 = 1$, if $127 \leqslant BP \leqslant 146$; 0, otherwise
$x_5 = 1$, if $147 \leqslant BP \leqslant 166$; 0, otherwise
$x_6 = 1$, if $167 \leqslant BP$; 0, otherwise

Note that the interpretation of the regression coefficients depends critically on the 0/1 coding of the x's. This particular coding is standard in the computer program GLIM (Baker & Nelder, 1978); other programs in packages such as BMDP and SAS may use alternative parameterizations of the same model.

Table 7-1. Observed and fitted numbers of coronary heart disease (CHD) cases by serum cholesterol (SC) and blood pressure (BP)

SC (mg/100cc)	BP (mm Hg)	Total (n)	CHD cases (d)[a]	SC alone	BP alone	SC + BP	Risk 100p(x)	Lower limit[b] 100p_L(x)	Upper limit 100p_U(x)
<200	<127	119	2	4.48	5.83	3.55	3.0	0.8	10.2
	127–146	124	3	4.67	6.26	3.55	2.9	0.8	9.5
	147–166	50	3	1.88	4.46	2.49	5.0	1.3	17.1
	167+	26	4	0.98	4.39	2.41	9.3	2.5	28.6
200–219	<127	88	3	2.77	4.31	2.14	2.4	0.5	10.4
	127–146	100	2	3.15	5.05	2.34	2.3	0.5	9.6
	147–166	43	0	1.35	3.84	1.75	4.1	0.9	16.9
	167+	23	3	0.72	3.89	1.76	7.7	1.7	28.3
220–259	<127	127	8	8.38	6.23	6.50	5.1	1.9	13.3
	127–146	220	11	14.51	11.10	10.83	4.8	2.1	11.3
	147–166	74	6	4.88	6.61	6.23	8.4	3.1	21.1
	167+	49	6	3.23	8.28	7.45	15.2	6.0	33.6
260+	<127	74	7	10.61	3.63	7.81	10.5	4.1	24.6
	127–146	111	12	15.91	5.60	11.28	10.2	4.4	21.7
	147–166	57	11	8.17	5.09	9.53	16.7	6.8	35.4
	167+	44	11	6.31	7.44	12.38	28.1	12.9	50.8
Totals		1329	92	92.00	92.00	92.00			

[a]Number of CHD cases.
[b]95% confidence limits based on equation (5).

Table 7-2 shows the results of the fit. The score tests were calculated in GLIM using Pregibon's (1982) method. The three test statistics for SC ($\beta_1 = \beta_2 = \beta_3 = 0$) and BP ($\beta_4 = \beta_5 = \beta_6 = 0$) effects have comparable and highly significant values. The inadequacy of either single-factor model (SC alone or BP alone) is evident from the fitted values shown in Table 7-1 and the deviances in Table 7-2. Using the model with BP effects only, the observed versus fitted numbers of CHD cases according to the four levels of SC are 12 versus 20.94, 8 versus 17.09, 31 versus 32.22, and 41 versus 21.76, which is clearly discrepant. The observed and fitted totals within each factor level agree for any model that includes that factor, in accordance with equation (2).

Examination of the regression coefficients suggests that there may be little or no difference in CHD risk between the first two levels of each factor, but that the risk increases substantially and linearly as SC is elevated beyond 220 mg/100 cc or BP beyond 147 mm Hg. As the confidence bounds in Table 7-1 make clear, however, these limited data are compatible with a wide variety of dose-response relations; one should resist concluding that the apparent "threshold" effects are real without further study.

Table 7-2. Results of fitting linear logistic models to Table 7-1 data

Model (terms)	Degrees of freedom (DF)	Deviance
Constant only (x_0)	15	58.73
SC alone (x_0, x_1, x_2, x_3)	12	26.80
BP alone (x_0, x_4, x_5, x_6)	12	35.16
SC + BP ($x_0 - x_6$)	9	8.08

	Test statistics (3 DF)		
Hypothesis	Deviance	Score	Wald
SC effects ($\beta_1 = \beta_2 = \beta_3 = 0$)	27.08	28.88	26.28
BP effects ($\beta_4 = \beta_5 = \beta_6 = 0$)	18.72	22.01	20.44

Parameter estimates and covariances for full model

Regression coefficients		Estimated covariance matrix						
		β_0	β_1	β_2	β_3	β_4	β_5	β_6
β_0	−3.482	0.1216						
β_1	−0.208	−0.0860	0.2175					
β_2	0.562	−0.0833	0.0875	0.1231				
β_3	1.344	−0.0828	0.0876	0.0879	0.1176			
β_4	−0.041	−0.0492	−0.0014	−0.0068	−0.0050	0.0922		
β_5	0.532	−0.0494	−0.0023	−0.0042	−0.0067	0.0538	0.1105	
β_6	1.200	−0.0479	−0.0026	−0.0062	−0.0089	0.0540	0.0341	0.1069

Since the CHD risk is rather low overall, and in view of the 0/1 coding of the x's already mentioned, one may interpret the regression coefficients roughly as log-relative risks (see next section). The risk for 220–259 mg/100 cc SC is thus approximately $\exp(\hat{\beta}_2) = \exp(0.562) = 1.75$ times as great as for someone with the lowest level of SC, whereas the risk for someone in the highest BP category is $\exp(1.2) = 3.3$ times that of someone in the lowest BP category. Since there are no interaction (cross-product) terms in the linear logistic equation, the individual risks multiply when the joint relative risks for combinations of SC and BP are estimated. These vary over a tenfold range from 2.3 to 28.1 percent (see Table 7-1). Introduction of interaction terms would allow more flexible modeling of the joint risks at the cost of greater instability in the fitted model. However, the deviance of the final model (8.1 on 9 DF) suggests that the no-interaction (multiplicative) hypothesis is consistent with these data.

THE LOGISTIC MODEL AND TIME-DEPENDENT OUTCOMES

Logistic regression developed as a way of modeling disease risk over a defined study period as a function of multiple risk factors. This development preceded and in many ways contributed to the proportional hazards (PH) regression model (Cox, 1972) which is today the standard method for regression analysis of survival and disease incidence data. In retrospect it is easy to point out several problems with logistic modeling of time-dependent outcomes that largely have been overcome by the related techniques of survival analysis.

Problems with Time-Related Outcomes

One clear drawback to the logistic model as used in this first example is that it refers to the risk or probability of disease development over a defined interval of time, yet time is not explicitly accounted for. It is assumed implicitly that everyone is available for follow-up for the entire study interval. While this assumption may be reasonably accurate when the interval is short, say no more than a year or two, it breaks down when one considers longer periods. Some subjects will almost certainly be removed from risk during extended periods, by death due to competing causes or by loss to follow-up. Obvious biases can arise if follow-up times vary according to the levels of the risk factors under study, for example because these same risk factors are related to competing illnesses or to a subject's propensity to remain "on-study."

Another difficulty with a logistic analysis of time-dependent outcomes is that the estimated regression coefficients depend on the length of the study interval. Coefficients from study periods of different length are not comparable. Furthermore, the model is inconsistent in the sense that two logistic models applied to (sub)intervals of time do not result in a logistic model for the entire period. Suppose that a study period of four years' duration is divided into two intervals of two years each. Denote by $p_1(x)$ the probability of CHD diagnosis over the first interval, and by $p_2(x)$ the analogous probability for the second interval *conditional* on disease-free survival to the start of the second interval. If these two probabilities satisfy logit $p_1(x) = x^t\beta_1$ and logit $p_2(x) = x^t\beta_2$, then the probability of disease development over the entire four year interval, which is given by

$$p(x) = 1 - [1 - p_1(x)] \cdot [1 - p_2(x)]$$

does *not* satisfy logit $p(x) = x^t\beta$ for any β.

The Discrete-Time Proportional Hazards Model

Various suggestions have been made to overcome these difficulties and at the same time preserve as much as possible of the logistic structure. Farewell (1977) developed a hybrid model that seems particularly applicable to studies of genetic risk factors with diseases of delayed onset. He postulated a logistic model for the probability of disease susceptibility and an exponential distribution $(f(t) = \lambda e^{-\lambda t})$ for the age at disease onset for members of the susceptible subgroup. Other approaches assumed that the logistic model applied to conditional disease risk over intervals. Myers, Hankey, and Mantel (1973) considered a series of unit time intervals indexed by $j = 1, \dots, J$. With $p_j(x)$ denoting the probability of response in the jth interval, conditional on still being at risk at its start, they assumed that logit $p_j(x) = x^t\beta$ independently of j. Woodbury, Manton, and Stallard (1981) made a similar assumption of constant-response probabilities over intervals and derived an approximate formula for converting the logistic regression coefficients for a study period of length one so that they applied to a shorter or longer period.

Much greater flexibility is provided by Cox's (1972) discrete-time proportional hazards model, where the conditional probabilities of disease development are assumed to satisfy

$$\text{logit } p_j(x) = \alpha_j + x^t\beta \tag{6}$$

The α_j represent (logit transforms of) the conditional probabilities of response during the J time intervals for someone with a standard ($x = 0$) set of regression variables. The linear predictor $x^t\beta$ is interpreted as the logarithm of the relative risk (rate ratio) of disease relative to $x = 0$. The term *proportional hazards* stems from the fact that the (odds) ratio of disease probabilities for two individuals with risk variables x_1 and x_2, respectively, namely

$$\frac{p_j(x_1)[1 - p_j(x_2)]}{[1 - p_j(x_1)]p_j(x_2)} = \exp\{(x_1 - x_2)^t\beta\} \tag{7}$$

does not depend on the time interval j.

This logit model suffers from the same inconsistency noted earlier regarding the combination of conditional probabilities of response over two intervals. To resolve this difficulty, Prentice and Gloeckler (1978) started with the continuous-time survival model (see section "The Continuous-Time Proportional Hazards Model") and derived the relation

$$\text{clog } p_j(x) = \alpha_j + x_j^t\beta \tag{8}$$

where *clog* denotes the complementary log-log transform defined by $clog(p) = \log[-\log(1 - p)]$. Since the probability of disease-free survival over two subintervals is $[1 - p_1(x)] \cdot [1 - p_2(x)] = \exp[-(e_1^\alpha + e_2^\alpha)e^{x^t\beta}]$, the *clog* transform of the disease probability over these two intervals is also linear in x. In view of the fact that logit $p \approx clog\, p \approx \log p$ for small p, however, it makes little difference in practice whether logits or *clogs* are used, provided that the time intervals are short.

Depending on the quantity of data and especially the number of disease cases, ten to twenty or more discrete time intervals may be used, each with its own α_j parameter. Subjects who do not develop the disease of interest are generally assumed to be withdrawn alive at the end of an interval. Thus a person contributes a factor $1 - p_j(x)$ to the likelihood function for *each* of the intervals over which he or she was followed if the disease of interest did not develop, and a factor $p_j(x)$ if the disease did develop in some interval. (A refinement (Thompson, 1977) is to use a contribution of $\sqrt{1 - p_j(x)}$ for any interval during which the subject is withdrawn from study while still disease free.) The analysis is easily performed using GLIM or other programs that facilitate logistic regression. One simply creates a separate data record for each time interval over which each individual is followed on study. The usual standard-errors output by GLIM or other programs are valid under model (6), even though each subject may contribute several data records, since the output depends only on correct specification of the likelihood function.

Time-Dependent Covariables

An important feature of longitudinal epidemiologic studies is the accumulation of time-oriented histories of personal habits and risk factor measurements for each individual. One wishes to use the entire time history in predictions of future disease risk (Wu & Ware, 1979). This is accomplished in practice by creation of covariables whose values change with time. Time-dependent covariables may represent current measurements on risk factors, past measurements, or summaries of the entire history. Problems of interpretation may arise, of course, if one attempts to include several highly correlated time-dependent covariables in the model, as with any model in which there is a high degree of colinearity. Also, when applied in the context of an intervention trial, some of the time-dependent measurements may best be regarded as outcome variables that are intermediate in the causal pathway between the intervention and disease. Although their inclusion in the model may provide important information about mechanisms, the covariable adjusted-treatment coefficient would not adequately express the effect of intervention on disease (Kalbfleisch & Prentice, 1980, Section 5.3.2).

Time-dependent covariables are easily accommodated in discrete-time proportional hazards analyses. One simply allows the regression variables to change values with time interval as well as with individual. The same computational considerations apply as discussed in the past section, namely creation of a separate data record for each time interval over which an individual is observed. (See the example that follows the next section.) Of course inclusion of time-dependent covariables in the model destroys the proportionality expressed in equation (7). In fact, the inclusion of cross-product terms involving (fixed) risk factor variables and time is a useful method of testing the proportional hazards assumption.

It is of historical interest that the Framingham investigators utilized the discrete-time proportional hazards approach to analysis of their time-dependent data long before the relevant statistical theory was developed (Feinleib, 1985).

The Continuous-Time Proportional Hazards Model

Cox's (1972) continuous-time model for the regression analysis of censored survival data follows directly from (6) or (8) by letting the number of time intervals increase in such a way that their lengths decrease to zero. The role of the $p_j(x)$ is played by a function $\lambda(t; x)$ that represents the instantaneous rate of disease development (incidence rate) at time t for someone with explanatory variables x who is alive and well just prior to t. The model is written

$$\lambda(t; x) = \lambda_0(t)\exp(x^t\beta) \tag{9}$$

where in place of the α_j parameters one has a "nuisance" function $\lambda_0(t)$ that represents the unknown incidence rate for someone with $x = 0$. Note that $\exp[(x_1 - x_2)^t\beta]$ now represents the ratio of instantaneous incidence rates for subjects with covariables x_1 and x_2. This ratio is constant under the assumed model, unless of course the covariables are allowed to depend on time: $x = x(t)$.

Techniques of estimation of the regression coefficients β and the hazard or incidence rate function λ_0 in (9) are discussed at length in texts by Kalbfleisch and Prentice (1980) and Cox and Oakes (1984), which should be consulted for details. Briefly, at each time t at which someone in the study develops the disease of interest, one forms a "risk set" $R = R(t)$ consisting of all those still alive, disease free, and under observation at that time. There is a contribution to the partial likelihood (Cox, 1975) function from R equal to

$$\frac{\exp(x^t\beta)}{\Sigma_{l \varepsilon R}\exp(x_l^t\beta)} \tag{10}$$

where the numerator x refers to the individual who developed the disease. If more than one person develops the disease at t, a suitable approximation to the likelihood arises from allowing a separate contribution of the form (10) for each one. Once $\hat{\beta}$ is obtained, via maximization of the product of such terms, a nonparametric estimate of the reference cumulative incidence function $\Lambda_0(t) = \int_0^t \lambda_0(s)ds$ is given by

$$\hat{\Lambda}_0(t) = \sum_{t_i \leqslant t} \frac{d_i}{\Sigma_{l \varepsilon R(t_i)}\exp(x_l^t\hat{\beta})} \tag{11}$$

where the t_i denote times at which disease cases are diagnosed and the d_i denote the number of cases ($d_i \geqslant 1$) diagnosed at those times (Breslow, 1974). If $\hat{\beta} = 0$, equation (11) reduces to the standard actuarial estimate of cumulative incidence for a homogeneous sample. Note that here i indexes individual times of diagnosis, and that when $\hat{\beta} = 0$ the denominator sum in (11) equals the total number at risk at t_i.

Provided that ten or twenty time intervals are used to cover the study period, β estimates based on the discrete time models (6) or (8) should be little different from those based on the partial likelihood (9). Even though quite different estimation strategies are involved, the basic model structure is the same.

Example

A public-use tape containing data from the first eighteen years of follow-up (exams 1–10) of the Framingham study was kindly supplied by Dr. Robert Garrison of the U.S. National Center for Health Statistics. Records were extracted for 874 men who were 40 through 62 years of age at the time of the first exam, had no evidence of CHD at that time, and had known baseline values for systolic blood pressure, serum cholesterol, smoking habits, and relative weight. These four variables and age were used in their original continuous form in the statistical analyses. See the appendix for SAS commands used in these analyses.

Table 7-3 presents a life table analysis of the risk of CHD over this eighteen-year period for the cohort of 874 men. The cumulative probability (risk) of CHD was estimated by actuarial methods to be 26.1 percent, compared with the crude figure of 209 of 874, or 23.9 percent, which fails to account for withdrawals from risk of CHD due to deaths from other causes. Table 7-4 contrasts the regression coefficients and standard errors estimated by the three procedures. The simple logistic regression analysis of the 874 data records based on equation (1) involved estimation of the "grand mean" $\hat{\beta}_0 = -6.998$ in addition to the five regression coefficients. Thus the logit transform of CHD risk for a "modal" subject (age 50, BP = 147, SC = 220, 10 cigarettes/day, relative weight 100) is $-6.998 + 50(0.0312) + 147(0.0115) + 220(0.00599) + 10(0.0135) +$

Table 7-3. Life table analysis of coronary heart disease (CHD) risk between exams 1 and 10 for 874 Framingham men aged 40 to 62 in 1948

Time interval (exam numbers)	Number at risk at start	Number of CHD cases	Number died other causes	Cumulative risk (%)	
				Observed[a]	Expected[b]
1–2	874	17	7	1.9	1.6
2–3	850	16	13	3.8	3.2
3–4	821	29	7	7.2	6.2
4–5	785	18	14	9.4	8.1
5–6	753	31	21	13.2	11.5
6–7	701	24	18	16.2	14.3
7–8	659	26	21	19.5	17.5
8–9	612	22	18	22.5	20.3
9–10	572	26	17	26.1	23.8
Total	6627	209	136	26.1	23.8

[a]Actuarial risk for entire sample.

[b]Estimated from α_j parameters in model (6) for a "modal" subject.

Table 7-4. Comparison of regression coefficients and standard errors estimated by three different methods for coronary heart disease (CHD) risk in Framingham

Variable		Simple logistic regression	Discrete-time proportional hazards	Continuous-time proportional hazards
Age (years)	Coeff	0.0312	0.0416	0.0400
	SE	0.0133	0.0118	0.0115
Blood pressure	Coeff	0.0115	0.0122	0.0116
(mm Hg)	SE	0.0036	0.0031	0.0030
Serum cholesterol	Coeff	0.00599	0.00498	0.00475
(mg/100cc)	SE	0.00184	0.00154	0.00149
Cigarettes	Coeff	0.0135	0.0157	0.0150
(N per day)	SE	0.0060	0.0050	0.0049
Relative weight	Coeff	0.0103	0.0093	0.0089
(%)	SE	0.0060	0.0052	0.0050

$100(0.0103) = -1.265$, corresponding to a CHD risk of 22.0 percent for the eighteen-year period. The second column of Table 7-4 presents results for the discrete-time proportional hazards model defined by equation (6). For this analysis 6627 data records were created, this being the total number of periods over which the 874 men were followed (see Table 7-3). Each such record contained an indicator of the time interval (1–9), a binary outcome variable denoting whether or not a CHD event occurred in that interval, and the five regression variables that were measured at the start of the study. In addition to the β coefficients shown, nine α_j parameters were estimated and used to obtain the final column shown in Table 7-3. The same logistic regression program was used for these two analyses (see appendix).

The final column of Table 7-4 shows regression coefficients estimated by the continuous-time proportional hazards model. These agree quite closely with coefficients for the corresponding discrete-time model, as expected since the basic model structures are the same. They differ somewhat more from those in the first column, which represent the logarithm of the odds ratios of disease development over the entire study period rather than the multiplicative effect of the covariables on instantaneous rates of disease assumed constant over time. The time variable was the duration of follow-up since enrollment in the study. The effects of the aging of the cohort with increasing follow-up are reflected in the $\hat{\alpha}_j$ parameters (Table 7-3, column 6) and the nonparametric cumulative incidence function (not shown, but see equation (11)).

Further analyses were undertaken using the time sequence of covariable measurements to exploit more fully the information in the longitudinal data base and to illustrate the ease of handling time-dependent covariables with the discrete-time proportional hazards model. These analyses used data for males who were aged 40–69 at the time of exam three, who had no prior history of CHD at that time, and who had known values for the relevant covariables for at least one of the first three exams. Follow-up started at exam three. When covariable measurements were missing for a particular exam, the last recorded value was used. This was of particular importance for cigarette smoking, which was not recorded at the second, third, and sixth exams. It is of interest to compare the results shown in column one of Table 7-5, with those shown in columns two and three. When blood pressure and serum cholesterol measurements for the current and preceding exams are both included in the model, only the coefficients for the earlier exam are statistically significant. There is no doubt that the earlier measurement is of greater value in predicting CHD events. Similarly, when the sequence of three exam measurements is used, the best prediction equation gives essentially no weight to the current values and approximately equal weight (blood pressure) or a 2:1 weight (serum cholesterol) to the two earlier values. Of course, the relative weights are not well determined due to the high degree of colinearity. Nonetheless, these results confirm those reported earlier for serum cholesterol in Framingham by Wu and Ware (1979) and for blood pressure among Hiroshima survivors by Prentice and colleagues (1982). The latter speculate that treatment for hypertension may bring blood pressure under control without a corresponding reduction in immediate CHD risk. Note that the coefficient of age decreases slightly as past measurements of

Table 7–5. Regression analysis of time-dependent risk factors for coronary heart disease in Framingham using discrete-time proportional hazards model

		Model		
		Current covariables	Current and preceding exam	Current and 2 preceding exams
Variable[a]				
Age (t)[b]	Coeff	0.0465	0.0447	0.0439
	SE	0.0088	0.0089	0.0089
Cigarettes (t)	Coeff	0.0161	0.0161	0.0161
	SE	0.0040	0.0040	0.0040
RW (t)	Coeff	0.0132	0.0127	0.0124
	SE	0.0044	0.0045	0.0045
BP (t)	Coeff	0.0121	0.0000	0.0013
	SE	0.0024	0.0042	0.0043
BP $(t - 1)$	Coeff	—	0.0153	0.0108
	SE	—	0.0042	0.0051
BP $(t - 2)$	Coeff	—	—	0.0070
	SE	—	—	0.0045
SC (t)	Coeff	0.0057	0.0010	0.0001
	SE	0.0013	0.0022	0.0023
SC $(t - 1)$	Coeff	—	0.0061	0.0046
	SE	—	0.0021	0.0025
SC $(t - 2)$	Coeff	—	—	0.0033
	SE	—	—	0.0022

[a]RW, relative weight; BP, blood pressure; SC, serum cholesterol.
[b]t = current exam (at beginning of risk period; $t - 1$ = preceding exam; $t - 2$ = exam prior to preceding exam.

SC and BP are included in the analysis, indicating that some of the age effect may be accounted for by the relation between aging and increasing SC and BP values that are more accurately measured when results from two or more exams are used.

Poisson Regression Analysis of Grouped Data

Poisson regression is useful and appropriate when the regression variables are relatively few and discrete and when the study is large, for example when the number of subjects is in the tens or hundreds of thousands. Methods that use individual data records in iterative calculations are computationally burdensome and may not be feasible in such circumstances. With the Poisson approach, the time-covariable space is partitioned into J regions, within the jth of which the (instantaneous) disease incidence rate is assumed to be a constant λ_j. Such regions might be constructed, for example, by age, calendar year, duration of employment, cumulative exposure, and smoking history. Each subject may contribute person-years of observation time to several regions as he or she is followed forward in time; the main computational difficulty is the determination of the person-year totals (Clayton, 1982). The summary data consist of triples (d_j, n_j, x_j), where d_j now denotes the number of disease cases diagnosed in the jth region, n_j denotes the person-years denominator, and x_j is the vector of regression variables. Berry (1983), Breslow et al. (1983), and Frome (1983) have provided introductory accounts of this methodology.

The likelihood function is formally specified by taking the d_j to have independent Poisson distributions with means $n_j \lambda_j$. The standard log-linear model is

$$\log \lambda_j = x_j^t \beta \tag{12}$$

which again specifies multiplicative combination of relative risks. The score equations are given by (2) with λ substituted for p, and the information matrix is $\mathscr{I} = (X^t V X)$ where now V is diagonal with variances $\text{var}(d_j) = n_j \lambda_j$ on the diagonal. The log likelihood is $L(\beta) = \Sigma_j (d_j \log \lambda_j n_j - n_j \lambda_j)$. With these minor changes, virtually all the estimation and testing procedures described in the section "Fitting the Logistic Model" apply. Moreover, provided that the d_j are small in comparison with the n_j, the Poisson likelihood analysis is well approximated by that for linear logistic regression where the d_j are treated as binomial with denominators n_j and the probabilities p_j satisfy the linear logistic equation. Our next example illustrates this fact.

Example

Kahn (1966) presented data on CHD mortality from the Dorn study of smoking and mortality among U.S. veterans. Deaths and person-years were classified according to two levels of attained age (55–64 and 65–74); four levels of amount smoked (1–9, 10–20, 21–39, and 40+ cigarettes/day); five levels of time since smoking stopped (0, 1–4, 5–9, 10–14, and 15+ years) and four levels of age started smoking (11–14, 14–19, 20–24, and 25+ years). Thus there were

Table 7-6. Deviances from fitting log-linear Poisson and linear logistic regression models to grouped data from Dorn's study of smoking and mortality among U.S. veterans

Factor(s) in model[a]	N of parameters (K)	Degrees of freedom	Deviance Logit model	Deviance Poisson model	Deviance + 2K Poisson model
GM	1	159	835.8	827.2	829.2
AGE	2	158	465.8	461.1	465.2
AGE+AMT	5	155	305.0	302.1	312.1
AGE+AMT+STOP	9	151	203.7	201.8	219.8
AGE+AMT+STOP+BEG	12	148	183.0	181.4	205.4
AGE+AMT·STOP	24	136	158.7	157.4	205.4
AGE+AMT·STOP+AGE ·BEG+AGE·AMT+AMT ·BEG+AGE·AMT·BEG	48	112	123.3	122.2	218.2

[a]GM, grand mean; AGE, attained age; AMT, amount smoked; STOP, years stopped smoking; BEG, age began smoking.

$J = 2 \times 4 \times 5 \times 4 = 160$ regions defined by four factors, two of which (attained age and numbers of years stopped smoking) were time dependent. These data were analyzed under the logistic model by Kullback and Cornfield (1976).* We repeated their analyses, obtaining slightly different results, and also analyzed the data by Poisson regression.

Table 7-6 reports the deviances obtained under a variety of models chosen to show the most important main and interaction effects. Kullback and Cornfield (1976) demonstrated that all four factors contributed substantially to the explanation of CHD mortality, and that there was a statistically significant interaction between amount smoked and years since smoking was stopped. They also concluded that the three-factor interaction (attained age × amount smoked × age began smoking), while marginally significant, was probably "the kind of nominally significant result that one finds in examining numerous effects, none of which is real." The deviances in Table 7-6 support these conclusions. Moreover, using a variable selection scheme based on adding twice the degrees of freedom to the deviance for each model (see the section "Selection of Variables for Analysis"), we conclude that the simple linear model and the two-factor interaction model are essentially equivalent in terms of predicting CHD mortality.

Table 7-7 reports the regression coefficients for the no-interaction model. These show the important effect of age and the tendency for CHD mortality to increase with amount and duration of smoking. The effect of stopping smoking, while very significant, does not demonstrate a clear trend; the reduction for

*There is a disparity between the number of person-years reported in their Table 1 and those given by Kahn (1966) for the category age 55–64; smoked 21–39 cigarettes/day; stopped for 1–4 years; began at age 20–24. We have used Kahn's figure of twenty three deaths and 2049 person-years for this category.

Table 7-7. Parameter estimates ($\pm$ standard errors) for regression coefficients for log-linear model fitted to Dorn data

Factor[a]	Level	Regression coefficient $\pm$ SE	
		Logit model	Poisson model
GM		-4.840 ± 0.548	-4.848 ± 0.545
AGE	65–74	0.484 ± 0.235	0.479 ± 0.234
AMT	10–20/Day	0.214 ± 0.039	0.212 ± 0.039
	21–39/Day	0.359 ± 0.041	0.355 ± 0.041
	40+/Day	0.448 ± 0.051	0.443 ± 0.051
STOP	1–4 years	-0.304 ± 0.070	-0.301 ± 0.070
	5–9 years	-0.120 ± 0.044	-0.119 ± 0.044
	10–14 years	-0.139 ± 0.050	-0.138 ± 0.050
	15+ years	-0.330 ± 0.037	-0.327 ± 0.037
BEG	15–19 years	-0.080 ± 0.043	-0.079 ± 0.043
	20–24 years	-0.147 ± 0.045	-0.145 ± 0.044
	25+ years	-0.185 ± 0.048	-0.183 ± 0.048

[a]GM, grand mean; AGE, attained age; AMT, amount smoked; STOP, years stopped smoking; BEG, age began smoking.

stopping fifteen or more years is little different from that of stopping for only one to four years, although the latter effect is not very accurately estimated. Examination of the two-factor interactions (not shown) suggests that the effect of stopping smoking is largely confined to those who had smoked at least ten cigarettes per day. The agreement between the results of the linear logistic and Poisson regression analyses is excellent.

GOODNESS OF FIT, VARIABLE SELECTION, AND MODEL STABILITY

An important aspect of fitting statistical models to data is the selection of regression variables to enter into the model equation in order to explain adequately the observed variation in response, and the elimination of variables whose presence is unnecessary or redundant and merely serves to increase the error of statistical prediction. One also wants to identify observations whose presence has a profound effect on the estimated regression coefficients or that are "outliers" in the sense of failing to conform to a model that fits the rest of the data well. Substantial progress has been made in recent years in adapting "diagnostic" procedures originally developed for least-squares regression problems to the maximum likelihood fitting of logistic models. This section reviews these developments, concentrating on the situation where response is defined as the probability of disease occurrence during a single study period. Analogous procedures are available for Poisson regression analysis of grouped incidence data. Extensions to the discrete- and continuous-time survival models are available also, but they are somewhat more complicated (Storer & Crowley, 1985).

Assessing Goodness of Fit

The simplest method of assessing goodness of fit with grouped data is to compare the observed and fitted values, d_i and $\hat{d}_i = n_i\hat{p}_i$ (cf. Table 7-1). The deviance or Pearson chi-square statistics should be supplemented by an examination of the individual residuals $d_i - \hat{d}_i$, which are usually standardized by division by $[n_i\hat{p}_i(1 - \hat{p}_i)]^{1/2}$ or in other ways as described later in this chapter (see "Deletion Diagnostics"). Graphic methods for examination of such residuals are well developed (Cook & Weisberg, 1982).

If the data are sparse, however, such residual analyses and especially the deviance are uninformative regarding goodness of fit. A better strategy is to add to the model equation additional regression variables that may represent, for example, nonlinear effects of continuous risk factors or interactions between different risk factors, testing each such addition for its contribution to the reduction in deviance. This approach detects particular types of departures from the fitted model. For a more global evaluation of the fit, we partition the risk factor space into relatively homogeneous regions and test the effect of adding to the model a set of regression variables that take on distinct values within each of them. The score test is of particular interest here since it compares the observed with the expected number of cases within each region (Tsiatis, 1980). Some authors have suggested basing the regions on the fitted probabilities of response, for example dividing the sample by deciles of risk and comparing observed and expected numbers in each decile (Lemeshow & Hosmer, 1982; Truett, Cornfield, & Kannel, 1967). In our experience, however, this approach has not been as informative as when the regions are defined to contain nearby values of x. Landwehr, Pregibon, and Shoemaker (1984) proposed a graphic method for use in this context.

Example

To examine the goodness of fit of the simple linear logistic model to the data on 874 Framingham men (Table 7-4, column 1), we initially partitioned the covariable space into $J = 192$ regions based on two levels of age (40–49 vs. 50–62 years); four levels of blood pressure (see Table 7-1); four levels of serum cholesterol (see Table 7-1); three levels of smoking (0, 1–20, 21 + cigarettes/day) and two levels of relative weight ($< 100, \geq 100$). However, since there were only 209 CHD events to distribute into the 192 cells, the data were too sparse to evaluate the fit. Consequently we collapsed the regions so as to consider only two or three variables at a time. Comparison of the observed values with those derived from the continuous analysis within discrete categories of blood pressure × serum cholesterol and blood pressure × smoking × age confirmed the goodness of fit of the continuous model.

Table 7-8 illustrates the comparison of observed and fitted numbers of cases when subjects are classified by their estimated CHD risk according to the logistic model. The classification by actual estimated risk appears more informative than the classification by decile of risk. For example, it shows that the distribution of estimated risks, which ranged from 7.3 to 65.8 percent, is skewed to the right. The rather aberrant value of 6 cases observed versus 15.5

Table 7-8. Comparison of observed and fitted numbers of coronary heart disease (CHD) cases for 874 Framingham men

By decile of risk

Decile (approx.)	Number of men	Number of CHD cases		Average risk for decile (%)
		Observed	Fitted	
1	87	8	10.5	12.0
2	88	14	13.3	15.2
3	88	6	15.5	17.6
4	88	25	17.3	19.6
5	88	23	19.0	21.6
6	88	22	20.6	23.4
7	88	23	22.5	25.6
8	88	27	25.0	28.4
9	88	31	29.0	32.9
10	83	30	36.3	41.7
Total	874	209	209.0	23.9

By estimated risk

Estimated risk	Number at risk	Number of CHD cases	
		Observed	Fitted
0	0	—	—
5	14	0	1.3
10	112	13	14.9
15	197	35	34.8
20	233	56	52.5
25	145	43	39.8
30	72	21	23.2
35	47	18	17.5
40	29	10	12.1
45	12	7	5.8
50	6	1	3.1
55	3	3	1.7
60	3	1	1.9
65	1	1	0.7

expected for the third decile of risk is difficult to interpret. Summary chi-square comparisons of the observed and fitted values based on Tsiatis' (1980) procedure are $\chi_9^2 = 16.8$ ($p = 0.05$) for decile of risk and $\chi_{12}^2 = 10.7$ ($p = 0.55$) for estimated risk.

Goodness-of-Link Tests

If the model appears not to fit without the introduction of complicated interaction terms, the problem may be with the logistic function itself. Some other transformation relating the linear predictors $x^t\beta$ to the response probabilities p could result in a simpler and more interpretable model equation. A common approach to this problem is to imbed the basic model (1) into a more general structure

$$g(p; \tau) = x^t\beta \tag{13}$$

where g is a family of transformations indexed by a parameter τ. (In some cases τ is a vector with components $\tau_1, \tau_2, \ldots$). g is termed a *link function* since it specifies the relation between the response probability and the linear predictor. This model has tolerance distribution interpretation similar to that discussed following equation (1).

Several families of link functions have been proposed for binomial response probabilities that include the logit model as a special case. Prentice's (1976) family includes the inverse normal (probit) and inverse extreme value links. That proposed by Copenhaver and Mielke (1977) contains the inverse double exponential and linear links, but is restricted to functions (like the logit) that are symmetric: $g(1 - p) = -g(p)$. Pregibon's (1980) family includes both symmetric and nonsymmetric links; Whittemore's (1983) is designed to discriminate between the logit and "one-hit" dose-response functions. Other suggestions have been made by Aranda-Ordaz (1981) and Guerrero and Johnson (1982).

Breslow and Storer (1985) proposed a family of models for binary response data that directs specific attention at the epidemiologic measure of relative risk. It cannot be expressed exactly in the form (13), but instead is written

$$\theta = \text{logit } p = \alpha + \log R(x^t\beta; \tau) \tag{14a}$$

where $R(x^t\beta; \tau)$ is a family of log relative risk functions specified by

$$\log R(x^t\beta; \tau) = \begin{cases} \dfrac{(1 + x^t\beta)^\tau - 1}{\tau} & \tau \neq 0 \\[2mm] \log(1 + x^t\beta) & \tau = 0 \end{cases} \tag{14b}$$

The logit model arises when $\tau = 1$, whereas the additive relative risk function $1 + x^t\beta$ occurs at $\tau = 0$. The additive formula is preferred by some epidemiologists. It facilitates low-dose linear extrapolation and leads to less extreme estimators of relative risk for large values of continuous covariables or joint exposure to several covariables.

This formulation implicitly assumes that the study period is short enough that the odds ratios $\{p(x)/[1 - p(x)]\} \div \{p(0)/[1 - p(0)]\}$ can be interpreted as relative risks. Otherwise, equation (14) can be used in conjunction with the discrete-time proportional hazards model (6). Related work is by Thomas (1981) and Barlow (1985). Breslow and Storer (1985) presented a set of GLIM macros to implement their procedure.

Estimation of the link parameter(s) and testing for departure from the standard logit model is easier than one might think using flexible programs such as GLIM. The trick is to express the regression model in terms of θ, the "natural parameter" of the binomial distribution ($\theta = \log \lambda$ for Poisson regression). As shown by Cox (1984) and Jorgensen (1984), solution of the likelihood equations for the general model is accomplished via the iterative scheme

$$\Delta \hat{\beta} = (Z^t V Z)^{-1} Z^t V y \qquad (15)$$

where now $Z = \partial \theta / \partial \beta$, y is a "working" vector with components $(d - np)/v$, and β is an augmented parameter vector that includes the coefficients of the regression variables x as well as the parameters in the link function. Score tests for the logit model, termed goodness-of-link tests by Pregibon (1980), are constructed by adding derived regression variables of the form $\partial \theta / \partial \tau$ to the basic model equation, where τ is set equal to its value for the logit link, and testing for the significance of their effect. Further details and examples of this approach are given by Atkinson (1985) and Breslow (1986).

Example

The data shown in Table 7-9 were obtained from those in Table 7-1 by collapsing the first two levels of serum cholesterol (SC) and blood pressure (BP), respectively. Our initial results showed the CHD rates to be lower for the second levels of SC and BP than for the baseline levels, and we wished to avoid

Table 7-9. Fitting of additive and multiplicative relative risk models to Cornfield's coronary heart disease (CHD) data

Risk factor		Observed data		Fitted cases		Fitted relative risk	
SC (mg/100cc)	BP (mmHg)	Total (n)	CHD cases (d)[a]	Mult model	Add RR model	Mult model	Add RR model
<220	<147	431	10	11.55	9.32	1.0	1.0
	147–166	93	3	4.26	4.13	1.74	2.06
	167+	49	7	4.19	6.52	3.40	6.79
220–259	<147	347	19	17.35	18.78	1.91	2.53
	147–166	74	6	6.22	5.55	3.33	3.59
	167+	49	6	7.43	7.76	6.49	8.32
260+	<147	185	19	19.10	22.46	4.18	6.12
	147–166	57	11	9.52	7.95	7.29	7.18
	167+	44	11	12.37	9.33	14.21	11.91
Deviance (df = 4)				3.39	3.21		
Chi square (df = 4)				3.64	3.25		

[a]Number of CHD cases.

problems in the additive relative risk model caused by regression variables with negative coefficients.

Four "dummy" regression variables were defined to identify the third and fourth levels of SC and BP. The multiplicative model based on the standard logistic equation (1) fit well, with a deviance of 3.4 on $9 - 5 = 4$ degrees of freedom. Nevertheless, to see whether the data strongly supported a multiplicative in preference to an additive relationship, we varied the τ parameter in equation (14b) over the range -0.4 to 1.0 in increments of 0.1. The resulting deviances (Figure 7-1) indicate that the best fitting model is intermediate between additive and multiplicative, both of which fit the data reasonably well. Nevertheless, there are substantial differences between them in estimated relative risks. When the other factor is at its reference level, the relative risks estimated for the additive model are more extreme: 6.79 for $167 +$ mm Hg BP and 6.12 for $260 +$ mg/100 cc SC, versus 3.40 and 4.18, respectively, for the multiplicative model. However, the relative risk estimated for the highest risk category is only $11.91 = 6.79 + 6.12 - 1$ for the additive model versus $3.40 \times 4.18 = 14.21$ for the multiplicative model. Wald's test does not work well with the additive model and Barlow's (1985) reparameterization is preferred.

The goodness-of-link test allows us to assess the logit link without actually carrying out the laborious calculations required for Figure 7-1. After fitting the logistic model, we construct a new variable

$$z = \partial\theta/\partial\tau = (1 + x^t\hat{\beta})[\log(1 + x^t\hat{\beta}) - 1]$$

The score (goodness-of-link) test for z yields $\chi_1^2 = 0.97$. Its regression coefficient of -0.83 gives a "first step" estimate of τ of $1 - 0.83 = 0.17$. In fact, as shown in Figure 7-1, the minimum deviance 2.38 occurs at $\tau = 0.37$. The deviance test for the logit model is thus $3.39 - 2.38 = 1.01$, in good agreement with the score test.

Selection of Variables for Analysis

Appropriate selection of variables for entry into the model equation requires a clear understanding of the subject matter and of the goals of the analysis. If the study has been designed to elucidate the relationship between the disease outcome and one particular risk factor, the main problem will be confounding of that relationship by other variables that are causally related to disease and that are associated with the risk factor in the source population. We have argued elsewhere (Breslow, 1982) that one should include in the regression equation the major known causal determinants of disease, whether or not these appear to confound the association in the sample data. Primary interest is in the regression coefficient of the putative risk factor after adjustment for variables that are conceded a priori to be important determinants of disease. When the risk factor of interest is binary, the propensity score (Rosenbaum & Rubin, 1984) appears to offer a simple and efficient means of adjusting simultaneously for the effects of a number of confounding variables. Generally, one does not want to include in the model equation variables that are intermediate in the causal pathway between risk factor and disease, lest the intermediates carry some of the "weight" that rightfully belong to the risk factor. Causal models based on simultaneous

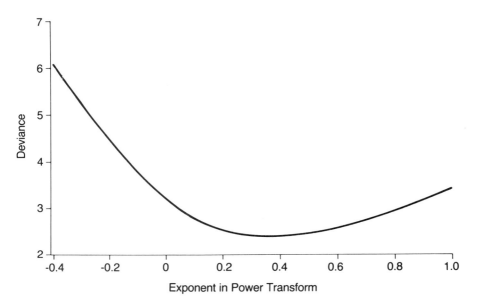

Figure 7–1. Deviances for a family of log relative risk functions fitted to the data shown in Table 7-9.

structural equations that attempt to account for such intermediate causation are discussed elsewhere in this monograph (Chapters 3, 6, and 15).

When the study is not designed to investigate a sharply focused hypothesis, but instead explores the relationship between the disease and a number of potential risk factors, the process of variable selection is more problematic. A first step is usually to reduce a large number of candidate variables to a smaller set for meaningful analysis. When several highly correlated variables are all measuring essentially the same biologic process, it is preferable to construct a single index to represent that process rather than having to pick and choose among competing variables. Once a priori reasoning has reduced the number of candidate variables as far as possible, efficient screening algorithms are available that identify sets of variables with small deviances among sets of the same size (Lawless & Singhal, 1978). To compare prediction error between variable sets of different sizes, several lines of investigation suggest penalizing the deviance by a quantity that depends on the number of estimated parameters (Atkinson, 1980; Efron, 1986). In particular, Efron (1986) demonstrated that the expected downward bias in the observed deviance based on K regression variables, when thought of as a measure of the prediction error when the logistic discriminant is used to predict disease outcomes in a new sample, is approximately $2K$. Thus a reasonable criterion for use in selecting the "best" model is dev $+ 2K$. Rather than simply identifying the single model that minimizes this criterion, however, it is preferable to present several alternative models if each of these have approximately the same degree of (bias corrected) prediction error. This emphasizes the uncertainty inherent in the variable selection process and also permits informed judgment based on knowledge of the subject matter to be used in making a final choice of model equation. The dev $+ 2K$ criterion was illustrated in the section "Example" under "The Logistic Model."

Deletion Diagnostics

A desirable property of any fitted model is that the estimated regression coefficients and test statistics are reasonably insensitive to minor perturbations in the data from which they were derived. One wants to be warned if any individual observations have an excessive influence on the fitted model or are outliers in the sense of being poorly fitted. A number of diagnostic aids have been developed for least-squares regression models that identify such influential or outlying observations. By exploiting the relationship between maximum likelihood estimation and weighted least squares, methods derived for ordinary regression may be shown to apply also, at least approximately, to logistic regression. These developments are summarized well by Pregibon (1981) and by Cook and Weisberg (1982).

In what follows we consider an "observation" to be the triple (d_i, n_i, x_i). (Thus for grouped data where $n_i > 1$, each cell constitutes the observation.) The quantities of greatest use in assessing model stability are the residuals $r_i = d_i - n_i \hat{p}_i$ and the diagonal elements h_i of the projection ("hat") matrix $H = V^{1/2} X^t (X^t V X)^{-1} X V^{1/2}$ (see the section "Maximum Likelihood Estimation"). The h_i identify "influential" observations in the sense of d_i having a large effect on the fitted value $n_i \hat{p}_i$. They sum to K, the number of parameters estimated, and larger values tend to be associated with observations having "extreme" covariables x_i (Pregibon, 1981).

Both r_i and h_i enter into the formula

$$\hat{\beta}_{(i)}^1 = \hat{\beta} - \frac{(X^t V X)^{-1} x_i r_i}{1 - h_i} \tag{16}$$

used to approximate the change in the estimated regression coefficients occasioned by deletion of the ith observation. (This is derived from [3] by starting from $\hat{\beta}$ and taking one step in the iterative estimation procedure toward $\hat{\beta}_{(i)}$, the actual coefficient with the ith observation deleted.) A useful summary of the approximate changes in all the coefficients is given by "Cook's distance"

$$c_i^1 = (\hat{\beta}_{(i)}^1 - \hat{\beta})^t (X^t V X)(\hat{\beta}_{(i)}^1 - \hat{\beta}) = \frac{r_i^2 h_i}{v_i (1 - h_i)^2} \tag{17}$$

where $v_i = n_i \hat{p}_i (1 - \hat{p}_i)$ is the estimated variance. Williams (1987) derived an approximation to the change in deviance from deletion of the ith observation:

$$r_{U_i} = \text{sign}(d_i - n_i \hat{p}_i) \left\{ \frac{dev_i^2 + h_i r_i^2}{[v_i (1 - h_i)]} \right\}^{1/2} \tag{18}$$

where $dev_i^2 = -2\{d_i \log(n_i \hat{p}_i / d_i) + (n_i - d_i) \log[n_i(1 - \hat{p}_i)/(n_i - d_i)]\}$ is the contribution of the ith observation to the deviance ($dev_i^2 = -2n_i \log(1 - \hat{p}_i)$ if $d_i = 0$ and $dev_i^2 = -2n_i \log(\hat{p}_i)$ if $d_i = n_i$). Cook and Weisberg (1982) recommended that the adjusted residuals $s_i = r_i/[v_i(1 - h_i)]^{1/2}$ and h_i be used and interpreted as one does for the corresponding quantities in ordinary regression.

Example

Figure 7-2 illustrates a number of the diagnostics available for logistic regression with data from Table 7-1. The sixteen observations correspond to the sixteen rows of that table. Most of the larger h_i values (Figure 7-2, first panel) are concentrated among observations numbered 9 through 16, where there are larger numbers of CHD events. The second panel presents Cook's distance as defined by equation (17). The largest changes in the β coefficients, relative to their covariance structure, are occasioned by deletion of observations number 1, 7, 15, and 16. Examination of the one-step approximations $\hat{\beta}_{(i)}^1 - \hat{\beta}$ (equation [16]) shows that removal of the first observation causes the estimate of the grand mean to increase by about 0.32. This is compensated, however, by a decline of approximately 0.23 in each of the serum cholesterol coefficients and of

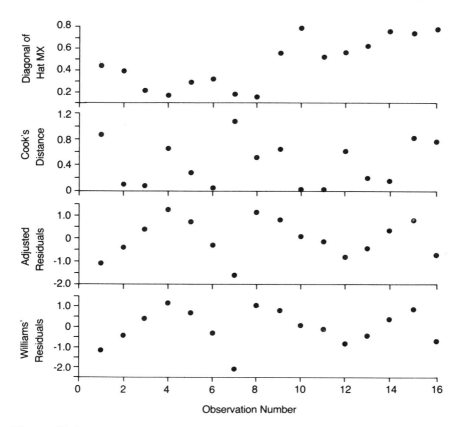

Figure 7-2. Regression diagnostics calculated from the data in Table 7-1: diagonal element of the hat matrix; Cook's distance; studentized residuals; Williams' residuals. See text for discussion.

0.13 in each of the blood pressure coefficients, with the result that the fitted values in the remaining cells are little affected. This example points up an inherent instability in logistic models in situations where the disease rate in the reference category is poorly determined due to a small number of disease events in that category. Observation 7 is the only one where no CHD events were observed. Its elimination would increase $\hat{\beta}_1$ by about 0.32 and $\hat{\beta}_5$ by 0.15, these coefficients corresponding to the relevant levels of SC and BP, but would leave the other β's essentially unchanged. Deletion of the last observation, corresponding to the highest level of SC and BP, would reduce $\hat{\beta}_6$ by 0.17. If one could be certain of the correct parametric form, some of the instability could be avoided by use of linear models in continuous covariables or some transform of them in place of the discrete variables used here.

The last two panels of Figure 7-2 present the adjusted or "studentized" residuals s_i and Williams' approximate residuals r_{U_i} (equation [18]). Whereas the first two panels are concerned more with observations that strongly influence the coefficients estimated under the model, the last two are oriented toward identifying outliers that are poorly fit by it. The two sets of residuals are remarkably close, the largest discrepancy being for observation 7, which also has the largest (in absolute value) residual: $s_7 = -1.61$ and $r_{U_7} = -2.08$. As noted previously, this observation is also relatively influential in terms of Cook's measure. On the other hand, the last observation is influential without any suggestion that it is also an outlier ($s_{16} = r_{U_{16}} = -0.73$). None of the diagnostic measures are sufficiently extreme as to lead to serious concern about the fit.

EXTENSIONS OF LOGISTIC REGRESSION

In this concluding section we review briefly several extensions of logistic modeling that are applicable to the assessment of chronic disease risk.

Case-Control Sampling

The logistic analysis of time-dependent outcomes may require a large number of data records due to the size of the initial cohort or, in the case of discrete proportional hazards analyses, may necessitate incorporation of a new record for each time interval over which a subject is followed (equation [6]). The computing time required for the iterative fitting process effectively rules out exploratory interactive analyses, even if only a small fraction of the data records refer to the event of interest. In the section, "The Discrete-Time Proportional Hazards Models," for example, only 209 of the 6627 data records used in the logistic analysis of conditional response probabilities were "positive" for the CHD outcome.

Several investigators (Mantel, 1973; Siegel & Greenhouse, 1973) have pointed out that unbiased estimates of relative risk may be obtained by fitting the logistic model using the records for the cases plus those of a "control" sample. This may be a random sample from the records for the noncases, or where appropriate, a stratified random sample of the records for each time interval. In the Framingham example, we could select seventeen control records from the $847 - 17 = 857$ noncases in the first time interval, sixteen controls from the $850 - 16 = 834$ noncases in the second, and so on for a total of 209 "controls," some of which may refer to the same subject. The formal mathematical justification for this procedure (Prentice & Pyke, 1979) is closely related to Cornfield's (1951) original demonstration that relative risks could be estimated from case-control studies. It depends critically on the fact that log-odds ratios (differences in the logit transforms of probabilities) for disease as a function of exposure are identical to the corresponding log odds ratios for exposure as a function of disease.

Case-control sampling is of particular interest when the values of some of the regression variables are not immediately available in the original data set but necessitate expensive laboratory tests on stored serum samples, abstracting of data from medical records, or interviews with (proxy) subjects. A variation of this approach whereby the control sample is selected at the outset of the study, and followed over time, is termed by Prentice (1986) a case-cohort design. It requires that account be taken of the correlations between the likelihood contributions for each time interval (or for each "risk set" in case of a continuous-time proportional hazards analysis).

Extraneous Variation (Overdispersion)

When fitting logistic or log-linear Poisson regression models to grouped data, especially when there are a large number of events so that the individual cell probabilities are well estimated, the discrepancies between observed and fitted numbers may be so large that they are not reasonably ascribed to chance. However, the pattern of residuals may appear random rather than due to one or two outliers, and is not explained by the introduction of further covariables into the model. This suggests the presence of an extraneous source of variation beyond the binomial or Poisson sampling errors that are explicitly taken into account. Tests of significance and confidence intervals that fail to account for the lack of fit may be seriously misleading.

More general models have been proposed to overcome this problem. These models incorporate an additional parameter to represent the degree of overdispersion. For example, assuming that the response probabilities within each cell are drawn from a beta distribution whose mean satisfies the logistic regression equation, one arrives at a beta-binomial model that may be analyzed using parametric maximum likelihood (Crowder, 1978). Regrettably, the computations are rather complex. Alternatively one may start with the mean-variance function of the beta binomial, namely $n_i p_i (1 - p_i) + n_i(n_i - 1)\sigma^2 p_i(1 - p_i)$, and jointly estimate the overdispersion parameter σ^2 and the regression coefficients β using a combination of quasi-likelihood and method-of-moments estimation procedures (Williams, 1982). An analogous procedure is available for Poisson regression (Breslow, 1984). These latter procedures are reasonably robust to misspecification of the mean-variance equation and are nearly as efficient as the parametric beta-binomial approach so far as β estimation is concerned (Moore, 1985). The theory of generalized linear models itself provides for an unknown scale parameter in the mean-variance function, but this formulation is not suggested by any probability model for the data.

Dependent Outcomes

So far in this chapter we have tacitly assumed that the binary or binomial outcome variables are statistically independent. Even though the same subject may contribute more than one data record to the analyses that incorporate time, survival analysis considerations show that the likelihood function is identical to that based on independent outcomes so long as a single binary outcome is measured for each subject. On the other hand, if the binary outcomes are measured repeatedly over time for each subject, or if the subjects are sampled in clusters (e.g., families in a genetic analysis), methods are needed that account for intrasubject or intrafamilial correlations.

Korn and Whittemore (1979) developed an autoregressive model based on the logistic function for the analysis of data from panel studies of the acute health effects of air pollution. The data consist of a series of binary observations d_{ij} for the jth time point on the ith individual with $d_{ij} = 1$ or 0 according to whether or not the health outcome of interest (e.g., asthmatic attack) occurs at that time, and a time-dependent vector x_j of exogenous variables (e.g., measures of air pollution constituents). The conditional probabilities of an adverse health outcome on the jth day, given the past, are specified by the modulated Markov model

$$\text{logit pr}(d_{ij} = 1 \mid d_{i1}, \dots, d_{j-1}) = a_0^i + a_1^i d_{i,j-1} + x_j^t \beta^i$$

Separate α^i and β^i are estimated for each individual and, taking account of the fact that they may be estimated with variable precision, these coefficients are averaged over individuals to measure the health effects. A more comprehensive approach treats the parameters as random variables drawn from a multivariate normal or other joint distribution, and attempts maximum likelihood estimation on the basis of the integrated likelihood (Stiratelli, Laird, & Ware, 1984).

Two other groups of researchers have developed models for the marginal response probabilities $p_{ij} = \text{pr}(d_{ij} = 1)$ that account for the correlations between outcomes recorded on the same subject (or family in the case of genetic analyses). In their pedigree analysis of binary traits, Hopper, Hannah, and Mathews (1984) expressed the joint probability of the outcomes $d_i = (d_{i1}, \dots, d_{iJ_i})$, where J_i is the size of the ith pedigree, in terms of the J_i marginal probabilities and the $J_i(J_i - 1)/2$ correlations. Since these $J_i(J_i + 1)/2$ parameters do not uniquely determine the joint distribution unless $J_i = 2$, they postulated a log-linear model for the joint probabilities such that second- and higher order interactions are zero. The marginal probabilities are modeled as functions of explanatory variables that depend on both subject and time via the logistic equation with nonrandom coefficients:

$$\text{logit } p_{ij} = \beta_0 + x_{ij}^t \beta \tag{19}$$

The correlations may also depend on characteristics associated with each subject or family. However, this approach is cumbersome, requires access to computer programs for general likelihood maximization, and is of uncertain robustness with regard to misspecification of the covariances.

A more promising and general method based on the theory of generalized linear models has recently been proposed in a series of papers by Zeger, Liang, and Self (1985), Zeger and Liang (1986), and Liang and Zeger (1986). This approach is reviewed in Chapter 8.

Nonparametric Logistic Regression

The advent of low-cost computing has stimulated the development of a number of computer-intensive approaches for relaxing the linearity assumptions inherent in the basic logistic model (1) so as to allow a smooth, nonparametric characterization of the response survace. Hastie and Tibshirani (1986) described a generalized additive model that is applicable to logistic regression as well as to other generalized models. The linear predictor $\beta_0 + \beta_1 x_1 + \cdots + \beta_k x_k$ in (1) is replaced by the sum $\beta_0 + S_1(x_1) + \cdots + S_k(x_k)$, where the S_K are smooth functions that are estimated nonparametrically. The degree of smoothness is selected to minimize the squared error of prediction. Thus there is an additive combination of effects from different regression variables (on the logit scale), but the effects themselves are arbitrary smooth functions of their quantitative arguments.

Figure 7-3 illustrates this approach with the Framingham data used for the simple logistic regression analysis shown in the first column of Table 7-4. These plots were obtained using a "span" of 0.25 for each variable, meaning that 25 percent of the data were used to estimate the regression curve at each covariable value. Most of the smooths, with the possible exception of cigarette smoking, demonstrate a reasonably linear structure. The difference in deviance between the linear and smooth fits was 34.0 with a difference in effective "degrees of freedom" (as described by Hastie and Tibshirani) of 19.4. The sampling distribution for such deviance differences, however, is known to be more dispersed than chi square and there is at present no way to assess the statistical significance of the deviance difference by reference to a tabled distribution. In fact, the cross-validated fit to these data chose spans of 1.0 for each variable, meaning that it agreed perfectly with the linear logistic model.

An alternative approach based on penalized maximum likelihood estimation (Good & Gaskins, 1971) has been proposed by O'Sullivan, Yandell, and Raynor (1986). It avoids the assumption of additivity altogether. In place of the linear predictor $x^t\beta$, the covariable function that arises as the approximate solution to the maximization problem takes the form (essentially) of a sum of polynomials of low degree that are analogous to the spline functions that occur in nonparametric least-squares regression. These authors used cross validation to select the degree of smoothing.

The nonparametric approach is of great benefit in suggesting possible transformations of the data to achieve linearity. On the other hand, problems of statistical inference for such algorithms have yet to be worked out.

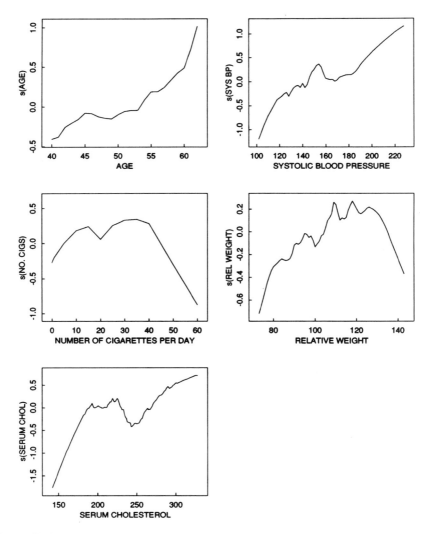

Figure 7–3. Logistic regression smooths estimated from data on 874 Framingham men 40 through 62 in 1948 using the method of Hastie and Tibshirani (1986). "Span" = 0.25 for each variable (25% of data used to estimate regression curve at each covariable value).

Appendix
SAS Commands Used to Produce
the Results Shown in Table 7-4

```
DATA TEMP; SET SASDATA. CHD;
   CHD = .; IF AC365 = 0 THEN CHD = 0;
          IF AC365 > = 2 AND AC365 = <10 THEN CHD = 1;
```

```
   AGE = AC305;
   BP = AC15;
   SC = AC75;
   CI = AC135;
   RW = AC5;
PROC LOGIST PCOV CT;      (SIMPLE LOGISTIC REGRESSION)
   MODEL CHD = AGE BP SC CI RW;
   DATA; SET SASFILE. CHD;
   J2 = 0; J3 = 0; J4 = 0; J5 = 0; J6 = 0; J7 = 0; J8 = 0; J9 = 0;
   IF J = 2 THEN J2 = 1;
   IF J = 3 THEN J3 = 1;
   IF J = 4 THEN J4 = 1;
   IF J = 5 THEN J5 = 1;
   IF J = 6 THEN J6 = 1;
   IF J = 7 THEN J7 = 1;
   IF J = 8 THEN J8 = 1;
   IF J = 9 THEN J9 = 1;
PROC LOGIST PCOV CT;      (DISCRETE TIME PROPORTIONAL HAZARDS)
   MODEL CHD = J2 J3 J4 J5 J6 J7 J8 J9 AGE BP SC SI RW;
DATA; SET TEMP;
   TIME = .;     IF AC365 = 0 AND AC388 = 0 THEN TIME = AC314 − AC305;
   IF AC365 = 0 THEN AC365 = 11; IF AC388 = 0 THEN AC388 = 11;;
     IF MIN(AC365, AC388) = 2 THEN TIME = AC306 − AC305;
     IF MIN(AC365, AC388) = 3 THEN TIME = AC307 − AC305;
     IF MIN(AC365, AC388) = 4 THEN TIME = AC308 − AC305;
     IF MIN(AC365, AC388) = 5 THEN TIME = AC309 − AC305;
     IF MIN(AC365, AC388) = 6 THEN TIME = AC310 − AC305;
     IF MIN(AC365, AC388) = 7 THEN TIME = AC311 − AC305;
     IF MIN(AC365, AC388) = 8 THEN TIME = AC312 − AC305;
     IF MIN(AC365, AC388) = 9 THEN TIME = AC313 − AC305;
     IF MIN(AC365, AC388) = 10 THEN TIME = AC314 − AC305;
PROC SORT;
   BY DESCENDING TIME;      (PROPORTIONAL HAZARDS)
PROC PHGLM PCOV;
   EVENT CHD;
   MODEL TIME = AGE BP SC CI RW;
```

ACKNOWLEDGMENTS

I am indebted to John Cologne and Yoicki Ii for computational assistance. This work was supported in part by USPHS Grant CA 40644.

REFERENCES

Aranda-Ordaz FJ (1981). "On two families of transformations to additivity for binary response data." *Biometrika* 68:357–363.

Atkinson AC (1980). "A note on the generalized information criterion for choice of a model." *Biometrika* 67:413–418.

Atkinson AC (1985). *Plots, Transformations and Regression.* Oxford, Clarendon Press.

Baker RJ, Nelder JA (1978). *The GLIM System, Release 3.* Oxford, Numerical Algorithms Group.

Barlow WE (1985). "General relative risk models in stratified epidemiologic studies." *Applied Statistics* 34:246–257.

Berkson J (1944). "Application of the logistic function to bio-assay." *Journal of the American Statistical Association* 39:357–365.

Berry C (1983). "The analysis of mortality by the subject-years method." *Biometrics* 39:173–184.

Bishop YMM, Fienberg SE, Holland PW (1975). *Discrete Multivariate Analysis.* Cambridge, Mass., MIT Press.

Breslow NE (1974). "Covariance analysis of grouped survival data." *Biometrics* 30:89–100.

Breslow NE (1982). "Design and analysis of case-control studies." *Annual Review of Public Health* 3:29–54.

Breslow NE (1984). "Extra-Poisson variation in log-linear models." *Applied Statistics* 33:38–44.

Breslow NE (1986). "Use of the power transform to discriminate between additive and multiplicative models in epidemiologic research." In Moolgavkar S, Prentice RL (eds), *Modern Statistical Methods in Chronic Disease Epidemiology.* New York, Wiley.

Breslow NE, Storer BE (1985). "General relative risk functions for case-control studies." *American Journal of Epidemiology* 122:149–162.

Breslow NE, et al. (1983). "Multiplicative models and cohort analysis." *Journal of the American Statistical Association* 78:1–12.

Clayton DG (1982). "The analysis of prospective studies of disease aetiology." *Communications in Statistics–Theory and Methods* 11:2129–2155.

Cook RD, Weisberg S (1982). *Residuals and Influence in Regression.* London, Chapman and Hall.

Copenhaver, TW, Mielke PW (1977). "Quantit analysis: A quantal assay refinement." *Biometrics* 33:175–171.

Cornfield J (1951). "A method of estimating comparative rates from clinical data: Applications to cancer of the lung, breast and cervix." *Journal of the National Cancer Institute* 11: 1269–1275.

Cornfield J (1962). "Joint dependence of risk of coronary heart disease on serum cholesterol and systolic blood pressure: A discriminant function analysis." *Federation Proceedings* 21:58–61.

Cox CL (1984). "Generalized linear models—the missing link." *Applied Statistics* 33:18–24.

Cox DR (1958). "The regression analysis of binary sequences." *Journal of the Royal Statistical Society B* 20:215–242.

Cox DR (1970). *Analysis of Binary Data.* London, Chapman and Hall.

Cox DR (1972). "Regression models and life tables (with discussion)." *Journal of the Royal Statistical Society B* 34:187–220.

Cox DR (1975). "Partial likelihood." *Biometrika* 62:269–276.

Cox DR, Hinkley DV (1974). *Theoretical Statistics.* London, Chapman and Hall.

Cox DR, Oakes D (1984). *Analysis of Survival Data.* London, Chapman and Hall.

Crowder MJ (1978). "Beta-binomial ANOVA for proportions." *Applied Statistics* 19:240–250.

Efron B (1986). "How biased is the apparent error rate of a prediction rule?" *Journal of the American Statistical Association* 81:461–470.

Farewell VT (1977). "A model for a binary variable with time censored observations." *Biometrika* 64:43–46.

Feinleib M (1985). "The Framingham study: Sample selection, follow-up and methods of analysis." *National Cancer Institute Monograph* 67:59–64.

Finney DJ (1952). *Probit Analysis*, 2nd ed. London, Cambridge University Press.

Frome EL (1983). "The analysis of rates using Poisson regression models." *Biometrics* 39:665–674.

Gabriel KR (1963). "Analysis of variance of proportions with unequal frequencies." *Journal of the American Statistical Association* 58:1133–1157.

Good IJ, Gaskins RA (1971). "Nonparametric roughness penalties for probability densities." *Biometrika* 58:255–277.

Grizzle JE, Starmer CF, Koch GG (1969). "Analysis of categorical data by linear models." *Biometrics* 2:489–504.

Guerrero VM, Johnson RA (1982). "Use of the Box-Cox transformation with binary response models." *Biometrika* 69:309–314.

Hastie TJ, Tibshirani RJ (1986). "Generalized additive models." *Statistical Science* 1:297–318.

Hauck WW (1983). "A note on confidence bands for the logistic response curve." *American Statistician* 37:158–160.

Hauck WW, Donner A (1977). "Wald's test as applied to hypotheses in logit analysis." *Journal of the American Statistical Association* 72:851–853, Corrigendum (1980) 75:482.

Hopper JL, Hannah MC, Mathews JD (1984). "Genetic analysis workshop II: Pedigree analysis of a binary trait without assuming an underlying liability." *Genetic Epidemiology* 1:183–188.

Ingram DD, Kleinman JC (1989). "Empirical comparisons of proportional hazards and logistic regression models." *Statistics in Medicine* 8:525–538.

Jorgensen S (1984). "The delta algorithm and GLIM." *International Statistical Review* 52:283–300.

Kahn HA (1966). "The Dorn study of smoking and mortality among US veterans: Report on eight and one-half years of observation." *Nation Cancer Institute Monograph* 19:1–126.

Kalbfleisch JD, Prentice RL (1980). *The Analysis of Failure Time Data*. New, Wiley.

Kaplan EL, Meier P (1958). "Nonparametric estimation from incomplete observation." *Journal of the American Statistical Association* 53:457–481.

Korn EL, Whittemore AS (1979). "Methods for analyzing panel studies of acute health effects of air pollution." *Biometrics* 35:795–802.

Ku HH, Kullback S (1974). "Loglinear models in contingency tables analysis." *American Statistician* 28:115–122.

Kullback S, Cornfield J (1976). "An information theoretic contingency table analysis of the Dorn study of smoking and mortality." *Computers and Biomedical Research* 9:409–437.

Landwehr JM, Pregibon D, Shoemaker A (1984). "Graphical methods for assessing logistic regression models." *Journal of the American Statistical Association* 79:61–83.

Lawless JF, Singhal K (1978). "Efficient screening of non-normal regression models. *Biometrics* 34:318–327.

Lemeshow S, Hosmer DW (1982). "A review of goodness-of-fit statistics for use in the development of logistic regression models." *American Journal of Epidemiology* 115:92–106.

Liang KY, Zeger SL (1986). "Longitudinal data analysis using generalized linear models." *Biometrika* 73:13–27.

McCullagh P, Nelder JA (1983). *Generalized Linear Models.* London, Chapman and Hall.

Mantel N (1973). "Synthetic retrospective studies and related topics." *Biometrics* 29:479–486.

Moore DF (1985). PhD diss., University of Washington, Seattle.

Myers MH, Hankey BF, Mantel N (1973). "A logistic regression model for use with response-time data involving regressor variables." *Biometrics* 29:257–269.

O'Sullivan F, Yandell BS, Raynor WS Jr (1986). "Automatic smoothing of regression functions in generalized linear models." *Journal of the American Statistical Association* 81:96–103.

Pregibon D (1980). "Goodness of link tests for generalized linear models." *Applied Statistics* 29:15–24.

Pregibon D (1981). "Logistic regression diagnostics." *Annals of Statistics* 9:705–724.

Pregibon D (1982). "Scores tests in GLIM." In Gilchrist R (ed), *GLIM 82: Proceedings of the International Conference on Generalised Linear Models.* New York, Springer-Verlag, pp 87–97.

Prentice RL (1976). "Generalization of the probit and logit models for dose response curves." *Biometrics* 32:761–768.

Prentice RL (1986). "A case-cohort design for epidemiologic cohort studies and disease prevention trials." *Biometrika* 73:1–11.

Prentice RL, Gloeckler LA (1978). "Regression analysis of grouped survival data with application to breast cancer development." *Biometrics* 34:57–67.

Prentice RL, Pyke R (1979). "Logistic disease incidence models and case-control studies." *Biometrika* 66:403–411.

Prentice RL, Shimizu Y, Lin CH, Peterson AV, Kato H, Mason MW, Szatrowski TP (1982). "Serial blood pressure measurements and cardiovascular disease in a Japanese cohort." *American Journal of Epidemiology* 116:1–28.

Rao, CR (1965). *Linear Statistical Inference and Its Applications.* New York, Wiley.

Rosenbaum PR, Rubin DB (1984). "Reducing bias in observational studies using subclassification on the propensity score." *Journal of the American Statistical Association* 79:516–524.

Siegel DG, Greenhouse SW (1973). "Multiple relative risk functions in case-control studies." *American Journal of Epidemiology* 97:324–331.

Stiratelli R, Laird N, Ware J (1984). "Random effects models for serial observations with binary response." *Biometrics* 40:961–971.

Storer BE, Crowley J (1985). "A diagnostic for Cox regression and general conditional likelihoods." *Journal of the American Statistical Association* 80:139–147.

Thall PF (1988). "Mixed Poisson likelihood regression models for longitudinal interval count data." *Biometrics* 44:197–209.

Thomas DC (1981). "General relative risk models for survival time and matched case-control analysis." *Biometrics* 37:673–686.

Thompson WA Jr (1977). "On the treatment of grouped observations in life studies." *Biometrika* 33:463–470.

Truett J, Cornfield J, Kannel W (1967). "A multivariate analysis of the risk of coronary heart disease in Framingham." *Journal of Chronic Disease* 20:511–524.

Tsiatis AA (1980). "A note on a goodness-of-fit test for the logistic regression model." *Biometrika* 67:250–251.

Vaeth M (1985). "On the use of Wald's test in exponential families." *International Statistical Review* 53:199–214.

Walker SH, Duncan DB (1967). "Estimation of the probability of an event as a function of several independent variables." *Biometrika* 54:167–179.

Whittemore A (1983). "Transformations to linearity in binary response." *SIAM Journal of Applied Mathematics* 43:703–710.

Williams DA (1982). "Extra-binomial variation in logistic linear models." *Applied Statistics* 31:144–148.

Williams PA (1987). "Generalized linear model diagnostics using the deviance and single case deletions." *Applied Statistics* 36:181–191.

Woodbury MA, Manton KG, Stallard E (1981). "Longitudinal models for chronic disease risk." *American Journal of Epidemiology* 10:187–197.

Wu M, Ware JH (1979). "On the use of repeated measurements in regression analysis with dichotomous responses." *Biometrics* 35:513–521.

8

Generalized Linear Models for Longitudinal Data
Application: Xerophthalmia in Indonesia

LAWRENCE MOULTON, SCOTT ZEGER,
AND KUNG-YEE LIANG

Investigators are often interested in examining the relationship between a response (Y) and a set of explanatory variables (X). When the responses are independent, a class of regression models known as *generalized linear models* (*GLMs*) (McCullagh & Nelder, 1989) provides great flexibility for such an investigation. GLMs include linear models for approximately Gaussian (normal) Y's, logit and probit regression for binary responses, log-linear models for counts, proportional odds models for ordered categorical data, and proportional hazards models for survival times. These methods and others share a common formulation, theory, and algorithm for estimation (e.g., GLIM, [Baker & Nelder, 1986]. In short, regression techniques for independent data are well developed.

In longitudinal studies, repeated observations on a subject tend to be correlated. This time dependence must be taken into account to make valid inferences about the relationship of Y with X; the standard GLM analyses are not appropriate. Extensions of ordinary linear models for longitudinal data are well developed because of the mathematical tractability of the multivariate Gaussian distribution. (For a review of these models, see Ware, 1985.) However, extensions of models for discrete and other non-Gaussian responses are in their infancy. The problem is more difficult because the regression and time-dependence parts of a model for discrete data do not separate as they do in the Gaussian case. In fact, the interpretation of the regression coefficients depends on the assumed form for the time dependence. Three approaches to non-Gaussian longitudinal data have been suggested: transitional, mixed, and marginal models (Ware, Lipsitz, & Speizer, 1988). In a transitional model, the conditional distribution of a response given its past is expressed as a function of the X's and past Y's. Autoregressive time series models and Markov chains are examples. In mixed models (e.g., Stiratelli, Laird, & Ware, 1984), subject-specific parameters are assumed to follow a distribution across the population with expectation that depends on X. In marginal models, the cross-sectional average or marginal expectation of Y is described as a function of X. Zeger, Liang, and Albert (1988) and Zeger (1988) have discussed these three approaches.

This chapter illustrates the application of marginal models to a data set on the health status of Indonesian children. Our methods are extensions of GLMs to longitudinal data and hence are applicable to a variety of discrete and continuous responses common in biomedical research. The marginal approach focuses on the dependence of Y on X and treats the time dependence as a nuisance. The parameters characterize the dependence on X of the population-averaged response rather than the response for a single subject as in mixed models. Marginal models have been discussed previously by Zeger, Liang, and Self (1985); Liang and Zeger (1986); Moulton and Zeger (1989) and Wei and Stram (1988). The next section introduces the data set and establishes notation. Subsequent sections describe a simple but effective special case called the "independence" working model that can be used with minor changes to existing software; discuss models that explicitly account for time dependence; and consider several robustness issues.

APPLICATION DATA SET AND NOTATION

Our study population consisted of 3111 Indonesian children between the ages of 2 and 8 living in six villages located in Purwakarta, West Java, Indonesia (Government of Indonesia and Helen Keller International, 1980). Medical examinations were first performed on them in March, 1977, and the children were reexamined at three-month intervals over a period of one and one-half years, permitting a maximum of $T = 7$ observations on each child. The response variable of interest, xerophthalmia, is an ocular conjunctivitis caused by a deficiency of vitamin A. If untreated it can lead to severe corneal damage and blindness. The primary objective of our analysis was to identify risk factors for xerophthalmia. We screened a variety of covariates including age and weight-for-height, and retained diarrheal and respiratory disease variables for further analysis. These diseases may deplete a child's vitamin A stores, and their effect on the risk of xerophthalmia was thus of great interest.

The marginal model for the probability of xerophthalmia is the logistic regression:

$$\text{logit}[\text{prob}(XER = 1)] = \beta_1 \text{INT} + \beta_2 \text{DIA} + \beta_3 \text{RES} + \beta_4 \text{DIA*RES}$$

The coding is:

Variable	Meaning	Coding
XER	Evidence of xerophthalmia	No = 0/yes = 1
DIA	Diarrheal episode within last month	No = 0/yes = 1
RES	Respiratory infection at exam	No = 0/yes = 1

where $\text{INT} \equiv 1$ is the intercept term.

We now establish notation for an arbitrary GLM. We will assume (without loss of generality) that each of N individuals has the same number T of observations across time. Each response $y_{it}(i = 1, \ldots, N; \; t = 1, \ldots, T)$ is assumed to have error density given by

$$f_\phi(y_{it}; \theta_{it}) = \exp\left[\frac{y_{it}\theta_{it} - a(\theta_{it}) + b(y_{it}; \phi)}{\phi}\right]$$

where $\theta_{it} = h(\eta_{it})$, and $\eta_{it} = x'_{it}\beta$, where x_{it} is a $(p \times 1)$ vector of covariates. Note that the first two moments of y_{it} are

$$E(y_{it}) = \dot{a}(\theta_{it}) \qquad \text{var}(y_{it}) = \ddot{a}(\theta_{it})\phi$$

Furthermore, for each time point we define the matrices

$$\underset{N \times p}{X_t} = (x_{1t}, \ldots, x_{Nt})', \qquad \underset{N \times N}{V_t} = \text{diag}(\ddot{a}(\theta_{it})),$$

and

$$\underset{N \times N}{\Delta_t} = \text{diag}\left[\frac{\partial \theta_{it}}{\partial \eta_{it}}\right], \quad t = 1, \ldots, T.$$

Rearrangement of the elements of these matrices yields the matrices

$$\underset{T \times p}{X_i}, \; \underset{T \times T}{V_i}, \; \underset{T \times T}{\Delta_i}, \; i = 1, \ldots, N,$$

defined for each individual.

INDEPENDENCE WORKING APPROACHES

Independence Estimating Equations

This section describes an approach given in Zeger, Liang, and Self (1985) based on the "working" assumption that repeated responses for an individual are independent. The analysis proceeds "as if" the observations were independent, with the exception that a robust variance estimator is employed assuring consistent variance estimation regardless of the actual degree of dependence. The corresponding likelihood analysis solves the score equations:

$$\sum_{i=1}^{N} X'_i\Delta_i s_i = 0$$

where $s_i = (y_i - \dot{a}(\theta_i))$ is a vector of order $(T \times 1)$ for the ith individual. We'll call the solution of this equation the independence estimator $\hat{\beta}_I$. It characterizes the marginal expectation of the response and the covariates. If in fact the working assumption of independence were true, the variance of $\hat{\beta}_I$ could be consistently estimated by the inverse of the Fisher information matrix, $[H(\hat{\beta}_I)]^{-1} = [\Sigma_{i=1}^N (G'_i G_i)]^{-1}$, where $G_i = V_i^{1/2}\Delta_i X_i$. However, if there were dependence across time, this would not consistently estimate the variance of $\hat{\beta}_I$. A consistent estimator is given by

$$\text{var}(\hat{\beta}_I) = [H(\hat{\beta}_I)]^{-1}\left[\sum_{i=1}^{N} X_i'\Delta_i s_i s_i' \Delta_i X_i\right][H(\hat{\beta}_I)]^{-1}$$

Zeger (1988) and Liang and Zeger (1986) have shown $\hat{\beta}_I$ to be nearly efficient when the number of subjects is large, as is the case in many epidemiologic studies. This "independence" approach has the advantage of being readily implemented with standard software, for example SAS or the S system with its interface to GLIM (Chambers & Schilling, 1982).

Bootstrapping Functions of Time-Specific Coefficients

We now present another means of accounting for within-subject dependence without explicit estimation of the degree of correlation across time. Suppose that at each time point t we use the available observations to solve the score equations $X_t'\Delta_t s_t = 0$, thus obtaining the separate vectors of maximum likelihood estimates $\hat{\beta}_t$, $t = 1, \ldots, T$. There are numerous summary measures $\hat{\psi} \equiv \psi(\hat{\beta}_1, \ldots, \hat{\beta}_T)$ that may be of interest. When, as in the previous section, we assume there is an underlying β constant across time, we will want to calculate measures of central tendency of the $\hat{\beta}_t$, such as

$$\hat{\psi}_{mn} = \frac{1}{T}\sum_{t=1}^{T} \hat{\beta}_t \quad \text{or} \quad \hat{\psi}_{md} = \left[\begin{array}{ccc} \text{median}\,(\hat{\beta}_{1t}), & \ldots, & \text{median}\,(\hat{\beta}_{pt}) \\ t \in (1, \ldots, T) & & t \in (1, \ldots, T) \end{array}\right].$$

Or, if we wish to posit the nature of a possibly changing β, we can calculate the appropriate function of the $\hat{\beta}_t$. For example, if we are interested in linear trends of the coefficients over time, we can calculate

$$\hat{\psi}_{sl} = [\gamma_1, \ldots, \gamma_p]', \quad \text{where } \gamma_k = 12\left[\sum_t t\hat{\beta}_{kt} - \left(\frac{T+1}{2}\right)\sum_t \hat{\beta}_{kt}\right](T-1)T(T+1)$$

for the case of equally spaced time points.

The estimates $\hat{\beta}_t$ will be correlated when within-individual responses are correlated, and thus care must be taken in assessing the variability of a function $\hat{\psi}$. The elements of $\hat{\psi}_{mn}$ and $\hat{\psi}_{sl}$ will be asymptotically normally distributed, and if we had estimates of the pairwise covariances among the $\hat{\beta}_t$ we could estimate the variances of these functions and calculate Wald tests or confidence intervals. This will not, however, be the case for quantities such as $\hat{\psi}_{md}$, for which we resort to the bootstrap.

The bootstrap is a general technique for evaluating the variability in a statistic while making minimal assumptions about its distribution (Efron, 1979). There are several ways in which it may be applied. In the longitudinal data setting with missing data, we believe it is preferable to base the bootstrap on the empirical distribution function of each individual's complete data history (Moulton, 1986). Specifically, we use

$$\hat{F}: \text{mass } \frac{1}{N} \quad \text{at } (y_{i1}, \ldots, y_{iT}; x_{i1}, \ldots, x_{iT}) \qquad i = 1, \ldots, N$$

We thereby leave intact the dependence patterns within individuals, making no assumptions about their specific forms. The sampling distribution of $\hat{\psi}$ can be estimated by first drawing samples of size N from $\hat{F}$, obtaining replicated data sets $\{(y_t^{*b}, X_t^{*b}), t = 1, \ldots, T\}$, $b = 1, \ldots, B$. From each such "pseudo-data set" we can obtain a new set of time-specific β_t^{*b}, from which we calculate the quantities ψ^{*b}, $b = 1, \ldots, B$. The resulting distribution estimates the sampling distribution of $\hat{\psi}$. If only a standard deviation is required, $B = 100$ usually will suffice, while if we want to calculate percentile intervals, we will need to choose $B \geqslant 1000$. Considerable economy can be achieved by adopting a one-step approximation to the bootstrap distribution, which is used in our calculations (Moulton & Zeger, 1991).

Application of the Independence Techniques

The techniques of the foregoing sections capture the effect of dependence within sets of observations without explicit modeling of the dependence structure. We first compare inferences made about β through the use of $\hat{\beta}_I$ and $\hat{\psi}_{mn}$ and their estimated standard errors. The z statistics and confidence intervals for the logistic model parameters are given in Table 8-1. It is not surprising that the z-statistics are similar, for the two methods are asymptotically equivalent, and our N is quite large. The slight discrepancy between the two point estimates of β would diminish if we were to use means of the $\hat{\beta}_t$ weighted by the inverse of their variances instead of using equal weights. Variability is influenced by the substantial number of missing observations at each time point; an observation is defined as missing if at least one of the responses for XER, DIA, or RES was not known.

As can be seen in Table 8-2, the regression relationships at each of the seven time points were highly similar, without any clearly outlying coefficients. The $\hat{\psi}_{mn}$ and $\hat{\psi}_{md}$ estimates are therefore very close, although $\hat{\psi}_{md}$ has uniformly greater variability. This has been discussed by Moulton and Zeger (1989). $\hat{\psi}_{sl}$ represents the average change per observation time interval in the log odds ratio associated with each coefficient. For this data set, only the intercept term exhibited a significant change, with an estimated 11-percent average reduction in prevalence between observation times (95% CI: 8–14%).

Additional insight may be gained through plotting the sets of bootstrap coefficients $(\beta_t^{*b}, t = 1, \ldots, T)$ for each of many bootstrap replications. In Figure

Table 8–1. Independence estimates for the Indonesian xerophthalmia data[a]

Parameter	$\hat{\beta}_I$	SE	z	95%CI	$\hat{\psi}_{mn}$	SE	z	95%CI
INT[b]	−2.75	0.06	−48.2	(−2.86, −2.64)	−2.81	0.06	−46.6	(−2.92, −2.69)
DIA	1.33	0.11	12.0	(1.11, 1.55)	1.42	0.12	11.7	(1.18, 1.65)
RES	0.74	0.12	6.3	(0.51, 0.97)	0.66	0.13	5.0	(0.40, 0.92)
DIA*RES	−0.68	0.30	−2.3	(−1.27, −0.09)	−0.73	0.35	−2.1	(−1.43, −0.04)

[a] $\hat{\psi}_{mn}$ and SE based on 100 bootstrap replications.

[b] INT, intercept term; DIA, diarrheal episode in last month; RES, respiratory infection at time of examination.

Table 8-2. Maximum likelihood estimates (and asymptotic standard errors) for
the logistic regressions at each time point

Time	1	2	3	4	5	6	7
Sample size	2522	2035	1915	1741	2032	2197	2168
NT[a]	-2.29	-2.52	-2.87	-3.02	-2.92	-2.95	-3.04
	(0.07)	(0.09)	(0.11)	(0.12)	(0.11)	(0.10)	(0.11)
DIA	1.08	1.26	1.32	1.46	1.59	1.82	1.35
	(0.22)	(0.31)	(0.22)	(0.28)	(0.34)	(0.36)	(0.30)
RES	0.48	0.66	0.43	0.79	1.15	0.72	0.46
	(0.21)	(0.24)	(0.44)	(0.37)	(0.28)	(0.37)	(0.44)
DIA*RES	0.04	-1.19	-0.39	-0.04	-1.22	-0.69	-1.48
	(0.62)	(0.85)	(0.92)	(0.75)	(0.90)	(1.26)	(1.16)

NT, intercept term; DIA, diarrheal episode within last month; RES, respiratory infection at time of examination.

8-1 we see that the intercept (interpretable as log prevalence in the absence of the risk factors) decreases over the first four time points and then levels out. For the interaction term, however, there is a great deal more variability, especially at observation time 6. This is due to the fact that only four of the eighty-three observations with both DIA and RES present occurred at the sixth time point.

The methods give evidence of strong DIA and RES effects, with estimated odds ratios of about 4 for DIA and 2 for RES. The importance of the interaction term is less clear, for in spite of the large sample size it is not very statistically significant. Its estimate implies that there is virtually no increase in risk associated with respiratory infection for a child who has recently had diarrhea.

MODELING THE TIME DEPENDENCE

The techniques of the previous section yield asymptotically correct analyses regardless of the nature of the within-subject correlation structures. More efficient analyses of the data may be possible using the methods described in this section.

Weighted Least-Squares Estimation

The estimator $\hat{\psi}_{mn}$ presented previously is a simple average of the coefficient vectors estimated from the observations taken at each time point. In terms of efficiency, we can improve on this estimator by combining the estimates $\hat{\beta}_t$ through a weighted least-squares (WLS) calculation. The covariance matrix for any pair of vectors $(\hat{\beta}_t, \hat{\beta}_{t'})$ may be estimated consistently by

$$\widehat{\text{cov}}(\hat{\beta}_t, \hat{\beta}_{t'}) = (G_t'G_t)^{-1}G_t' \text{diag}(r_{it}r_{it'})G_{t'}(G_{t'}'G_{t'})^{-1}$$

where $G_t' = X_t'\Delta_t V_t^{1/2}$ and the r_{it} are the elements of the vector of Pearson residuals $r_t = V_t^{-1/2}s_t$.

This estimator may be derived either as the closed-form version of a

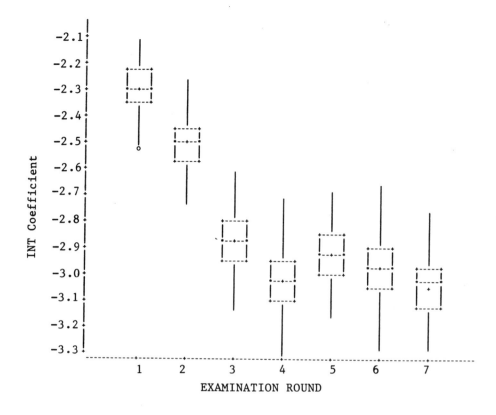

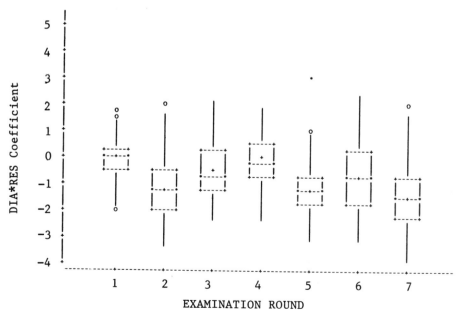

Figure 8–1. Box plots of 100 bootstrap coefficients by time point. INT, intercept term; DIA, diarrheal episode in last month; RES, respiratory infection at time of examination.

bootstrap approximation or as an extension of a robust variance estimator suggested by Huber (1967) (Moulton & Zeger, 1989). Thus the $(Tp \times Tp)$ covariance matrix $\hat{C}$ of the $(Tp \times 1)$ vector $\hat{b} = [\hat{\beta}'_1, \dots, \hat{\beta}'_T]'$ may be built from each of its T^2 submatrices $\widehat{\text{cov}}(\hat{\beta}_t, \hat{\beta}_{t'})$. The WLS estimator of the underlying β is given by

$$\hat{\beta}_M = (Z'\hat{C}^{-1}Z)^{-1}Z'\hat{C}^{-1}\hat{b}$$

where $\underset{Tp \times p}{Z} = (I_p, \dots, I_p)'$. The estimated variance of $\hat{\beta}_M$ is $(Z'\hat{C}^{-1}Z)^{-1}$. Note, however, that estimation of C will become unstable as the square of the length T of the series becomes large relative to N. In such a case it may be preferable to work separately with each variable's vector of time-specific coefficients and associated $T \times T$ covariance matrix, an approach adopted by Wei and Stram (1988). A GAUSS (Edlefsen & Jones, 1984) program to perform these analyses for the binary outcome case with logit link and complete data is provided in the appendix.

Missing data are handled easily under the assumption that observations are missing completely at random. When computing the $(p \times p)$ submatrix of $\hat{C}$ for a given pair (t, t') of time points, we merely ignore the pairs of observations for which at least one observation is missing. Let (c) indicate matrices that have been compressed by deleting elements corresponding to individuals for whom at least one observation is missing for the time points (t, t'). Then we may use

$$\widehat{\text{cov}}^{(c)}(\hat{\beta}_t, \hat{\beta}_{t'}) = (G'_t G_t)^{-1} X_t'^{(c)} \Delta_t^{(c)} V_t^{(c)} \, \text{diag}^{(c)}(r_{it} r_{it'}) V_{t'}^{(c)} \Delta_{t'}^{(c)} X_{t'}^{(c)} (G'_{t'} G_{t'})^{-1} \frac{N_t N_{t'}}{N_{tt'}^2}$$

where N_t and $N_{t'}$ are the numbers of valid observations at each time, $N_{tt'}$ is the number of valid pairs. Note that we are able to retain the original inverses of the estimated information matrices at both time points, which translates into higher efficiency.

The influence of individual observations on the estimate $\hat{\beta}_M$ is easily calculated. The approximate change in $\hat{\beta}_M$ corresponding either to the deletion of any given individual's entire set of observations, or to the deletion of any single observation, are respectively (here Δ means "change in")

$$\Delta_i \hat{\beta}_M^1 = (Z'\hat{C}^{-1}Z)^{-1}Z'\hat{C}^{-1}[\Delta_i \hat{\beta}_1^1 \cdots \Delta_i \hat{\beta}_T^1]'$$

$$\Delta_{it} \hat{\beta}_M^1 = (Z'\hat{C}^{-1}Z)^{-1}Z'\hat{C}^{-1}[0 \cdots 0 \, \Delta_i \hat{\beta}_t^1 \, 0 \cdots 0]'$$

where the one-step approximation given by Pregibon (1981) is performed for each time point (given here for a canonical link):

$$\Delta_i \hat{\beta}^1 = (X'VX)^{-1} x_i' \frac{y_i - \hat{y}_i}{1 - h_{ii}} \qquad i = 1, \dots, N$$

where h_{ii} is the ith diagonal element of $V^{1/2}X(X'VX)^{-1}X'V^{1/2}$. The elements of the $\Delta_i \hat{\beta}_M^1$ may be put on the same dimensionless scale by dividing them by the square roots of the diagonal elements of $(Z'\hat{C}^{-1}Z)^{-1}$. (For additional details, see Moulton, 1986.)

Generalized Estimating Equations

The estimation technique presented in the section "Independence Estimating Equations" can be generalized to include specification of an approximate correlation structure for the Y_i, the vectors of subjects' responses. We have $\text{cov}\,(Y_i) = V_i^{1/2}\text{corr}(Y_i)V_i^{1/2}\phi$. We can borrow strength across subjects to
$_{T \times T}$
estimate a common "working" correlation matrix $R(\alpha)$, characterized by a vector α of length m. With non-Gaussian responses, the actual correlation, like the variance, is usually a function of the mean. We can approximate the true correlation by a simpler form, $R(\alpha)$, without losing much efficiency. Defining $A_i = V_i^{1/2}R(\alpha)V_i^{1/2}\phi$, $D_i = V_i\Delta_i X_i$, the generalized estimating equations (GEEs) are defined to be

$$\sum_{1=i}^{N} D_i'A_i^{-1}s_i = 0$$

Note that when $R(\alpha)$ is the identity matrix these equations reduce to the independence equations given under "Independence Estimating Equations." The GEE can be solved by iterating between a modified Fisher scoring method for β and moment estimation of α and ϕ using the Pearson residuals $e_{it} = [y_{it} - \dot{a}(\hat{\theta}_{it})]/[\ddot{a}(\hat{\theta}_{it})]^{1/2}$ (Liang & Zeger, 1986). These are in general distinct from the r_{it} just defined in the previous section, as they are based on the data from all time points.

Being able to specify $R(\alpha)$ gives us great flexibility in model fitting. If we assume correlation is introduced by a random effect, that is, that each individul has a random response level (e.g., Laird & Ware, 1982), then we let $m = 1$ and use the working assumption that $\text{corr}(Y_{it}, Y_{it'}) = \alpha$ for all $t \neq t'$. This common correlation can be estimated simply by averaging all products of pairs of Pearson residuals (adjusting for deflation of the residuals):

$$\hat{\alpha} = \phi \sum_{i=1}^{N} \sum_{t>t'} \frac{e_{it}e_{it'}}{\left\{\dfrac{NT(T-1)}{2} - p\right\}}$$

When products are unavailable due to missing observations, the denominator is adjusted accordingly.

It may be that the degree of correlation is not constant across time, but is a function of the elapsed time between observations, in which case we may specify the elements of $R(\alpha)$ to be $\alpha_{|t-t'|}$. For the case of Gaussian response, this is the correlation structure of a stationary process. In this case, $E(e_{it}e_{it'}) = \alpha_{|t-t'|}$, and $E(\alpha)$ is a symmetric Toeplitz matrix, with each pair of subdiagonals estimated from

$$\hat{\alpha}_d = \sum_{|t-t'|=d} \frac{e_{it}e_{it'}}{2(T-d)} \qquad d = 1, \dots, T-1$$

If we do not wish to assume a particular correlation structure, we can use the information from all of the individuals to estimate separately each pairwise correlation; that is, we estimate each element of $R(\alpha)$, which now consists of

$m = T(T-1)/2$ distinct parameters. R can be estimated by

$$\frac{\phi}{N} \sum_{i=1}^{N} V_i^{-1/2} s_i s_i' V_i^{-1/2}$$

Although the asymptotic efficiency of our estimators can be high using this completely general form, caution must be applied in application when m is large relative to N, as was the case with the weighted least-squares method of the previous section.

Methods described in the foregoing two sections may be implemented by a compiled interactive FORTRAN77 program written by David Leon of the Population Council, and by an SAS/IML macro written by M. Rezaul Karim of The Johns Hopkins University, both available from Lawrence Moulton.

Application of Time-Dependent Models

Even though our data set has a maximum of only seven observations per subject, if we assume the subjects' observations share a common correlation structure we can take advantage of our large sample size to obtain an accurate assessment of it. We estimated the correlation for each pair of time points using all the nonmissing pairs of observations. The first line of Table 8-3 contains the medians of these correlations for each time lag. Also in Table 8-3 are the estimates of $R(\alpha)$ for the exchangeable and stationary working correlation structures; the stationary structure appears to be the most appropriate.

Table 8-4 contains the estimates obtained from applying the WLS method and the versions of the GEE approach, previously discussed, for stationary and exchangeable correlation. The GEE results under the two $R(\alpha)$ specifications are virtually identical and differ only slightly from the WLS estimates. The large sample size has masked efficiency differences, as all of the methods supply robust variance estimators that are consistent under any correlation structure.

Comparing the results displayed in Table 8-4 with those given in Table 8-1 we see that confidence intervals calculated using the methods of this section have uniformly smaller widths than the "independence" approaches. This accords with the higher efficiency associated with directly incorporating estimates of the degree of dependence across time. However, the differences in

Table 8–3. Estimated correlation structure of the Indonesian xerophthalmia data

	Observation time lag					
	1	2	3	4	5	6
Median of pairwise estimated correlations	0.48	0.40	0.31	0.35	0.33	0.27
Exchangeable correlation estimate of $R(\alpha)$	0.35	0.35	0.35	0.35	0.35	0.35
Stationary process estimate of $R(\alpha)$	0.46	0.36	0.29	0.30	0.30	0.24

Table 8–4. Dependence specification estimates for the Indonesian xerophthalmia data

Method	WLS[a]				GEE[b]: exchangeable correlation				GEE: autoregressive correlation			
Parameter	Est.	SE	Z	95% CI	Est.	SE	Z	95% CI	Est.	SE	Z	95% CI
INT[c]	-2.56	0.06	-42.1	(-2.68, -2.44)	-2.60	0.05	-48.1	(-2.70, -2.50)	-2.62	0.05	-48.8	(-2.73, -2.51)
DIA	1.22	0.11	11.2	(1.01, 1.44)	1.00	0.10	9.9	(0.80, 1.20)	0.97	0.10	9.6	(0.77, 1.17)
RES	0.86	0.11	7.6	(0.64, 1.09)	0.56	0.10	5.6	(0.36, 0.75)	0.56	0.10	5.7	(0.37, 0.76)
DIA*RES	-0.65	0.27	-2.4	(-1.19, -0.12)	-0.51	0.28	-1.8	(-1.06, 0.05)	-0.45	0.28	-1.6	(-1.00, 0.10)

[a]WLS, weighted least squares.
[b]GEE, generalized estimating equation.
[c]INT, intercept term; DIA, diarrheal episode in last month; RES, respiratory infection at time of examination.

interval width are quite small when we consider the high degree of correlation present in the data (Table 8-3). Again, the large sample size is responsible for the smallness of these observed differences.

We calculated the approximate contribution $\Delta_i \hat{\beta}_M^1$ of each child's entire set of observations to the WLS estimate $\hat{\beta}_M$, standardizing by the appropriate standard errors. The most extreme quantities were found for the interaction term DIA*RES. The twelve highest values correspond to children who at one time point had positive responses coded for XER, DIA, and RES, a profile that occurred in only 17 of the 14,610 nonmissing observations. Further investigation showed that two of these twelve children provided the only such profiles at the sixth and seventh time points; thus when their data are deleted, the DIA*RES parameter estimates from the logistic regressions fitted at these times diverge to minus infinity. This calls into question the stability of the overall interaction estimates to a greater degree than do their wide confidence intervals.

DISCUSSION

The statistical methods for the analysis of longitudinal data presented in this chapter are all concerned with modeling the marginal regression relationship between a response variable and a set of time-dependent covariates. In practice there are many situations (e.g., growth curve analysis) in which the coefficient vector β may also vary over time. We have already seen (under "Bootstrapping Functions...") how a bootstrap method can be used to investigate any function $\psi(\beta_1, \ldots, \beta_T)$. The GEE approach is also easily adapted to such a situation. For example, if we let $\beta_t = \gamma_0 + \gamma_1 t$, the degree of linear change over time can be evaluated as was done with the ψ_{sl} in the bootstrap method. The WLS method can accomplish the same goal by using the estimated covariance matrix $\hat{C}$ of the $\hat{\beta}_t$ to find the variance of any linear combination of the $\hat{\beta}_t$.

Although the Indonesian data set analyzed here consists of categorical variables, it is not amenable to a GSK analysis as described by Landis, Miller Davis, and Koch (1988) and by Koch et al. (1977). There is a small number of response profiles ($2^7 = 128$) relative to the number of children, but the time-dependent nature of the two covariates creates too many ($4^7 = 16,384$) potentially different subgroups to be considered as such.

As already discussed, the methods presented here are robust to misspecification of the dependence structure across time. One implication is that even though the methods have been conceived for observations that have the same interval spacings across subjects, this requirement may be relaxed. In the Indonesian data set, many of the observations in fact took place a month before or after the designated three-month interval, inducing many different correlation patterns between responses. This degree of variation, however, is minimal in view of the large sample size. Still, more work is needed to determine just how robust our methods will be for varying sample sizes and dependence structures.

The robust estimation of variance also protects us against other forms of model misspecification. Except for the bootstrap method, all of our methods make use of a robust variance estimator derived from a series expansion of the "working" score vector about the true parameter vector (Huber, 1967). Other examples of its application are found in White (1982), Pregibon (1983), and Royall (1986). When there is unexplained overdispersion, as is often the case with binomial and Poisson responses, the true variance matrix of the estimated coefficients is automatically consistently estimated. In the case of Gaussian response models, extra variance engendered by a random effect specified as fixed or by heterogeneity of errors is consistently taken into account.

Attrition of subjects is a major potential source of bias in longitudinal studies. In our analyses we have assumed the unobserved data to be missing completely at random. If, however, whether or not an observation is missing depends on variables of interest, bias in estimation of covariate effects is possible. Much investigation remains to be done on how different types of missing data situations are best handled.

A common problem in epidemiologic studies is that of exposure mis-classification. In the Indonesian data, for example, occurrence of diarrhea during the preceding month may have been underreported. The mean reported monthly incidence of 5.4 percent translates to an approximate average of $12(0.054) = 0.65$ episode per child-year, which seems a bit low. Suppose that 5 percent of the children classified as having had diarrhea actually did not, and that 10 percent of those from whom a negative response was obtained in fact had had an episode. This would yield a monthly incidence of 15 percent, for an average of about two episodes per child-year. A method provided by Reade and Kupper (1990) permits any of the methods of this chapter to estimate the bias in the estimate of β_{DIA} that would result from such a misclassification scenario. The binary variable DIA is merely replaced by $MDIA = 0.95(DIA) + 0.1(1 - DIA)$. Using MDIA in the WLS method (the other methods would give similar results), we get the overall estimate of the odds ratio $\exp(\hat{\beta}_{MDIA}) = 4.2$, compared with $\exp(\hat{\beta}_{DIA}) = 3.4$. The statistical significance remains unchanged, but the object is to evaluate the degree of potential bias caused by misclassification.

We remind the reader that there are many situations in which an analysis that models a marginal regression relationship will be less than satisfactory. The analysis of growth curves often calls for a mixed-effects model where each subject has a separate parameter vector. In many psychological or sociological studies a transitional model is needed to model directly the nature of change or correlation. Conditioning on past events may be particularly desirable when the phenomenon under study contains a feedback loop wherein the independent variable at one point in time depends on the "dependent" variable response at a previous time. For example, it may be that signs of xerophthalmia place a child into a higher risk category for future respiratory infection, as it indicates vitamin A depletion which in turn may lower resistance. In such a case, modeling only the marginal distribution would exaggerate the importance of respiratory infection as a cause of xerophthalmia. Only a conditional model could eliminate such a bias.

In summary, these methods are useful for a wide class of discrete and continuous outcomes. They are robust to several departures from the specified analytic model, the most important of which is the nature of the dependence among observations. Moreover, their close relationship to regression models for data collected at one point in time allows the use of current data-analytic techniques.

Appendix

```
/* This no-frills GAUSS(tm) program is for the case of repeated measures on a binary
response variable with no missing data.
    Logistic regression coefficients are calculated for data from each of T time points,
and then combined through a weighted least squares calculation as described in
the section "Weighted Least-Squares Estimation."
    The data is input from a GAUSS data set of the form:

                    y1 y2 ··· yT x1 x2 ··· xT

where the yt are the N × 1 response vectors at each time and the xt are the
corresponding N × np matrices of regressors. The first column of each x-matrix
should be a vector of ones for the intercept.
    Change the following line to indicate the number of time points: */
        T = 2;                          @ t = # of time points           @
new;
load dta = a:lgt.dta;                   @ get the file lgt.dta           @
    output file = lgt.out reset;
n = rows(dta); np = (cols(dta) − t)/t;  @ find # of individuals and      @
                                          parameters                     @
yy = dta[.,1:t];                        @ separate the y's from the x's  @
xx = dta[.,t + 1:t + t*np];

tt = 1;
do while tt < = t;                      @ loop over time points          @
y = yy[.,tt]; x = xx[.,(tt − 1)*np + 1:(tt − 1)*np + np];   @pick off y and x at time t@
b0 = zeros(np, 1);                      @ initialize before beginning iterations@
p = .5*ones(n,1);
db = 1; bf = 1; iter = 1;
                                        @ iter loop and convergence test @
do while (sumc((abs(db./bf) .> 1e − 4) > 0)) and (iter < 30);
rtv = sqrt(p.*(1 − p));
g = x.*rtv;
s = y − p;
r = s./rtv;                             @ r is vector of Pearson residuals @
bf = b0 + r/g;                          @ bf is current estimate of beta @
db = bf − b0;
p = 1/(1 + exp(−x*bf));
l = sumc(y.*ln(p) + (1 − y).*ln(1 − p));    @ calculation of the log-likelihood @
format 2,0;  "iteration" iter;          @ print relevant iteration info  @
format 12,6; "log lik"    l;
              "beta"         bf';
```

```
iter = iter + 1;    b0 = bf;                @ update beta                        @
endo;
var = invpd(g'*g); se = sqrt(diag(var));   @ var is inverse of the             @
                                           @ information matrix                 @
sdix = x.*s;                               @ sdix = diag(y − p) *x              @
@ concatenate results from each time point @
if tt = = 1;   tsdixv = sdix*var;   tb = bf;
   else;        tsdixv = tsdixv ~ (sdix*var);   tb = tb|bf;
endif;
format 12,6; ?; "Time = " tt;?;            @ print logistic regression          @
          "  Est. Beta = " bf';            @ results from this time             @
          "      S.E. = " se'; ?;
tt = tt + 1;
endo; ?;
    @ make C Inverse, with which to weight the betas from each time             @
    @ if get a non-positive definite matrix, go on to the alternate method      @
    ts2 = tsdixv'*tsdixv;
        trap 1;
      ci = invpd(ts2);
        if scalerr(ci); goto altern; endif;
      z = ones(t, 1).*.eye(np);            @ make z by stacking identities      @
      varo = invpd(z'*ci*z);               @ asymptotic variance of             @
        if scalerr(ci); goto altern; endif;
      b = varo*z'*ci*tb;                   @ the overall beta                   @
      seo = sqrt(diag(varo));
ast = chrs(ones(59,1)*42); ast;            @ output results                     @
      ?; "      Overall Beta = " b';
      ?; "S.E. of Overall Beta = " seo';
    ast;
altern:
    @ ignoring across-time coefficient covariances; use if ci too unstable      @
pp = 0; tseq = seqa(0,1,t); bfin = zeros(np,1); sefin = bfin;
do while pp < np; pp = pp + 1;             @ calculate separately for each parameter  @
      coord = pp + tseq*np;
      vto = submat(ts2,coord,coord); bt = submat(tb,coord,1);
      vti = invpd(vto);
      vtis = sumc(sumc(vti));
      bfin[pp,1] = sumc(vti*bt)/vtis;
      sefin[pp,1] = sqrt(1/vtis);
endo;
      ?; "      Alternate Beta = " bfin';
      ?; "  S.E. of Alt. Beta = " sefin';
ast;
```

ACKNOWLEDGMENTS

We thank Dr. Alfred Sommer of the International Center for Epidemiologic and Preventive Ophthalmology for providing the data on xerophthalmia in Indonesia. We also thank Paul Albert for expert programming support.

REFERENCES

Baker RJ, Nelder JA (1986). *The GLIM System, Release 3. Generalised Linear Interactive Modelling*. Oxford, Numerical Algorithms Group.

Chambers JM, Schilling JM (1982). "S and GLIM: An experiment in interfacing statistical systems." *GLIM Newsletter* 6:43–50.

Conaway MR (1989). "Analysis of repeated categorical measurements with conditional likelihood methods. *Journal of the American Statistical Association* 84:53–62.

Edlefsen LE, Jones SD (1984). *The GAUSS Programming Language*. Kent, Wash., Applied Technical Systems.

Efron B (1979). "Bootstrap methods: Another look at the jackknife." *Annals of Statistics* 7:1–26.

Government of Indonesia and Helen Keller International (1980). *Nutritional Blindness Prevention Project*. New York, Helen Keller International.

Huber PJ (1967). *The Behavior of Maximum Likelihood Estimates under Nonstandard Conditions*. Proceedings of the Fifth Berkeley Symposium on Mathematical Statistics and Probability. Berkeley and Los Angeles, University of California Press, Vol 1, pp 221–233.

Koch GG, Landis JR, Freeman JL, Freeman DH Jr, Lehnen RG (1977). "A general methodology for the analysis of experiments with repeated measurement of categorical data." *Biometrics* 33:133–158.

Laird NM, Ware JH (1982). "Random-effects models for longitudinal data." *Biometrics* 38:963–974.

Landis JR, Miller ME, Davis CS, Koch GG (1988). "Some general methods for the analysis of categorical data in longitudinal studies." *Statistics in Medicine* 7:109–138.

Liang K-Y, Zeger SL (1986). "Longitudinal data analysis using generalized linear models." *Biometrika* 73:13–22.

McCullagh P, Nelder JA (1989). *Generalized Linear Models*, 2nd ed. London, Chapman and Hall.

Moulton LH (1986). "Bootstrapping generalized linear models with application to longitudinal data." PhD diss., Johns Hopkins University.

Moulton LH, Zeger SL (1989). "Analyzing repeated measures on generalized linear models via the bootstrap." *Biometrics* 45:381–394.

Moulton LH, Zeger SL (1991). "Bootstrapping generalized linear models." *Computational Statistics and Data Analysis*, to appear.

Pregibon D (1981). "Logistic regression diagnostics.' *Annals of Statistics* 4:705–724.

Pregibon D (1983). "An alternative covariance estimated for generalized linear models." *GLIM Newsletter* 6:51–55.

Prentice RL (1988). "Correlated binary regression with covariates specific to each binary observation." *Biometrics* 44:1033–1048.

Reade SJ, Kupper, LL (1990). "Effects of exposure misclassification on regression analyses of epidemiologic follow-up study data." *Biometrics*, in press.

Royall RM (1986). "Model robust confidence intervals using maximum likelihood estimators." *International Statistical Review* 54:221–226.

Stiratelli R, Laird N, Ware JH (1984). "Random effects models for serial observations with binary response." *Biometrics* 40:961–971.

Ware JH (1985). "Linear models for the analysis of longitudinal studies." *American Statistician* 39:95–101.

Ware JH, Lipsitz S, Speizer FE (1988). "Issues in the analysis of repeated categorical outcomes." *Statistics in Medicine* 7:95–108.

Wei LJ, Stram, DO (1988). "Analysing repeated measures with possibly missing observations by modelling marginal distributions." *Statistics in medicine* 7:139–148.

White H (1982). "Maximum likelihood estimation of misspecified models." *Econometrica* 50:1–25.

Zeger SL (1988). "The analysis of discrete longitudinal data: Discussion." *Statistics in Medicine* 7:161–168.

Zeger SL, Liang K-Y, Albert P (1988). "Models for longitudinal data, a generalized estimating equation approach." *Biometrics* 44:1049–1060.

Zeger SL, Liang K-Y, Self SG (1985). "The analysis of binary longitudinal data with time independent covariates." *Biometrika* 72:31–38.

Zeger SL, Qaqish B (1988). "Markov regression models for time series: A quasi-likelihood approach." *Biometrics* 44:1019–1031.

9

Some Aspects of Weighted Least-Squares Analysis for Longitudinal Categorical Data
Application: Clinical Trial of Treatment for Skin Disorder

GARY KOCH, JULIO SINGER, AND MAURA STOKES
IN COLLABORATION WITH
GREGORY CARR, STEVEN COHEN, AND RONALD FORTHOFER

In the statistical literature, longitudinal studies encompass investigations of the behavior of one or more response variables along a specific dimension. Usually this dimension is time, but it can also be distance from some reference point or intensities of a particular stimulus. Some situations that represent longitudinal studies are the following:

1. Clinical trials to evaluate the nature of improvement over time for patients receiving treatment for a health disorder
2. Surveys to explore changes over time in the utilization pattern of health and social services
3. Surveys to investigate the effects of successively more compelling information in a sequence of questions in which respondents choose between alternative actions

This chapter describes ways of using weighted least-squares (WLS) methods to address statistical questions of interest for longitudinal studies with sufficiently large samples. This introductory section summarizes noteworthy features of longitudinal studies; a more comprehensive discussion of these issues is given elsewhere—for example, Cook and Ware (1983), Singer (1985), Ware (1985), and Koch, Elashoff, and Amara (1986), and their bibliographies. Technical aspects of weighted least-squares methodology are presented in the second section together with some comments on alternative statistical procedures. The application of WLS methods is illustrated through some examples in the third section. A relatively casual examination of the second section provides sufficient background for following the discussion of examples in the third section, and a careful reading of these examples will enhance understanding of the technical aspects of WLS methods.

Computing procedures for obtaining the results for the examples in the third section are described in the appendix.

As a further consideration it is appropriate to note that the characterization of longitudinal studies given here does not include follow-up studies for the time until the occurrence of some target event like death or failure. Statistical methods for such situations are beyond the scope of this chapter (see Cox & Oakes, 1984; Kalbfleisch & Prentice, 1980; Lee, 1980).

OBJECTIVES AND GENERAL METHODS

Some Statistical Objectives for Longitudinal Studies

The subjects in longitudinal studies often come from two or more subpopulations. The corresponding groups might be based on a randomly assigned experimental factor such as treatment in a clinical trial or a demographic characteristic such as sex; also, they might represent the cross-classification of two or more factors or explanatory variables. The subjects in each group have their responses observed for a sequence of distinct conditions over some underlying dimension; such conditions usually correspond to occasions or waves of measurement over time. Under this framework, some statistical objectives for analysis are as follows:

1. Comparisons among groups for the (across conditions) average distributions of responses (i.e., the evaluation of group effects)
2. Comparisons among conditions for the (across groups) average distributions of responses (i.e., the evaluation of condition effects)
3. Comparisons among groups for changes over conditions in the distributions of response variables (i.e., group × condition interaction)
4. Description of the pattern of variation of response distributions across groups and conditions
5. Description of the pattern of variation of response transition distributions across groups and conditions.

These objectives need to be addressed by methods that appropriately account for the multivariate structure of the data for the respective conditions. For categorical responses, this consideration implies that well-known methods such as logistic regression (see Imrey et al., 1981, 1982) or the Mantel-Haenszel procedure (see Mantel, 1963) have limited utility because of their univariate nature.

Sampling Process, Measurement Scale, and Data Structure

Sampling process considerations are important for any type of study because they identify the basis for inference from the observed data to the target population, that is, the population for which conclusions are to be formulated.

Three sampling processes that encompass most longitudinal studies are as follows:

1. Historical/observational enumerations of all subjects in a defined population through prospective and/or retrospective procedures (e.g., the administrative records for the experience of all patients treated for a specific disorder at a specific clinic during a specific time period)
2. Experiments with randomized allocation of subjects to treatments
3. Sample surveys based on probability random selection of subjects from the target population

Analyses that directly account for the sampling process and do not involve external assumptions about the distributions of the data are said to provide design-based inferences for the target population. Such methodology is often applied to sample surveys; an application involving weighted least squares is given in Koch and Stokes (1982) (see also the example in the section "Estimates from a National Survey"). Design-based inference is also occasionally of interest for comparisons among treatments for the population of all randomized subjects in an experiment. Analyses for this purpose can be undertaken with nonparametric randomization methods such as the Kruskal–Wallis (1953) statistic, the extended Mantel–Haenszel (Mantel, 1963) statistic, or their multivariate counterparts. An example illustrating the application of such methods to a longitudinal study is given in Koch, Carr, Amara, Stokes, and Uryniak (1990). However, usually the data from subjects in experiments are assumed to be representative of a broadly defined, conceptual (target) population through some statistical model for its probability distribution. Analyses of the resulting framework by maximum likelihood, weighted least squares, or some other appropriate method provide model-based inferences. Also, inferences pertaining to the assumed structure of a stochastic process such as a Markov chain are model based. A worthwhile advantage of model-based inferences is their broader scope (as encompassed by the conceptual population or process for which they are claimed), while a noteworthy limitation is the usually unknown validity of their underlying assumptions. Contrarily, design-based inferences have the advantage of being essentially assumption free, but they also have the limitation of applying only to the population actually encompassed by the (explicitly applied) sampling process. Thus each of these types of inference is of interest, and often analyses directed at both are desirable for complementary purposes (see Koch, Amara, Davis, & Gillings, 1982; Koch, Amara, & Singer, 1985; and Koch & Gillings, 1983, for further discussion of these issues).

The measurement scale of response variables expresses the nature of information available for statistical analysis. In this chapter attention is given primarily to categorical data, although the methodology discussed has some applicability to data with a continuous distribution. The scope of categorical data includes the following specific types of response variables:

1. Dichotomous classifications, for example the occurrence or not of a particular symptom
2. Nominal classifications (with no ordering among three or more outcomes), for example type of health service used

3. Ordinal classifications, for example excellent, good, fair, or poor relief of pain
4. Discrete enumerations, for example number of headaches during a week
5. Grouped data along a continuum, for example relative to a sequence of stimuli with increasing intensity, the interval between the lowest level for which an outcome occurs and the highest level for which it does not occur

In general the subpopulations can be based on either categorical or continuously distributed explanatory variables. Most applications of weighted least-squares methods, however, require a fixed set of subpopulations with moderately large groups of observed subjects. Thus in the subsequent discussion, subpopulations are assumed to be based on the cross-classification of categorical explanatory variables.

An important feature of the data structure for longitudinal studies is the number of conditions d for which subjects are observed. If d is relatively small (e.g., 12 or less), conditions can be viewed as a fixed factor. Analysis can then be undertaken to describe the pattern of variation of response distributions across both conditions and groups. Weighted least-squares methods are potentially useful for this purpose provided that consistent estimates for the covariance matrices of responses for the conditions can be constructed for the respective subpopulations. For such covariance matrix extimation to be feasible, the sample sizes (n_i) for all groups need to be sufficiently large; for example $n_i \geqslant (d + 25)$. When d is large (e.g., $d \geqslant 30$), analysis of conditions as a fixed factor may not be reasonable. For these situations, another methodology is needed, such as categorical data counterparts to the random-effects models and the autoregressive models, discussed in Ware (1985), (see also Liang & Zeger, 1986; Stiratelli, Laird, & Ware, 1984; and Zeger & Liang, 1986).

WEIGHTED LEAST-SQUARES METHODS

This section describes the technical background that pertains to the use of weighted least-squares methods for the analysis of longitudinal categorical data. For reference purposes, it is convenient to consider the data structure shown in Table 9-1. There, y_{ijk} represents the response of the kth subject in the ith group for the jth condition; $i = 1, 2, \ldots, s; j = 1, 2, \ldots, d; k = 1, 2, \ldots, n_i$. The possible outcomes of each y_{ijk} are indexed by $l = 0, 1, 2, \ldots, L$ for the classification of the corresponding subject into one of $(L + 1)$ categories of a binary $(L = 1)$, nominal, or ordinal scale. More generally, the set of possible outcomes can pertain to multivariate profiles of responses. For each group the n_i subjects are assumed to be representative of a corresponding infinite subpopulation in the sense of simple random sampling.

The statistical objectives outlined at the beginning of this chapter can be addressed through the testing of hypotheses or fitting of models for relevant summary functions of the data from the respective groups and conditions. For comparisons (1) through (3) and the pattern of variation description (4), attention can be restricted to the first-order marginal distributions of response

Table 9–1. Basic data array for longitudinal studies

Group	Subjects within groups	Conditions 1	2	...	d
1	1	y_{111}	y_{121}	...	y_{1d1}
1	2	y_{112}	y_{122}	...	y_{1d2}
$\vdots$	$\vdots$	$\vdots$	$\vdots$		$\vdots$
1	n_1	y_{11n_1}	y_{12n_1}	...	y_{1dn_1}
2	1	y_{211}	y_{221}	...	y_{2d1}
2	2	y_{212}	y_{222}	...	y_{2d2}
$\vdots$	$\vdots$	$\vdots$	$\vdots$		$\vdots$
2	n_2	y_{21n_2}	y_{22n_2}	...	y_{2dn_2}
$\vdots$	$\vdots$	$\vdots$	$\vdots$		$\vdots$
s	1	y_{s11}	y_{s21}	...	y_{sd1}
s	2	y_{s12}	y_{s22}	...	y_{sd2}
$\vdots$	$\vdots$	$\vdots$	$\vdots$		$\vdots$
s	n_s	y_{s1n_s}	y_{s2n_s}	...	y_{sdn_s}

at each condition, that is, to the $\phi_{ijl} = \mathrm{pr}(y_{ijk} = l)$. Analysis can then be undertaken in a spirit similar to that provided for continuously distributed data by multivariate analysis of variance methods.

The most straightforward situation involves an ordinally scaled (or binary) response for which there is interest in the variation of the mean scores $\mu_{ij} = \Sigma_{l=0}^{L} m_l \phi_{ijl}$ with respect to the values $m_0, m_1, \ldots, m_L$ across the groups and conditions; in the binary case, $m_0 = 0$, $m_1 = 1$ leads to $\mu_{ij} = \phi_{ij1}$. The hypotheses corresponding to the statistical objectives (1) through (3) can be expressed in terms of the (μ_{ij}) as follows:

$$H_{01}: \mu_{1j} = \mu_{2j} = \cdots = \mu_{sj} \quad j = 1, 2, \ldots, d$$

$$H_{02}: \mu_{i1} = \mu_{i2} = \cdots = \mu_{id} \quad i = 1, 2, \ldots, s \tag{1}$$

$$H_{03}: \mu_{1j} - \mu_{1d} = \mu_{2j} - \mu_{2d} = \cdots = \mu_{sj} - \mu_{sd} \quad j = 1, 2, \ldots, (d-1).$$

Alternatively, the hypothesis H_{03} of no interaction between groups and conditions can be formulated in terms of the additive model

$$H_{03}: \mu_{ij} = \mu + \xi_i + \tau_j \tag{2}$$

With the restrictions $\xi_1 = 0$ and $\tau_1 = 0$, μ denotes the reference mean for group 1 and condition 1, ξ_i represents the increment for the ith group, and τ_j represents the increment for the jth condition. When the model (2) provides a satisfactory description of the (μ_{ij}), the hypotheses of no differences among groups and no differences among conditions can be expressed as

$$H_{01}^*: \xi_1 = \xi_2 = \cdots = \xi_s = 0$$

$$H_{02}^*: \tau_1 = \tau_2 = \cdots = \tau_d = 0 \tag{3}$$

Other hypotheses can be specified to address the structure of group effects and condition effects, for example, the role of cross-classified factors.

Estimates of the (μ_{ij}) are obtained by computing the across-subjects means $(\bar{g}_{ij})$ of the finite scores (m_l) that is, $\bar{g}_{ij} = (\Sigma_{k=1}^{n_i} g_{ijk}/n_i)$, where $g_{ijk} = m_l$ for $y_{ijk} = l$. Let $\mathbf{g}_{i*k} = (g_{i1k}, \ldots, g_{idk})'$ denote the $(d \times 1)$ vector of response scores for the kth subject in the ith group; then $\bar{\mathbf{g}}_i = \Sigma_{k=1}^{n_i} (\mathbf{g}_{i*k}/n_i)$ represents the vector of mean scores at the d conditions for the ith group. When the sample sizes (n_i) are sufficiently large (e.g., $n_i \geqslant (d + 25)$), then the $(\bar{\mathbf{g}}_i)$ approximately have multivariate normal distributions; consistent estimates for the corresponding covariance matrices are the

$$\mathbf{V}_{g,i} = \frac{1}{n_i^2} \sum_{k=1}^{n_i} (\mathbf{g}_{i*k} - \bar{\mathbf{g}}_i)(\mathbf{g}_{i*k} - \bar{\mathbf{g}}_i)' \tag{4}$$

In (4) it is sometimes preferable to replace the divisor n_i^2 by $(n_i(n_i - 1))$ for moderate sample sizes; the divisor n_i^2 arises when $\bar{\mathbf{g}}_i$ and $\mathbf{V}_{g,i}$ are computed by matrix operations on the $(d + 1)$-dimensional contingency table for the cross-classification of the s groups with the $(L + 1)^d$ possible scores for the (g_{ijk}). An illustration of this computational framework is given later in this chapter ("Analysis of the Proportions Excellent") (See also Koch et al., 1977; Landis & Koch, 1979.)

Linear models like (2) for describing the variation among the (μ_{ij}) have the general form

$$\boldsymbol{\mu} = \mathbf{X}\boldsymbol{\beta} \tag{5}$$

where $\boldsymbol{\mu} = (\mu_{11}, \mu_{12}, \ldots, \mu_{1d}, \mu_{21}, \ldots, \mu_{sd})'$, $\mathbf{X}$ is a known (sd $\times$ t) model specification matrix with full rank $t \leqslant \mathrm{sd}$, and $\boldsymbol{\beta}$ is the $(t \times 1)$ vector of unknown parameters. The elements of $\boldsymbol{\beta}$ are coefficients of the corresponding columns of $\mathbf{X}$; for a model like (2) they would represent the parameters μ, (ξ_i), and (τ_j), and the rows of $\mathbf{X}$ would be indicator variables with the value 1 for the parameters that applied to the respective (μ_{ij}) and the value 0 otherwise. The weighted least-squares (WLS) estimator $\mathbf{b}$ for $\boldsymbol{\beta}$ is given by

$$\mathbf{b} = (\mathbf{X}'\mathbf{V}_{\bar{g}}^{-1}\mathbf{X})^{-1}\mathbf{X}'\mathbf{V}_{\bar{g}}^{-1}\bar{\mathbf{g}} \tag{6}$$

where $\bar{\mathbf{g}} = (\bar{\mathbf{g}}_1', \bar{\mathbf{g}}_2', \ldots, \bar{\mathbf{g}}_s')'$ is the composite vector of means $(\bar{g}_{ij})$ for all (group $\times$ condition) combinations; also, $\mathbf{V}_{\bar{g}}$ is the (sd $\times$ sd) block diagonal matrix with the $(\mathbf{V}_{g,i})$ as the diagonal blocks and hence is a consistent estimate for the covariance matrix of $\bar{\mathbf{g}}$. The minimized value for the weighted residual sums of squares

$$Q_W = (\bar{\mathbf{g}} - \mathbf{X}\mathbf{b})'\mathbf{V}_{\bar{g}}^{-1}(\bar{\mathbf{g}} - \mathbf{X}\mathbf{b}) \tag{7}$$

of differences between $\bar{\mathbf{g}}$ and its predicted value $\hat{\boldsymbol{\mu}} = \mathbf{X}\mathbf{b}$ provides a goodness-of-fit statistic for the model (5). When the (μ_{ij}) are compatible with (5), Q_W approximately has the chi-square distribution with (sd $-$ t) degrees of freedom (df). Some additional insight concerning Q_W is provided by its identity to the Wald statistic

$$Q_W = \bar{\mathbf{g}}'\mathbf{W}'(\mathbf{W}\mathbf{V}_{\bar{g}}\mathbf{W}')^{-1}\mathbf{W}\bar{\mathbf{g}}$$

where $\mathbf{W}$ is a full rank ((sd $-$ t) $\times$ sd) orthocomplement to $\mathbf{X}'$ (i.e., $\mathbf{W}\mathbf{X} = 0$); the matrix $\mathbf{W}$ specifies the constraint formulation $\mathbf{W}\boldsymbol{\mu} = \mathbf{0}$ of the model. (For further discussion, see Koch and Bhapkar, 1982.)

The WLS estimates $\mathbf{b}$ approximately have a multivariate normal distribution for which

$$\mathbf{V_b} = (\mathbf{X}'\mathbf{V}_{\bar{g}}^{-1}\mathbf{X})^{-1} \tag{8}$$

provides a consistent estimate of the covariance matrix (i.e., an estimate that is essentially the same as the actual covariance matrix of $\mathbf{b}$ for sufficiently large (n_i)); these properties follow from the approximate normality of $\bar{\mathbf{g}}$ (when the (n_i) are sufficiently large relative to potential skewness for distributions of elements of $\bar{\mathbf{g}}$) and the use of linear Taylor series methods along the lines shown in Koch, Imrey, et al. (1985). They are also a consequence of the identity of $\mathbf{b}$ to the Neyman (1949) minimum modified chi-square estimator of $\boldsymbol{\beta}$ in the $(d + 1)$-dimensional contingency table for summarizing the data (see Bhapkar, 1966; Koch et al., 1977; Koch, Imrey, et al., 1985). An additional point of interest is that replacement of $\mathbf{V}_{\bar{g}}$ in (6) by the (sd × sd) diagonal matrix $\mathbf{D}_n^{-1}$, where $\mathbf{n} = (n_1, \ldots, n_1, n_2, \ldots, n_2, \ldots, n_s, \ldots, n_s)'$ is the (sd × 1) vector of sample sizes for the respective (group × condition) combinations, yields the ordinary least-squares estimates $\tilde{\mathbf{b}}$ of $\boldsymbol{\beta}$. Although $\tilde{\mathbf{b}}$ is an unbiased estimator of $\boldsymbol{\beta}$, variances that apply to it are larger than those for its weighted least-squares counterpart $\mathbf{b}$; also, $\tilde{\mathbf{b}}$ does not have direct linkage to a goodness-of-fit statistic as $\mathbf{b}$ does for Q_W in (7).

For models considered to provide a satisfactory description of the variation in $\boldsymbol{\mu}$, evaluation can be given to hypotheses

$$H_{\text{OC}}: \mathbf{C}\boldsymbol{\beta} = \mathbf{0} \tag{9}$$

where $\mathbf{C}$ is a known $(c \times t)$ matrix with full rank c. Examples of such hypotheses include specifications that certain elements of $\boldsymbol{\beta}$ are 0 or that differences between elements of $\boldsymbol{\beta}$ are 0. Under H_{OC}, the test statistic

$$Q_C = \mathbf{b}'\mathbf{C}'(\mathbf{C}\mathbf{V}_b\mathbf{C}')^{-1}\mathbf{C}\mathbf{b} \tag{10}$$

approximately has the chi-square distribution with df $= c$. Another noteworthy feature of Q_C is that it represents the amount by which the goodness-of-fit statistic Q_W in (7) would increase if the model (5) were simplified by accounting for the constraints (9); that is, if $\mathbf{Z}'$ denotes a $((t - c) \times t)$ orthocomplement to $\mathbf{C}$, then the goodness-of-fit statistic (7) for the reduced model $\mathbf{X}_c = \mathbf{X}\mathbf{Z}$ is identical to $Q_{W'c} = (Q_W + Q_C)$. Thus the usage of $\mathbf{C}$ matrices to test hypotheses like (9) enables the evaluation of the compatibility of the (μ_{ij}) with reduced models without requiring the fitting of such models. Predicted values for $\boldsymbol{\mu}$ from the model (5) are obtained via

$$\hat{\boldsymbol{\mu}} = \mathbf{X}\mathbf{b} \tag{11}$$

a consistent estimate for their covariance matrix is

$$\mathbf{V}_{\hat{\mu}} = \mathbf{X}\mathbf{V}_b\mathbf{X}' \tag{12}$$

where $\mathbf{V}_b$ is the estimated covariance matrix (8) for $\mathbf{b}$. The predicted values $\hat{\boldsymbol{\mu}}$ are descriptively useful by expressing the relationship of $\bar{\mathbf{g}}$ to the components of $\mathbf{X}$. They also have smaller variances than their counterparts in $\bar{\mathbf{g}}$ because they are based on an estimation process for which sources of extraneous variability (i.e., the observed model constraints $\mathbf{W}\bar{\mathbf{g}}$) are eliminated.

The application of the WLS methodology in (5) through (10) to the hypotheses and models specified in (1) through (3) can be illustrated by considering the special case of $s =$ two groups and $d =$ three conditions. The framework for assessing the hypotheses (1) is the cell mean model $\mathbf{X} = \mathbf{I}_6$ where $\mathbf{I}_6$ is the (6×6) identity matrix. For $H_{01}, H_{02},$ and $H_{03},$ the respective $\mathbf{C}$ matrices for use in (10) are

$$\mathbf{C}_1 = \begin{bmatrix} 1 & 0 & 0 & -1 & 0 & 0 \\ 0 & 1 & 0 & 0 & -1 & 0 \\ 0 & 0 & 1 & 0 & 0 & -1 \end{bmatrix}$$

$$\mathbf{C}_2 = \begin{bmatrix} 1 & -1 & 0 & 0 & 0 & 0 \\ 1 & 0 & -1 & 0 & 0 & 0 \\ 0 & 0 & 0 & 1 & -1 & 0 \\ 0 & 0 & 0 & 1 & 0 & -1 \end{bmatrix}$$

$$\mathbf{C}_3 = \begin{bmatrix} 1 & -1 & 0 & -1 & 1 & 0 \\ 1 & 0 & -1 & -1 & 0 & 1 \end{bmatrix}$$

The additive model (2) has the specification

$$\boldsymbol{\mu} = \begin{bmatrix} \mu_{11} \\ \mu_{12} \\ \mu_{13} \\ \mu_{21} \\ \mu_{22} \\ \mu_{23} \end{bmatrix} = \begin{bmatrix} 1 & 0 & 0 & 0 \\ 1 & 0 & 1 & 0 \\ 1 & 0 & 0 & 1 \\ 1 & 1 & 0 & 0 \\ 1 & 1 & 1 & 0 \\ 1 & 1 & 0 & 1 \end{bmatrix} \begin{bmatrix} \mu \\ \xi_2 \\ \tau_2 \\ \tau_3 \end{bmatrix} = \mathbf{X}\boldsymbol{\beta}$$

Given that the means $\bar{\mathbf{g}} = (\bar{g}_{11}, \bar{g}_{12}, \bar{g}_{13}, \bar{g}_{21}, \bar{g}_{22}, \bar{g}_{23})'$ are compatible with the model (2), the hypotheses H_{01}^* and H_{02}^* in (3) are assessed through (10) with

$$\mathbf{C}_{1*} = [0 \quad 1 \quad 0 \quad 0] \qquad \mathbf{C}_{2*} = \begin{bmatrix} 0 & 0 & 1 & 0 \\ 0 & 0 & 0 & 1 \end{bmatrix}$$

For some situations there is interest in functions of the first-order marginal distributions (ϕ_{ijl}) other than the mean scores (μ_{ij}). Examples of such functions are the probabilities (ϕ_{ijl}) for a subset of the possible outcomes, logarithms of the odds $(\phi_{ijl}/\phi_{ijl'})$ for pairs of outcomes, and nonparametric rank measures of association (for which an illustrative description is given in the following "Analysis of Rank Measures of Association"). A concise expression for a set of u functions of the first-order marginal distributions is

$$\mathbf{F}(\boldsymbol{\phi}) = [F_1(\boldsymbol{\phi}), F_2(\boldsymbol{\phi}), \ldots, F_u(\boldsymbol{\phi})]'$$

where $\boldsymbol{\phi} = (\phi_{110}, \ldots, \phi_{11L}, \phi_{120}, \ldots, \phi_{12L}, \ldots, \phi_{1dL}, \phi_{210}, \ldots, \phi_{sdL})'$ is the compound vector of the $\{\phi_{ijl}\}$. In the subsequent discussion, the functions $\mathbf{F}(\boldsymbol{\phi})$ are assumed to have continuous partial derivatives through order 2 in the open region containing $\boldsymbol{\phi}$. The functions $\mathbf{F}(\boldsymbol{\phi})$ are estimated by $\mathbf{F} = \mathbf{F}(\mathbf{f})$ where $\mathbf{f}$ is the counterpart to $\boldsymbol{\phi}$ for the observed proportions f_{ijl} of the lth outcome at the jth condition for subjects in the ith group. More formally, the $\{f_{ijl}\}$ are the means of outcome indicator variables

$$y_{ijkl} = \begin{cases} 1 & \text{if } y_{ijk} = l \\ 0 & \text{if } y_{ijk} \neq l \end{cases}$$

for the respective subjects; that is, $f_{ijl} = (\Sigma_{k=1}^{n_i} y_{ijkl}/n_i)$. From the $((d(L+1) \times 1)$ vectors of response indicators

$$\mathbf{y}_{i*k*} = (y_{i1k0}, \ldots, y_{i1kL}, y_{i2k0}, \ldots, y_{idkL})'$$

the means $\mathbf{f}_i = (\Sigma_{k=1}^{n_i} \mathbf{y}_{i*k*}/n_i)$ are the respective components of the compound vector $\mathbf{f} = (\mathbf{f}_1, \mathbf{f}_2', \ldots, \mathbf{f}_s')'$.

When the sample sizes (n_i) are sufficiently large, the function estimates $\mathbf{F}$ approximately have a multivariate normal distribution on the basis of central limit theory and linear Taylor series methods. A consistent estimate for their covariance matrix is

$$\mathbf{V}_F = \mathbf{H}\mathbf{V}_f\mathbf{H}' \tag{13}$$

where $\mathbf{H} = [\partial\mathbf{F}(\mathbf{z})/\partial\mathbf{z}|\mathbf{z} = \mathbf{f}]$ and $\mathbf{V}_f$ is the $(\mathrm{sd}(L+1) \times (\mathrm{sd}(L+1))$ estimated covariance matrix for $\mathbf{f}$ with an analogous block diagonal structure to $\mathbf{V}_{\bar{g}}$ in (6); the diagonal blocks $\mathbf{V}_{f,i}$ of $\mathbf{V}_f$ have the same form as the $\mathbf{V}_{g,i}$ in (4) except that the $\{\mathbf{g}_{i*k}\}$ are replaced by the $\mathbf{y}_{i*k*}$ and the $\{\bar{\mathbf{g}}_i\}$ are replaced by the $\{f_i\}$; that is,

$$\mathbf{V}_{f,i} = \frac{1}{n_i^2} \sum_{k=1}^{n_i} (\mathbf{y}_{i*k*} - \mathbf{f}_i)(\mathbf{y}_{i*k*} - \mathbf{f}_i)' \tag{14}$$

Otherwise it is assumed that the function estimates $\mathbf{F}$ have been constructed so that $\mathbf{V}_F$ is nonsingular.

The use of weighted least-squares methods to fit linear models to the function estimates $\mathbf{F}$ is essentially the same as that summarized for the means $\bar{\mathbf{g}}$ in (6) through (12). Such models have the form

$$\mathbf{E}_A(\mathbf{F}) = \mathbf{F}(\boldsymbol{\phi}) = \mathbf{X}\boldsymbol{\beta} \tag{15}$$

where $\mathbf{E}_A(\ )$ denotes asymptotic expectation, $\mathbf{X}$ is the $(u \times t)$ model specification matrix with full rank $t \leqslant u$, and $\boldsymbol{\beta}$ is the $(t \times 1)$ vector of unknown parameters. When the $\mathbf{F}(\boldsymbol{\phi})$ are logarithms of the odds $(\phi_{ijl}/\phi_{ijl'})$, specification (15) is analogous to a log-linear model with respect to categorical explanatory variables (see Bishop, Fienberg, & Holland, 1975; Imrey et al., 1981, 1982). The WLS estimates $\mathbf{b}$ for $\boldsymbol{\beta}$ in (15) and their estimated covariance matrix $\mathbf{V}_b$ are obtained from (6) and (8) with $\bar{\mathbf{g}}$ replaced by $\mathbf{F}$ and $\mathbf{V}_{\bar{g}}$ replaced by $\mathbf{V}_F$; the application of these same modifications to (7) gives the Wald goodness-of-fit statistic for the model (15) with $\mathrm{df} = (u - t)$. No changes are needed for the methods in (9) and (10) for testing hypotheses; the predicted values $\hat{\mathbf{F}}$ with respect to the model (15) and their estimated covariance matrix $\mathbf{V}_f$ are obtained from (11) and (12) with $\hat{\boldsymbol{\mu}}$ replaced by $\hat{\mathbf{F}}$.

The previous description of weighted least-squares methods for functions of the first-order marginal distributions has straightforward extensions to functions of higher order marginal distributions. In this regard, the second-order marginal distributions of response for the respective pairs of conditions provide information for functions concerning response distribution transitions; thus they are relevant to statistical objective (5) in the section "Some Statistical Objectives for Longitudinal Studies." More specifically, let $\psi_{ijl,j'l'} = \text{pr}(y_{ijk} = l, y_{ij'k} = l')$ denote the joint probability of the lth outcome for the jth condition and the l'th outcome for the j'th condition for subjects in the ith group where $i = 1, 2, \ldots, s$; $j < j' = 1, 2, \ldots, d$; and $l, l' = 0, 1, 2, \ldots, L$. The functions

$$\theta_{ij'l':jl} = \frac{\psi_{ijl,j'l'}}{\sum\limits_{l=0}^{L} \psi_{ijl,j'l'}}$$

represent transition probabilities from the lth outcome at the jth condition to the l'th outcome at the j'th condition for $j < j'$. If $\boldsymbol{\theta}$ and $\boldsymbol{\psi}$ denote the vectors of transition probabilities and pairwise joint probabilities, respectively, then $\boldsymbol{\Theta} = \mathbf{F}(\boldsymbol{\psi})$ expresses the functional relationship of $\boldsymbol{\Theta}$ to $\boldsymbol{\psi}$. The sample counterparts $\mathbf{q}$ for estimating $\boldsymbol{\psi}$ are the within-group means of the indicator variables

$$y_{ijkl,j'l'} = \begin{cases} 1 & \text{if } y_{ijk} = l \text{ and } y_{ij'k} = l' \\ 0 & \text{if otherwise} \end{cases}$$

that is, $q_{ijl,j'l'} = (\sum_{k=1}^{n_i} y_{ijkl,j'l'}/n_i)$, and so the $(q_{ijl,j'l'})$ denote the observed proportions of the lth outcome at the jth condition and the l'th outcome at the j'th condition for subjects in the ith group. It then follows that the functions $\mathbf{F} = \mathbf{F}(\mathbf{q})$ are estimates of the transition probabilities $\boldsymbol{\theta}$. The availability of sufficient sample size for $\mathbf{F}$ approximately to have a multivariate normal distribution enables the use of weighted least-squares methods along lines analogous to (6) through (12) for analyses concerning $\boldsymbol{\theta}$. The functions $\mathbf{F}$ actually included in such analyses would be constructed so that the estimate from (14) for their covariance matrix would be nonsingular. Measures of association between responses for pairs of conditions are other functions of $\boldsymbol{\psi}$ that merit potential attention. For nominal (or binary) responses, such functions might be the log-odds ratios

$$\lambda_{ijl,j'l'} = \log_e \left\{ \frac{\psi_{ijl,j'l'}\psi_{ij0,j'0}}{\psi_{ijl,j'0}\psi_{ij0,j'l'}} \right\}$$

while for ordinal data they might be rank correlation coefficients for pairs of conditions.

At the most general level, consideration can be given to functions of the joint probabilities

$$\pi_{i,1} = \pi_{i,l_1 l_2, \ldots, l_d} = \text{pr}\{y_{i1k} = l_1, \ldots, y_{idk} = l_d\}$$

Sample estimates for the $(\pi_{i,1})$ are provided by the within-group means $p_{i,1}$ of the indicator variables

$$y_{i*kl} = \begin{cases} 1 & \text{if } y_{i1k} = l_1, \, y_{i2k} = l_2, \ldots, \, y_{idk} = l_d \\ 0 & \text{if otherwise} \end{cases}$$

that is, the $p_{i,1} = (\Sigma_{k=1}^{n_i} y_{i*kl}/n_i) = (n_{i,1}/n_i)$ are the observed proportions corresponding to the frequency $n_{i,1}$ of the lth response profile among the n_i subjects from the ith group. Also, the $(n_{i,1})$ comprise the $(d + 1)$th dimensional contingency table for the cross-classification of the s groups with the $(L + 1)^d$ possible response outcomes. Under the assumption that the subjects in each group are equivalent to simple random samples from corresponding infinite subpopulations, the $(n_{i,1})$ have the product multinomial distribution

$$\text{pr}[(n_{i,1})] = \prod_{i=1}^{s} n_i! \prod_{1} \left(\frac{\pi_{i,1}^{ni,1}}{n_{i,1}!} \right) \tag{16}$$

Let π denote the vector of joint probabilities $(\pi_{i,1})$; and let $\mathbf{F}(\pi)$ denote a set of functions that are of interest and have continuous partial derivatives through order 2 in an open interval containing π. An estimate for $\mathbf{F}(\pi)$ is $F = F(\mathbf{p})$ where $\mathbf{p}$ is the vector of observed proportions $(p_{i,1})$. When the sample sizes (n_i) are sufficiently large for $\mathbf{F}$ approximately to have a multivariate normal distribution, then weighted least-squares methods can be used to fit linear models with the form

$$\mathbf{E}_A\{\mathbf{F}\} = \mathbf{F}(\pi) = \mathbf{X}\boldsymbol{\beta} \tag{17}$$

The nature of such analysis would be similar to (6) through (12) with $\bar{\mathbf{g}}$ replaced by $\mathbf{F}$ and $\mathbf{V}_g$ replaced by the estimated covariance matrix $\mathbf{V}_F$ for $\mathbf{F}$. Moreover, the first-order marginal probabilities $\boldsymbol{\phi}$ or the second-order marginal probabilities $\boldsymbol{\psi}$ are functions of π, and so the previously described analyses pertaining to them are special cases of the general framework outlined here. For situations where all the cell frequencies $n_{i,1}$ are large (e.g., all $n_{i,1} \geq 5$), weighted least-squares methods are the same as the minimum modified chi-square methods of Neyman (1949); hence they are equivalent (in an asymptotic sense) to maximum likelihood methods, although such considerations are not necessary for their use in the specific situations discussed previously for functions of first- or second-order marginal distributions (see Bhapkar, 1966; Koch et al., 1977; Koch, Imrey, et al., 1985). Maximum likelihood methods involve the estimation of $\boldsymbol{\beta}$ in (17) by maximizing (16). When the number of outcomes l is not large, the computations to obtain maximum likelihood estimates $\boldsymbol{\beta}$ are usually feasible. (See Bishop et al., 1975, and Haber, 1985, for a discussion of maximum likelihood methods pertaining to models like (17) for linear functions $\mathbf{F}(\pi)$ such as the mean scores $\boldsymbol{\mu}$ or the first-order marginal distributions $\boldsymbol{\phi}$.) However, when the number of outcomes l is very large (e.g., ≥ 1000), the computation of maximum likelihood estimates relative to (16) might not be practically feasible. One way to address this issue is through simplification of the likelihood function on the basis of assumptions concerning the structure of the response distributions for the respective conditions; this might involve stochastic process models such as Markov chains. (For further discussion, see Bishop et al., 1975, Chapter 7.)

Another analysis strategy with potentially broad applicability involves the combined use of maximum likelihood and weighted least-squares methods. For each condition, maximum likelihood methods are used to fit logistic or log-linear models that describe the variation across groups. A consistent estimate is then constructed for the covariance matrix of the composite vector of estimated parameters for all conditions. The variation of the estimated parameters across conditions is analyzed by weighted least-squares methods. This combined (or two-stage) method requires only that the overall sample size $n = \Sigma_{i=1}^{S} n_i$ be sufficiently large to support approximate normality of the maximum likelihood estimates for each condition; whereas weighted least-squares methods have the more stringent requirement of large sample sizes (n_i) for each group separately. Also, the computations for maximum likelihood estimation for the response distribution at each condition separately are substantially more straightforward than those for the joint distribution for all conditions. Thus the two-stage method has the strongest advantages for analysis for the many situations with small sample sizes (n_i) for a large number of groups comprising a large overall sample size n and with a large number of possible outcomes $(L + 1)^d$ for the profile of responses. A principal difficulty in the use of the two-stage method is the construction of the estimated covariance matrix for the composite vector of estimated parameters for all conditions. For ordinal responses, Stram, Wei, and Ware (1988) have provided a method for obtaining this covariance matrix when the proportional odds (logistic) model described in McCullagh (1980) is fitted to each condition by maximum likelihood; also this method is applicable when there are randomly missing data for the responses at some conditions. An example illustrating this two-stage analysis for a longitudinal study with incomplete response vectors for some subjects is given in Wei et al. (1985). The section "Analysis of Proportional Odds Models" in this chapter deals with an example for which weighted least-squares methods are used to fit the proportional odds model. (For discussion of two-stage methods involving maximum likelihood and weighted least squares in other settings, see Imrey et al., 1981, 1982, and Koch, Amara, & Singer, 1985.) Discussion of other types of methods that are potentially useful for the analysis of longitudinal categorical data is given in Ochi and Prentice (1984), Stiratelli et al. (1984), Anderson and Pemberton (1985), Zeger, Liang, and Self (1985), Liang and Zeger (1986), and Zeger and Liang (1986).

Some additional aspects of weighted least-squares methods are worthy of attention. One is that ways of dealing with incomplete data are available for situations with sufficiently large sample sizes $\{n_i\}$ for the respective groups; these are described in Koch Imrey, and Reinfurt (1972) and Stanish, Gillings, and Koch (1978); an example illustrating their application is given in the later section "An Observational Study . . . ." Another is that weighted least-squares analyses are applicable to estimates from longitudinal studies for which the subjects are obtained by complex multistage sample surveys. In these situations, the function estimates and their covariance matrix are constructed in accordance with the survey. Additional discussion of such analysis is given in Koch et al. (1975), Freeman, Freeman, Brock, and Koch (1976), Landis, Lepkowski, Eklund, and

Stenhouwer (1982), and Koch, Imrey, et al., (1985). The application of weighted least-squares methods to longitudinal survey data is illustrated in the section "Estimates from a National Survey . . . ."

EXAMPLES

This section discusses the application of weighted least-squares methods to three examples. The first is a clinical trial with two treatment groups and four visits; analyses are undertaken for several types of functions. A national health survey is the source of the second example; consideration is given to estimated proportions for Medicaid coverage at two time points for four groups. The third example is based on an observational study concerning occurrences of colds for children during each of three years; methods for dealing with incomplete data are illustrated.

A Clinical Trial for a Skin Disorder

A single-center clinical trial was conducted to compare two treatments (active and placebo) for a population of subjects with a skin disorder. Their responses were evaluated at each of four visits as follows: D1 = three days, D2 = seven days, D3 = ten days, D4 = fourteen days. Each of the four response variables was expressed in terms of four ordinal categories: 0 = excellent, 1 = good, 2 = fair, 3 = poor. The case record data for the $n_1 = n_2 = 36$ subjects in each of the two treatment groups are displayed in Table 9-2. The marginal response distributions for each of the two treatment groups at each of the four visits are summarized in Table 9-3. For each treatment these distributions can be described as having larger proportions of excellent responses and smaller proportions of poor responses at the later visits; also, at each visit the distribution for active treatment is more favorable than that for placebo. Thus analysis can be anticipated to indicate strong treatment effects, strong visit effects, and minimal (treatment × visit) interaction.

Several ways of applying weighted least-squares methods to longitudinal data with ordinal response categories are illustrated for this example:

1. Analysis of the proportions of excellent responses
2. Analysis of mean scores for the integer scaling of 0, 1, 2, 3 for excellent, good, fair, poor, respectively
3. Analysis of nonparametric rank measures of association
4. Analysis of the proportional odds model

Functions for implementing these analyses are described; also their advantages and limitations are discussed.

Analysis of the Proportions Excellent

Analysis of the proportions of excellent responses can proceed in either of two equivalent ways. One is to transform the case record data in Table 9-2 to binary

Table 9-2. Data from clinical trial to compare active and placebo treatments for skin disorder[a]

	Active treatment					Placebo treatment			
Subject	D1[b]	D2	D3	D4		Subject	D1	D2	D3	D4
1	2[c]	1	1	1		1	2	1	1	1
2	1	1	1	0		2	1	1	0	0
3	1	1	1	1		3	2	2	2	1
4	0	1	0	1		4	1	1	0	1
5	2	1	1	0		5	2	1	1	0
6	1	1	0	2		6	1	1	1	0
7	2	1	1	0		7	1	1	1	1
8	1	0	1	0		8	2	2	2	1
9	1	1	1	0		9	3	1	2	1
10	1	0	1	0		10	1	1	0	1
11	1	0	1	1		11	0	1	0	1
12	1	1	0	1		12	2	1	1	1
13	2	1	1	1		13	1	0	0	0
14	1	0	0	0		14	1	1	2	1
15	2	1	2	1		15	2	1	1	1
16	2	1	0	0		16	1	0	1	1
17	1	2	1	1		17	2	2	2	1
18	2	2	2	1		18	1	1	1	0
19	0	0	0	0		19	2	1	2	1
20	1	1	1	0		20	2	2	2	1
21	2	0	1	1		21	3	1	2	1
22	1	1	2	0		22	1	1	0	0
23	1	0	0	0		23	2	2	2	0
24	1	0	0	0		24	1	1	0	0
25	1	0	1	0		25	2	2	1	1
26	1	1	1	1		26	2	1	2	0
27	2	1	2	1		27	2	2	2	1
28	2	1	1	1		28	2	0	1	2
29	1	2	1	1		29	2	1	1	1
30	0	0	0	0		30	2	0	2	0
31	0	1	0	1		31	2	1	1	0
32	1	1	1	0		32	1	1	0	1
33	1	0	0	0		33	2	1	1	1
34	0	0	0	0		34	2	2	2	1
35	1	0	0	0		35	2	2	1	1
36	1	2	1	1		36	2	1	1	1

[b]D1 = 3 days, D2 = 7 days, D3 = 10 days, D4 = 14 days are time points for response evaluation.
[c]Response outcomes are 0 = excellent, 1 = good, 2 = fair, 3 = poor.
[a]These data do not actually pertain to a skin disorder; they are from a study dealing with a different type of health condition. Their real nature cannot be specified because of confidentiality considerations.

indicators

$$g_{ijk} = \begin{cases} 1 & \text{if response } y_{ijk} = 0 \\ 0 & \text{if response } y_{ijk} = 1, 2, 3 \end{cases} \tag{18}$$

and then to determine the means $\bar{g}_{ij} = (\Sigma_{k=1}^{36} g_{ijk}/36)$ for each (treatment $\times$ visit)

Table 9-3. Response proportions from clinical trial for skin disorder

Response	Active treatment				Placebo treatment			
	3 days	7 days	10 days	14 days	3 days	7 days	10 days	14 days
Excellent	0.139	0.361	0.361	0.556	0.028	0.111	0.222	0.306
Good	0.583	0.528	0.528	0.417	0.333	0.639	0.417	0.667
Fair	0.278	0.111	0.111	0.028	0.583	0.250	0.361	0.028
Poor	0.000	0.000	0.000	0.000	0.056	0.000	0.000	0.000
Number of patients	36	36	36	36	36	36	36	36

and their estimated covariance matrix $\mathbf{V}_{\bar{g}}$; here

$$\mathbf{V}_{\bar{g}} = \begin{bmatrix} \mathbf{V}_{g,1} & 0_{4,4} \\ 0_{4,4} & \mathbf{V}_{g,2} \end{bmatrix} \tag{19}$$

is an (8×8) block diagonal matrix; $0_{4,4}$ denotes (4×4) matrices of 0's; $\mathbf{V}_{g,1}$ and $\mathbf{V}_{g,2}$ are the estimated covariance matrices for the two treatment groups. Results for $V_{g,1}$ and $\mathbf{V}_{g,2}$ from an expression like (4) are as follows:

$$\mathbf{V}_{g,1} = \begin{bmatrix} 33.22 & 9.22 & 24.65 & 1.71 \\ 9.22 & 64.09 & 25.51 & 29.15 \\ 24.65 & 25.51 & 64.09 & 13.72 \\ 1.71 & 29.15 & 13.72 & 68.59 \end{bmatrix} \times 10^{-4}$$

$$\mathbf{V}_{g,2} = \begin{bmatrix} 7.50 & -0.86 & 6.00 & -2.36 \\ -0.86 & 27.43 & 0.86 & 6.00 \\ 6.00 & 0.86 & 48.01 & 12.00 \\ -2.36 & 6.00 & 12.00 & 58.94 \end{bmatrix} \times 10^{-4} \tag{20}$$

The vector of means $\bar{\mathbf{g}}$ for the respective (treatment $\times$ visit) combinations is given by

$$\bar{\mathbf{g}} = (0.139, 0.361, 0.361, 0.556, 0.028, 0.111, 0.222, 0.306)' \tag{21}$$

The second way to obtain $\bar{\mathbf{g}}$ and $\mathbf{V}_{\bar{g}}$ is through matrix operations on the five-dimensional contingency table for the cross-classification of the two treatment groups with the 2^4 possible outcomes for the g_{ijk} at the four visits. The frequencies of response profile $\mathbf{l} = (l_1, l_2, l_3, l_4)'$ for group i subjects is

$$n_{i,1} = \sum_{k=1}^{36} (g_{i1kl_1} g_{i2kl_2} g_{i3kl_3} g_{i4kl_4}) \tag{22}$$

where the $\{g_{ijkl_j}\}$ are indicator variables defined by

$$g_{ijkl_j} = \begin{cases} 1 & \text{if } g_{ijk} = l_j \\ 0 & \text{if } g_{ijk} \neq l_j \end{cases}$$

for the possible outcomes $l = 0, 1$ of the $\{g_{ijkl_j}\}$.

Table 9-4. Contingency table for excellent response profiles at four time points

						Response profiles for visits										
3 days	0[a]	0	0	0	0	0	0	0	1	1	1	1	1	1	1	1
7 days	0	0	0	0	1	1	1	1	0	0	0	0	1	1	1	1
10 days	0	0	1	1	0	0	1	1	0	0	1	1	0	0	1	1
14 days	0	1	0	1	0	1	0	1	0	1	0	1	0	1	0	1

																	Total
Active	10	8	2	1	2	3	0	5	0	0	2	0	0	0	0	3	36
Placebo	19	6	3	3	2	1	0	1	0	0	1	0	0	0	0	0	36

[a]$0 =$ not excellent, $1 =$ excellent.

The $n_{i,1}$ are displayed in Table 9-4. The mean vector $\bar{\mathbf{g}}$ and its estimated covariance matrix $\mathbf{V}_{\bar{g}}$ are obtained from the proportions $\{p_{i,1} = n_{i,1}/n_i\}$ for the response profile distributions in the respective treatment groups by the matrix operations

$$\bar{\mathbf{g}} = \mathbf{Ap}, \quad \mathbf{V}_{\bar{g}} = \mathbf{AV}_p\mathbf{A}' \qquad (23)$$

Here $\mathbf{p} = (\mathbf{p}_1', \mathbf{p}_2')'$ with $\mathbf{p}_i = (p_{i,0000}, p_{i,0001}, \ldots, p_{i,1111})'$ is the composite vector of proportions; $\mathbf{V}_p$ is the (32×32) block diagonal estimated covariance matrix for $\mathbf{p}$ with the multinomial based, (16×16) diagonal blocks $\mathbf{V}_{p,i} = [\mathbf{D}_{p,i} - \mathbf{p}_i\mathbf{p}_i']/n_i$ for which $\mathbf{D}_{p,i}$ denotes the diagonal matrix with diagonal elements $\mathbf{p}_i$; and $\mathbf{A}$ is the (8×32) block diagonal matrix with (4×16) diagonal blocks

$$\mathbf{A} = \begin{bmatrix} 0 & 0 & 0 & 0 & 0 & 0 & 0 & 0 & 1 & 1 & 1 & 1 & 1 & 1 & 1 & 1 \\ 0 & 0 & 0 & 0 & 1 & 1 & 1 & 1 & 0 & 0 & 0 & 0 & 1 & 1 & 1 & 1 \\ 0 & 0 & 1 & 1 & 0 & 0 & 1 & 1 & 0 & 0 & 1 & 1 & 0 & 0 & 1 & 1 \\ 0 & 1 & 0 & 1 & 0 & 1 & 0 & 1 & 0 & 1 & 0 & 1 & 0 & 1 & 0 & 1 \end{bmatrix} \qquad (24)$$

It is appropriate to note that the results for $\bar{\mathbf{g}}$ and $\mathbf{V}_{\bar{g}}$ from the case record framework and the contingency table framework are identical. For most applications, the computational procedures for the case record framework are more convenient and straightforward; as discussed under "Weighted Least-Squares Methods," the contingency table framework is useful when the number of time points d and the number of response outcomes L are sufficiently small that the number of response profiles $(L + 1)^d$ is not excessively large (e.g., $d \leqslant 6$ and $L \leqslant 3$ so that $(L + 1)^d \leqslant 81$).

Since there is not an a priori model for the means $\bar{\mathbf{g}}$, the statistical significance of treatment effects, visit effects, and (treatment × visit) interaction is initially assessed through the cell mean (or identity) model $\mathbf{X}_I = \mathbf{I}_8$. For this model, the estimated parameters and their estimated covariance matrix are

$$\mathbf{b}_I = \bar{\mathbf{g}} \qquad \mathbf{V}_{b,I} = \mathbf{V}_{\bar{g}} \qquad (25)$$

Hypotheses for sources of variation pertaining to $\mathbf{b}_I$ are specified through $\mathbf{C}$ matrices as in (9), and the corresponding Wald test statistics are computed (10);

results are shown in Table 9-5. The conclusions from Table 9-5 are that treatment effects and visit effects are significant ($p \leqslant 0.01$) and their interaction is clearly nonsignificant ($p \geqslant 0.25$).

Since there is no interaction between treatment effects and visit effects, the means $\bar{\mathbf{g}}$ are compatible with the main effects model

$$
E(\bar{\mathbf{g}}) =
\begin{bmatrix}
1 & 0 & 0 & 0 & 0 \\
1 & 0 & 1 & 0 & 0 \\
1 & 0 & 0 & 1 & 0 \\
1 & 0 & 0 & 0 & 1 \\
1 & 1 & 0 & 0 & 0 \\
1 & 1 & 1 & 0 & 0 \\
1 & 1 & 0 & 1 & 0 \\
1 & 1 & 0 & 0 & 1
\end{bmatrix}
\begin{bmatrix}
\beta_{\mathrm{ME},1} \\
\beta_{\mathrm{ME},2} \\
\beta_{\mathrm{ME},3} \\
\beta_{\mathrm{ME},4} \\
\beta_{\mathrm{ME},5}
\end{bmatrix}
= \mathbf{X}_{\mathrm{ME}} \boldsymbol{\beta}_{\mathrm{ME}}
\tag{26}
$$

For this model $\beta_{\mathrm{ME},1}$ represents the predicted proportion excellent for active treatment at three days, $\beta_{\mathrm{ME},2}$ represents the effect for placebo, and $\beta_{\mathrm{ME},3}$, $\beta_{\mathrm{ME},4}$, $\beta_{\mathrm{ME},5}$ represent the effects for seven days, ten days, and fourteen days. The weighted least-squares estimates for the parameter vector $\boldsymbol{\beta}_{\mathrm{ME}}$ and its estimated covariance matrix are obtained via (6) and (8); the results are

$$
\mathbf{b}_{\mathrm{ME}} =
\begin{bmatrix}
0.175 \\
-0.160 \\
0.126 \\
0.197 \\
0.324
\end{bmatrix}
$$

$$
\mathbf{V}_{b,\mathrm{ME}} =
\begin{bmatrix}
25.91 & -23.51 & -6.95 & -2.58 & -11.70 \\
-23.51 & 27.80 & 1.14 & 1.20 & 5.34 \\
-6.95 & 1.14 & 24.54 & 5.18 & 13.88 \\
-2.58 & 1.20 & 5.18 & 21.74 & 7.59 \\
-11.70 & 5.34 & 13.88 & 7.59 & 39.62
\end{bmatrix} \times 10^{-4}
\tag{27}
$$

Table 9–5. Results of hypothesis tests from cell mean model for excellent response proportions

Source of variation	C matrix		Q_C	df	Approximate p value
Treatment effects (averaged over time)	$[1 \quad 1 \quad 1 \quad 1 \; -1 \; -1 \; -1 \; -1]$		9.03	1	<0.010
Visit effects (averaged over treatment)	$\begin{bmatrix} -1 & 1 & 0 & 0 & -1 & 1 & 0 & 0 \\ -1 & 0 & 1 & 0 & -1 & 0 & 1 & 0 \\ -1 & 0 & 0 & 1 & -1 & 0 & 0 & 1 \end{bmatrix}$		37.02	3	<0.010
No treatment × visit interaction	$\begin{bmatrix} -1 & 1 & 0 & 0 & 1 & -1 & 0 & 0 \\ -1 & 0 & 1 & 0 & 1 & 0 & -1 & 0 \\ -1 & 0 & 0 & 1 & 1 & 0 & 0 & -1 \end{bmatrix}$		1.95	3	0.584

The standard errors of the elements of $\mathbf{b}_{ME}$ are the square roots of the respective diagonal elements of $\mathbf{V}_{b,ME}$; the off-diagonal elements of $\mathbf{V}_{b,ME}$ enable the determination of standard errors of linear functions of $\mathbf{b}_{ME}$ such as differences between day effects. The Wald goodness-of-fit statistic for the model $\mathbf{X}_{ME}$ is the same as the no-interaction test statistic in Table 9-5, but its method of computation is (7); the nonsignificance ($p \geqslant 0.25$) of this criterion supports use of the model $\mathbf{X}_{ME}$.

Test statistics for treatment effects and visit effects with respect to the model $\mathbf{X}_{ME}$ are obtained via (10); results are shown in Table 9-6. They indicate that treatment effects and visit effects are significant ($p < 0.01$); also, for each treatment group, the proportions for excellent response can be interpreted as increasing linearly over days of the successive visits, since the test statistic for lack of linearity for visit effects is nonsignificant ($p \geqslant 0.25$).

The simplification of visit effects to a linear structure is specified through the final model

$$
E\{\bar{\mathbf{g}}\} = \begin{bmatrix} 1 & 0 & 3 \\ 1 & 0 & 7 \\ 1 & 0 & 10 \\ 1 & 0 & 14 \\ 1 & 1 & 3 \\ 1 & 1 & 7 \\ 1 & 1 & 10 \\ 1 & 1 & 14 \end{bmatrix} \begin{bmatrix} \beta_{F1} \\ \beta_{F2} \\ \beta_{F3} \end{bmatrix} = \mathbf{X}_F \boldsymbol{\beta}_F \tag{28}
$$

For this model β_{F1} represents the predicted proportion excellent for active treatment at 0 days, β_{F2} represents the effect for placebo, and β_{F3} represents the "linear" effect of visits. The weighted least-squares estimates for the parameter vector $\boldsymbol{\beta}_F$ and its estimated covariance matrix are

$$
\mathbf{b}_F = \begin{bmatrix} 0.092 \\ -0.161 \\ 0.029 \end{bmatrix} \quad \mathbf{V}_{b,F} = \begin{bmatrix} 31.28 & -24.32 & -1.4751 \\ -24.32 & 27.61 & 0.3639 \\ -1.4751 & 0.3639 & 0.2356 \end{bmatrix} \times 10^{-4} \tag{29}
$$

Table 9–6. Results of hypothesis tests from main effects model for excellent response proportions

Source of variation	C matrix					Q_C	df	Approximate p value
Treatment effects	[0	1	0	0	0]	9.21	1	<0.010
Visit effects	[0 0 0	0 0 0	1 0 0	0 1 0	0 0 1]	35.56	3	<0.010
Lack of linearity over days for visit effects	[0 0	0 0	-7 -11	4 0	0 4]	0.07	2	0.964

The use of the final model $\mathbf{X}_F$ is supported by the nonsignificance ($p \geqslant 0.25$) of the Wald goodness-of-fit statistic $Q_W(\mathrm{df} = 5) = 2.02$.

Predicted values from the final model are obtained for the means $\bar{\mathbf{g}}$ by (11); their estimated standard errors are the square roots of the diagonal elements of (12). These quantities are displayed in Table 9-7 with the observed means $\bar{\mathbf{g}}$ and their standard errors. Since the predicted values are based on an estimation process for which sources of extraneous variability (i.e., (treatment × visit) interaction and lack of linearity of visit effects) are eliminated, their standard errors are smaller than their observed counterparts in $\bar{\mathbf{g}}$. They also provide a clearer description of the relationship of the excellent response proportions to treatment and visit.

Analysis of Mean Scores

A straightforward summary function that encompasses all possible outcomes of the response distribution for subjects in the ith group at the jth visit is the mean score $\bar{g}_{ij} = (\Sigma_{k=1}^{36} g_{ijk}/36)$ with respect to the integer scaling $g_{ijk} = y_{ijk} = 0, 1, 2, 3$ for excellent, good, fair, and poor, respectively. These mean scores are the linear functions

$$\bar{g}_{ij} = 0f_{ij0} + 1f_{ij1} + 2f_{ij2} + 3f_{ij3} \tag{30}$$

of the proportions $f_{ijl} = (\Sigma_{k=1}^{36} y_{ijkl}/36)$ where

$$y_{ijkl} = \begin{cases} 1 & \text{if response } y_{ijk} = l \\ 0 & \text{if response } y_{ijk} \neq l \end{cases} \tag{31}$$

The (f_{ijl}) comprise the first-order marginal distributions shown in Table 9-3 for the $j = 1, 2, 3, 4$ visits of subjects in the $i = 1, 2$ treatment groups. From expression (30) it follows that

$$\bar{g}_{ij} = f_{ij3} + (f_{ij2} + f_{ij3}) + (f_{ij1} + f_{ij2} + f_{ij3}) \tag{32}$$

and so variation among the $\{\bar{g}_{ij}\}$ would reflect tendencies for consistent

Table 9-7. Observed and final model predicted proportions excellent, and standard errors

Treatment	Visit	Observed excellent		Predicted excellent	
		Proportion	SE	Proportion	SE
Active	3 days	0.139	0.058	0.178	0.050
	7 days	0.361	0.080	0.294	0.047
	10 days	0.361	0.080	0.381	0.050
	14 days	0.556	0.083	0.497	0.060
Placebo	3 days	0.028	0.027	0.018	0.024
	7 days	0.111	0.052	0.134	0.025
	10 days	0.222	0.069	0.220	0.034
	14 days	0.306	0.077	0.336	0.050

increases in the probabilities of poorer responses relative to successive binary splits of the response outcomes.

The means scores $(\bar{g}_{ij})$ from the integer scaling 0, 1, 2, 3 and their estimated covariance matrix from an expression like (4) are shown for each treatment group in Table 9-8. These results were computed by direct operations on case record data for the (g_{ijk}); alternatively they could have been obtained by matrix operations like (23) on the five-dimensional contingency table for the cross-classification of the two treatment groups with the 4^4 possible outcomes for the (g_{ijk}) at the four visits (although only the twenty-five possible outcomes that actually occurred for the seventy-two subjects under study need to be taken into account).

Let $\bar{g}$ denote the vector of mean scores for the respective (treatment × visit) combinations, and let $V_{\bar{g}}$ denote its block-diagonal estimated covariance matrix. The elements of $\bar{g}$ are given in the third column of Table 9-8; the upper and lower diagonal blocks of $V_{\bar{g}}$ are given in columns five through eight of Table 9-8. Statistical tests for treatment effects, visit effects, and (treatment × visit) inter-action are undertaken for the cell mean (or identity) model $X_I = I_8$ through the same C matrices as those shown in Table 9-5. The results are $Q_C(\text{df}=1)=13.90$ for treatment effects, $Q_C(\text{df}=3)=107.35$ for visit effects, and $Q_C(\text{df}=3)=3.06$ for (treatment × visit) interaction. Thus both treatment effects and visit effects are significant ($p < 0.01$), whereas their interaction is not ($p \geqslant 0.25$). The latter finding implies that the variation among the mean scores $\bar{g}$ can be described by the main effects model X_{ME} with the same structure shown in (26). From (6) and (8), the weighted least-squares estimates b_{ME} for the parameter vector β_{ME} and its estimated covariance matrix are

$$
b_{ME} = \begin{bmatrix} 1.236 \\ 0.362 \\ -0.486 \\ -0.475 \\ -0.824 \end{bmatrix}
$$

$$
V_{b,ME} = \begin{bmatrix} 74.95 & -45.75 & -31.12 & -17.24 & -41.28 \\ -45.75 & 95.11 & -13.15 & 2.8 & -8.0 \\ -31.12 & -13.15 & 73.62 & 24.87 & 44.27 \\ -17.24 & 2.8 & 24.87 & 44.29 & 15.62 \\ -41.28 & -8.0 & 44.27 & 15.62 & 74.64 \end{bmatrix} \times 10^{-4} \tag{33}
$$

Results of statistical tests with respect to the main effects model X_{ME} through C matrices like those in Table 9-6 are $Q_C(\text{df}=1)=13.76$ for treatment effects and $Q_C(\text{df}=3)=116.67$ for time effects; both are significant ($p < 0.01$). Thus the conclusions from the analysis of the mean scores with respect to the integers 0, 1, 2, 3 are similar to those reported in the section "Analysis of the Proportions Excellent."

Table 9–8. Estimated means and covariance matrix for 0, 1, 2, 3 scaling of response categories from clinical trial for skin disorder

Treatment	Visit	Mean	SE	Covariance matrix × 10⁴			
Active	3 days	1.139	0.105	110.4	32.8	63.7	12.6
	7 days	0.750	0.107	32.8	113.8	52.1	48.2
	10 days	0.750	0.107	63.7	52.1	113.8	17.4
	14 days	0.472	0.092	12.6	48.2	17.4	84.7
Placebo	3 days	1.667	0.104	108.0	28.3	90.0	20.6
	7 days	1.139	0.097	28.3	95.0	48.7	10.7
	10 days	1.139	0.125	90.0	48.7	156.7	18.4
	14 days	0.722	0.084	20.6	10.7	18.4	71.2

Analysis of Rank Measures of Association

For each visit the marginal distributions $(f_{ij0}, f_{ij1}, f_{ij2}, f_{ij3})$ provide information on which treatment comparisons can be based. A general way to account for the ordinal nature of the response categories in these distributions is through nonparametric rank measures of association between treatment and response. A function of the (f_{ijl}) that is similar in spirit to the Mann–Whitney (1947) statistic for the jth visit is

$$G_j = \sum_{l=0}^{3} f_{1jl}\left[\left(\sum_{l'=l}^{3} f_{2jl'}\right) - 0.5 f_{2jl}\right] \tag{34}$$

This function describes the probability with which a subject randomly selected for active treatment has more favorable response at the jth visit than a subject randomly chosen for placebo when ties are randomly broken with probability $(1/2)$. The (G_j) lie in the range $[0, 1]$; under the hypothesis of no difference between treatments, their expected values are 0.5. It follows that substantial departures of the (G_j) from 0.5 are indicative of treatment differences at the corresponding visits, and heterogeneity of such tendencies across visits is indicative of (treatment × visit) interaction.

The vector $\mathbf{G} = (G_1, G_2, G_3, G_4)'$ of rank measures of association may be computed by compound function operations

$$\mathbf{G} = \mathbf{A}_3(\exp(\mathbf{A}_2[\log_e(\mathbf{A}_1 \mathbf{f})]\}) \tag{35}$$

where $\mathbf{f} = (f_{110}, f_{111}, f_{112}, f_{113}, f_{120}, \ldots, f_{243})'$ is the (32 × 1) vector of marginal proportions in Table 9-3; also **exp** (or $\log_e$) are operators that exponentiate (or form natural logarithms) of the elements of vectors, and

1. $\mathbf{A}_1$ is a linear transformation matrix that forms nonzero values of the (f_{1jl}) and the $[(\Sigma_{l'=l}^{3} f_{2jl'}) - 0.5 f_{2jl}]$.
2. $\mathbf{A}_2$ is a linear transformation matrix that provides the sum of logarithms of the (f_{1jl}) and the $[(\Sigma_{l'=l}^{3} f_{2jl'}) - 0.5 f_{2jl}]$ and thereby the logarithms of their products.

3. A_3 is a linear transformation matrix that provides the sum of the $\{f_{1jl}[\Sigma_{l'=1}^{3}(f_{2jl'}) - 0.5f_{2jl}]\}$.

The specification (35) for G is useful because it enables the linear Taylor series-based estimate V_G for the covariance matrix of G to be obtained by the straightforward matrix multiplication operations

$$V_G = HV_f H' \qquad (36)$$

where $H = A_3 D_{a_2} A_2 D_{a_1}^{-1} A_1$ with $a_1 = A_1 f$ and $a_2 = \exp\{A_2[\log_e(A_1 f)]\}$; V_f is the estimated covariance matrix for f from an expression such as (14). (For additional discussion of the use of specifications like (35) as a way to obtain estimated covariance matrices like (36), see Koch et al., 1977; also for rank measures of association see Koch, Imrey, et al., 1985; Semenya, Koch, Stokes & Forthofer, 1983. Another method is in Carr, Hafner, and Koch, 1989.)

The rank measures of association G and their estimated covariance matrix V_G are shown in Table 9-9. The homogeneity of the (G_j) across the respective visits can be assessed through the goodness of fit of the model

$$E_A(G) = \begin{bmatrix} 1 \\ 1 \\ 1 \\ 1 \end{bmatrix} \beta = X\beta \qquad (37)$$

where $E_A( )$ denotes the asymptotic expected value; the parameter β represents the common value over time of the measures of association (G_j) under the model. The Wald goodness-of-fit statistic from (7) for the model (37) is $Q_W(\mathrm{df}=3)=2.28$; its nonsignificance $(p \geqslant 0.25)$ supports use of the model and thereby the interpretation that the (G_j) are homogeneous across visits. Thus with respect to the measures of association (G_j) between treatment and response, there is no (treatment × visit) interaction.

The weighted least-squares estimate b from (6) and its estimated standard error from (8) are

$$b = 0.659 \qquad SE(b) = 0.040 \qquad (38)$$

A test for the hypothesis of no difference between treatments is provided by comparing b with 0.50 through the chi-square statistic

$$Q_C(\mathrm{df}=1) = \left[\frac{b - 0.500}{SE(b)}\right]^2 = 15.80 \qquad (39)$$

Table 9–9. Estimated rank measures of association between treatment and response from clinical trial for skin disorder

Visit	G	SE	Covariance matrix × 10^4			
3 days	0.703	0.055	29.95	8.55	20.68	6.00
7 days	0.655	0.056	8.55	31.08	12.80	11.83
10 days	0.642	0.060	20.68	12.80	35.80	6.98
14 days	0.622	0.058	6.00	11.83	6.98	33.38

This result is significant ($p < 0.01$). The estimate $b = 0.659$ can be interpreted as indicating that the probability is about 0.66 for a randomly selected active treatment subject to have more favorable response at any particular visit j than a placebo counterpart.

Analysis of Proportional Odds Models

The description of the structure of response distributions with ordinal categories like those in Table 9-3 is often of interest in its own right as well as for providing a framework for comparisons. One useful strategy for addressing this analysis objective is the fitting of proportional odds models. For cross-sectional studies, multiple regression types of proportional odds models have been discussed in Walker and Duncan (1967), McCullagh (1980), McCullagh and Nelder (1983), and Agresti (1984); their extension to longitudinal studies and other situations with repeated measurements of response on the same subject has been described by Stram, Wei, and Ware (1988).

The proportional odds model can be fitted to the marginal distributions $(f_{ij0}, f_{ij1}, f_{ij2}, f_{ij3})$ for the respective (treatment × visit) combinations in Table 9-3 by WLS methods through the cumulative logits

$$F_{ij1} = \log_e \left(\frac{f_{ij0}}{f_{ij1} + f_{ij2} + f_{ij3}} \right)$$

$$F_{ij2} = \log_e \left(\frac{f_{ij0} + f_{ij1}}{f_{ij2} + f_{ij3}} \right) \tag{40}$$

Since poor response never occurred for active treatment patients and only rarely occurred for placebo patients, consideration is not given to the logit function for "at least fair versus poor." More generally, the occurrence of 0 values for any of the (f_{ijl}) induces potential computational problems in the use of weighted least-squares methods to fit the proportional odds model, for example, 0 divide or $\log\{0\}$ operations or singularities in the estimated covariance matrix of the (F_{ijl}). For the logit functions specified in (40), such computational problems do not occur because all of the (f_{ij0}), (f_{ij1}), and $(f_{ij2} + f_{ij3})$ are strictly positive. Otherwise, maximum likelihood methods for fitting the proportional odds model are usually less susceptible to computational dilemmas from 0 values than weighted least-squares methods (although for this example the pooling of "fair and poor" would still be appropriate).

The (16 × 1) vector of cumulative logits

$$\mathbf{F} = (F_{111}, F_{112}, F_{121}, F_{122}, \ldots, F_{242})' \tag{41}$$

can be computed by the compound function operations

$$\mathbf{F} = \mathbf{A}_2 \log_e (\mathbf{A}_1 \mathbf{f}) \tag{42}$$

Here $\mathbf{f}$ is the (32 × 1) vector of marginal proportions shown following (35); also

1. $\mathbf{A}_1$ is a linear transformation matrix that provides the (f_{ij0}), the $(f_{ij1} + f_{ij2} + f_{ij3})$, the $(f_{ij0} + f_{ij1})$, and the $(f_{ij2} + f_{ij3})$.
2. $\mathbf{A}_2$ is a linear transformation matrix that provides the (F_{ij1}) and the (F_{ij2}) through differences of the logarithms of the functions $\mathbf{a}_1 = \mathbf{A}_1 \mathbf{f}$.

As noted previously, specification (42) is useful with respect to the computation of the linear Taylor series-based estimate $\mathbf{V}_F$ for the covariance matrix of $\mathbf{F}$; this estimate is given by

$$\mathbf{V}_F = \mathbf{H}\mathbf{V}_f\mathbf{H}' = \mathbf{A}_2\mathbf{D}_{\mathbf{a}_1}^{-1}\mathbf{A}_1\mathbf{V}_f\mathbf{A}_1'\mathbf{D}_{\mathbf{a}_1}^{-1}\mathbf{A}_2' \tag{43}$$

where $\mathbf{V}_f$ is the estimated covariance matrix for $\mathbf{f}$ from an expression like (14). The proportional odds model is specified for $\mathbf{F}$ as

$$\mathbf{E}_A(\mathbf{F}) = \begin{bmatrix} 1 & 0 & 0 & 0 & 0 & 0 & 0 & 0 & 0 \\ 0 & 1 & 0 & 0 & 0 & 0 & 0 & 0 & 0 \\ 1 & 0 & 1 & 0 & 0 & 0 & 0 & 0 & 0 \\ 0 & 1 & 1 & 0 & 0 & 0 & 0 & 0 & 0 \\ 1 & 0 & 0 & 1 & 0 & 0 & 0 & 0 & 0 \\ 0 & 1 & 0 & 1 & 0 & 0 & 0 & 0 & 0 \\ 1 & 0 & 0 & 0 & 1 & 0 & 0 & 0 & 0 \\ 0 & 1 & 0 & 0 & 1 & 0 & 0 & 0 & 0 \\ 1 & 0 & 0 & 0 & 0 & 1 & 0 & 0 & 0 \\ 0 & 1 & 0 & 0 & 0 & 1 & 0 & 0 & 0 \\ 1 & 0 & 0 & 0 & 0 & 0 & 1 & 0 & 0 \\ 0 & 1 & 0 & 0 & 0 & 0 & 1 & 0 & 0 \\ 1 & 0 & 0 & 0 & 0 & 0 & 0 & 1 & 0 \\ 0 & 1 & 0 & 0 & 0 & 0 & 0 & 1 & 0 \\ 1 & 0 & 0 & 0 & 0 & 0 & 0 & 0 & 1 \\ 0 & 1 & 0 & 0 & 0 & 0 & 0 & 0 & 1 \end{bmatrix} \begin{bmatrix} \beta_{P1} \\ \beta_{P2} \\ \beta_{P3} \\ \beta_{P4} \\ \beta_{P5} \\ \beta_{P6} \\ \beta_{P7} \\ \beta_{P8} \\ \beta_{P9} \end{bmatrix} = \mathbf{X}_P\mathbf{\beta}_P \tag{44}$$

where $\mathbf{E}_A(\ )$ denotes asymptotic expectation; the parameters β_{P1} and β_{P2} represent predicted logits for active treatment at three days; β_{P3}, β_{P4}, β_{P5}, β_{P6}, β_{P7}, β_{P8}, β_{P9} represent increments at seven days, ten days, and fourteen days of active treatment and three days, seven days, ten days, and fourteen days of placebo treatment, respectively. The goodness of fit of this model is supported by the nonsignificance ($p \geqslant 0.25$) of the Wald goodness-of-fit statistic $Q_W(\mathrm{df} = 7) = 7.23$, as obtained via (7). This result can be interpreted as indicating that the effects of treatment and of days are the same for the two types of logged odds shown in (40).

The hypothesis of no (treatment $\times$ visit) interaction can be assessed by using (10) with

$$C = \begin{bmatrix} 0 & 0 & 1 & 0 & 0 & 1 & -1 & 0 & 0 \\ 0 & 0 & 0 & 1 & 0 & 1 & 0 & -1 & 0 \\ 0 & 0 & 0 & 0 & 1 & 1 & 0 & 0 & -1 \end{bmatrix} \tag{45}$$

Since $Q_C(\mathrm{df} = 3) = 3.46$ is nonsignificant ($p \geqslant 0.25$), the functions $\mathbf{F}$ can be interpreted as being compatible with the main effects proportional odds model

$$
\mathbf{E}_A(\mathbf{F}) =
\begin{bmatrix}
1 & 0 & 0 & 0 & 0 & 0 \\
0 & 1 & 0 & 0 & 0 & 0 \\
1 & 0 & 0 & 1 & 0 & 0 \\
0 & 1 & 0 & 1 & 0 & 0 \\
1 & 0 & 0 & 0 & 1 & 0 \\
0 & 1 & 0 & 0 & 1 & 0 \\
1 & 0 & 0 & 0 & 0 & 1 \\
0 & 1 & 0 & 0 & 0 & 1 \\
1 & 0 & 1 & 0 & 0 & 0 \\
0 & 1 & 1 & 0 & 0 & 0 \\
1 & 0 & 1 & 1 & 0 & 0 \\
0 & 1 & 1 & 1 & 0 & 0 \\
1 & 0 & 1 & 0 & 1 & 0 \\
0 & 1 & 1 & 0 & 1 & 0 \\
1 & 0 & 1 & 0 & 0 & 1 \\
0 & 1 & 1 & 0 & 0 & 1
\end{bmatrix}
\begin{bmatrix}
\beta_{PM1} \\
\beta_{PM2} \\
\beta_{PM3} \\
\beta_{PM4} \\
\beta_{PM5} \\
\beta_{PM6}
\end{bmatrix}
= \mathbf{X}_{PM}\boldsymbol{\beta}_{PM}
\tag{46}
$$

For this model, β_{PM1} and β_{PM2} represent predicted logits for active treatment at three days, β_{PM3} represents the effect of placebo, and β_{PM4}, β_{PM5}, and β_{PM6} represent the effects of seven days, ten days, and fourteen days. The Wald goodness-of-fit statistic for this model, $Q_W(\mathrm{df} = 10) = 10.69$, is nonsignificant ($p \geqslant 0.25$). The weighted least-squares estimates for the parameter vector $\boldsymbol{\beta}_{PM}$ and its estimated covariance matrix are obtained via (6) and (8); the results are

$$
\mathbf{b}_{PM} =
\begin{bmatrix}
-1.99 \\
0.65 \\
-1.26 \\
1.67 \\
1.55 \\
2.38
\end{bmatrix}
$$

$$
\mathbf{V}_{b,PM} =
\begin{bmatrix}
10.65 & 6.85 & -4.00 & -4.60 & -3.59 & -7.35 \\
6.85 & 7.30 & -4.90 & -2.37 & -1.58 & -3.15 \\
-4.00 & -4.90 & 10.30 & -1.36 & -0.90 & -1.61 \\
-4.60 & -2.37 & -1.36 & 7.01 & 3.07 & 6.07 \\
-3.59 & -1.58 & -0.90 & 3.07 & 4.30 & 3.93 \\
-7.35 & -3.15 & -1.61 & 6.07 & 3.93 & 12.37
\end{bmatrix}
\times 10^{-2}
\tag{47}
$$

Test statistics for treatment effects and visit effects are undertaken with respect to model (46) with

$$C = [0 \quad 0 \quad 1 \quad 0 \quad 0 \quad 0] \qquad C = \begin{bmatrix} 0 & 0 & 0 & 1 & 0 & 0 \\ 0 & 0 & 0 & 0 & 1 & 0 \\ 0 & 0 & 0 & 0 & 0 & 1 \end{bmatrix} \qquad (48)$$

respectively; the corresponding results $Q_C(\text{df} = 1) = 15.52$ and $Q_C(\text{df} = 3)$ = 67.73 are both significant ($p < 0.01$). Thus the conclusions of the proportional odds model analysis agree with those from the methods discussed in the sections "Analysis of Proportions Excellent," Analysis of Mean Scores," and "Analysis of Rank Measures of Association." Finally, predicted values for the (F_{ijl}) can be obtained by (11). These quantities can then be further transformed to predicted values for the proportions of patients with excellent response, good response, and fair or poor response; standard errors for these quantities can be computed through the application of appropriate matrix operations to the estimated covariance matrix (12) of the predicted values for the (F_{ijl}). (For additional discussion of such operations, see Imrey et al. 1981, 1982, or Koch, Imrey, et al., 1985.)

Discussion

The foregoing analyses of the proportions for excellent response and the mean scores were easier to apply than those for the rank measures of association and the proportional odds model. The results for the proportions excellent and the rank measures of association have a more straightforward interpretation than those for the mean scores and for the proportional odds model. A potential limitation of the mean scores is that integer scaling may not suitably describe the response categories. The estimated parameters from the proportional odds model have the awkward feature of corresponding to multipliers for the odds for responses above each particular outcome versus responses below. Since the mean scores and the rank measures of association involve all response outcomes, the sample sizes for approximate normality do not need to be as large as those for the proportions excellent or proportional odds models. A noteworthy advantage of the proportional odds model over the other methods is its capability for characterizing the structure of response distributions, but unsatisfactory goodness of fit can contradict its usage. Thus each of the four methods of analysis have useful features and limitations, which are relevant to the choice among them. For the example considered in this chapter, all of them were applicable and yielded similar conclusions.

An additional consideration is that the illustrated methods can be used to encompass responses at a baseline time prior to treatment in a spirit similar to covariance analysis (see Koch et al., 1982, for related discussion).

Estimates from a National Survey Concerning Health Services

Comprehensive data on health insurance coverage and the utilization, costs, and sources of payment associated with health services were obtained for the United

States through the National Medical Care Expenditure Survey (NMCES). This survey had a stratified, multistage, area probability design with the further complication of two components that corresponded to two independently drawn samples of households by two different survey research groups. The sampling specifications of NMCES called for the selection of approximately 14,000 households to represent the noninstitutionalized civilian population of the United States. Longitudinal data were obtained from the households in NMCES so that evaluation would be feasible for population characteristics for which changes over time occur. Data collection for the core health care measures was to be applied to the same panel of sample households in five rounds of interviewing, with 1977 as the reference period. Short recall periods of two to three months in duration were generally implemented to minimize reporting errors of omission. Additional aspects of NMCES are discussed in Cohen (1982).

This example is concerned with estimates from NMCES for the proportions of the U.S. noninstitutionalized population with Medicaid coverage. The estimated proportions with Medicaid coverage at two time points (period 1 for the first quarter, January–March 1977 and period 2 for December 31, 1977) are shown in Table 9-10 for four groups (i.e., population domains); these groups correspond to the cross-classification of sex (male, female) and residential area (SMSA [standard metropolitan statistical area], non-SMSA). The estimated covariance matrix for the proportions with Medicaid is also shown in Table 9-10. The results in Table 9-10 were obtained from the data for those subjects who completed all interviews in NMCES; the approximately 11 percent of subjects who did not participate in one or more interviews were computationally managed as total nonrespondents. Adjustments for nonresponse were applied to the NMCES sample weights through which the estimation process for the proportions with Medicaid accounted for the structure of the survey design. The determination of the estimated covariance matrix in Table 9-10 involved the use

Table 9-10. Estimated proportions with Medicaid for the noninstitutionalized population of the United States during 1977, and corresponding estimated covariance matrix[a]

Sex	Residential area[b]	Time	Estimated proportions ($\times 10^2$)	Estimated covariance matrix $\times 10^4$							
Male	SMSA	Period 1	6.25	0.27	0.25	0.00	0.00	0.31	0.27	0.00	0.00
Male	SMSA	Period 2	5.74	0.25	0.26	0.00	0.00	0.29	0.28	0.00	0.00
Male	Non-SMSA	Period 1	5.34	0.00	0.00	0.39	0.26	0.00	0.00	0.48	0.33
Male	Non-SMSA	Period 2	4.85	0.00	0.00	0.26	0.31	0.00	0.00	0.30	0.36
Female	SMSA	Period 1	9.80	0.31	0.29	0.00	0.00	0.42	0.36	−0.01	−0.01
Female	SMSA	Period 2	8.44	0.27	0.28	0.00	0.00	0.36	0.38	−0.01	−0.01
Female	Non-SMSA	Period 1	8.23	0.00	0.00	0.48	0.30	−0.01	−0.01	0.68	0.45
Female	Non-SMSA	Period 2	7.07	0.00	0.00	0.33	0.36	−0.01	−0.01	0.45	0.55

[a]Results are based on the National Medical Care Expenditure Survey (NMCES) for the United States.
[b]SMSA denotes standard metropolitan statistical area.

of linear Taylor series methods for survey data along the lines discussed in Woodruff (1971).

Let $\mathbf{F}$ denote the vector of estimated proportions with Medicaid in the order shown in Table 9-10, and let $\mathbf{V}_F$ denote its corresponding estimated covariance matrix. The large sample size of NMCES supports the view that $\mathbf{F}$ has an approximately multivariate normal distribution for which the covariance matrix is known through $\mathbf{V}_F$. On this basis, weighted least-squares analyses can be applied to the estimated proportions with Medicaid in a spirit similar to that in (6) through (12).

A preliminary evaluation is undertaken for the sex, residential area, and time period sources of variation for the estimated proportions with Medicaid through the cell mean (or identity) model $\mathbf{X}_I = \mathbf{I}_8$. Hypotheses pertaining to this model are specified through $\mathbf{C}$ matrices as in (9), and results from Wald test statistics such as in (10) are shown in Table 9-11. The conclusions from Table 9-11 are that the sources of variation for sex, time, and (sex × time) interaction are significant ($p \leqslant 0.01$), whereas those for residential area and its interactions with sex and time are all nonsignificant ($p \geqslant 0.150$).

A reduced model of interest involves components for sex, residential area, time, and (sex × time); it has the specification

$$\mathbf{F} \triangleq \begin{bmatrix} 1 & 0 & 0 & 0 & 0 \\ 1 & 0 & 0 & 1 & 0 \\ 1 & 0 & 1 & 0 & 0 \\ 1 & 0 & 1 & 1 & 0 \\ 1 & 1 & 0 & 0 & 0 \\ 1 & 1 & 0 & 1 & 1 \\ 1 & 1 & 1 & 0 & 0 \\ 1 & 1 & 1 & 1 & 1 \end{bmatrix} \begin{bmatrix} b_{R1} \\ b_{R2} \\ b_{R3} \\ b_{R4} \\ b_{R5} \end{bmatrix} = \mathbf{X}_R \mathbf{b}_R \qquad (49)$$

where b_{R1} denotes the predicted value for males in SMSA areas at period 1, b_{R2} is the increment for females, b_{R3} is the increment for non-SMSA area, b_{R4} is the increment for period 2, and b_{R5} is the interaction increment for females at period

Table 9–11. Results of hypothesis tests from cell mean model for estimated proportions with Medicaid

Source of variation[a]	C matrix								Q_C	df	Approx. p value
Sex (S)	[1	1	1	1	−1	−1	−1	−1]	205.72	1	<0.010
Residential area (R)	[1	1	−1	−1	1	1	−1	−1]	2.01	1	0.157
Time (T)	[1	−1	1	−1	1	−1	1	−1]	11.19	1	<0.001
S × R	[1	1	−1	−1	−1	−1	1	1]	1.86	1	0.173
S × T	[1	−1	1	−1	−1	1	−1	1]	16.79	1	<0.001
R × T	[1	−1	−1	1	1	−1	−1	1]	0.04	1	0.835
S × R × T	[1	−1	−1	1	−1	1	1	−1]	0.20	1	0.651

[a]The contrast for sex is an average over (R × T), the contrast for residential area is an average over (S × T), and the contrast for time is an average over (S × R); the (S × R) interaction is an average over T, the (S × T) interaction is an average over R, and the (R × T) interaction is an average over S.

2. The notation $\triangleq$ expresses equivalence relative to sampling variability and replaces $E_A(\ )$ so as to avoid controversy over the compatibility of a vector of finite population parameters with a reduced model (see Koch, Imrey, et al., 1985, for further discussion). The Wald goodness-of-fit statistic in the sense of (7) for model (49) is $Q_W(df = 3) = 2.42$; its nonsignificance ($p = 0.491$) supports use of the model. The weighted least-squares estimates $\mathbf{b}_R$ and their estimated covariance matrix are

$$\mathbf{b}_R = \begin{bmatrix} 0.0611 \\ 0.0328 \\ -0.0054 \\ -0.0052 \\ -0.0077 \end{bmatrix}$$

$$\mathbf{V}_{b,R} = \begin{bmatrix} 25.95 & 2.42 & -23.59 & -1.84 & -1.32 \\ 2.42 & 3.92 & -0.04 & -0.22 & -1.13 \\ -23.59 & -0.04 & 50.02 & 0.18 & 1.08 \\ -1.84 & -0.22 & 0.18 & 2.52 & 0.20 \\ -1.32 & -1.13 & 1.08 & 0.20 & 3.14 \end{bmatrix} \times 10^{-6}$$

As was the case for the preliminary model, the statistical test for the (sex × time) interaction is significant (with $Q_C(df = 1) = 19.01$, $p < 0.010$) and that for area is nonsignificant (with $Q_C(df = 1) = 0.58$, $p = 0.444$). The estimates from the reduced model can be interpreted as indicating that the estimated proportions with Medicaid are higher for females than for males and higher for period 1 than for period 2, and that the difference between time periods is larger for females than males.

An Observational Study Concerning Health Status of Children

This example is based on an observational study that was undertaken to evaluate the association of geographic area with aspects of the respiratory status of children. A response measure of interest was the classification of presence or absence of a cold for each child for each of three consecutive years from reports during the fall, winter, and spring. The response profiles for some children, however, were incomplete in the sense of having missing classifications for one or two of the three years. The different patterns of incomplete data give rise to additional groups beyond the one with responses for all three years. These groups are considered to represent the same population. The observed distributions for the different types of response patterns are shown in Table 9-12 for the cross-classification of children according to sex (male, female) and two areas (area 1, area 2).

Estimates for the proportions of children with colds can be constructed for those years that are encompassed by each of the different types of data patterns; for example, all three years for those children with responses for all three years,

Table 9–12. Frequencies of response profiles for presence or absence of colds during three years

Presence of colds			Area 1		Area 2	
Year 1	Year 2	Year 3	Male	Female	Male	Female
Yes	Yes	Yes	80	109	59	94
Yes	Yes	No	46	48	31	31
Yes	No	Yes	38	39	22	11
Yes	No	No	61	47	30	32
No	Yes	Yes	57	45	35	28
No	Yes	No	60	43	15	21
No	No	Yes	59	47	41	30
No	No	No	121	79	55	45
Yes	Yes	—	20	34	44	34
Yes	No	—	14	10	23	17
No	Yes	—	14	19	28	10
No	No	—	39	28	41	28
Yes	—	Yes	16	13	7	9
Yes	—	No	5	8	4	4
No	—	Yes	15	14	10	6
No	—	No	13	9	16	6
—	Yes	Yes	47	60	26	23
—	Yes	No	32	15	26	11
—	No	Yes	32	30	23	11
—	No	No	50	39	22	7
Yes	—	—	141	170	129	133
No	—	—	191	155	140	91
—	Yes	—	87	91	65	85
—	No	—	83	84	88	51
—	—	Yes	156	173	129	116
—	—	No	173	152	167	113

years 1 and 2 for those children who only have missing data for year 3, and so on. These estimates can be combined through the weighted least-squares methods described in Koch et al. (1972). More specifically, let the seven types of data patterns be indexed by $h = 1$ for all three years, 2 for years 1 and 2, 3 for years 1 and 3, 4 for years 2 and 3, 5 for year 1, 6 for year 2, and 7 for year 3; then the proportions $(\bar{g}_{hij})$ with colds for the applicable years j from the hth data type for the ith (area × sex) can be represented by

$$\bar{\mathbf{g}}_i = (\bar{g}_{1i1}, \bar{g}_{1i2}, \bar{g}_{1i3}, \bar{g}_{2i1}, \bar{g}_{2i2}, \bar{g}_{3i1}, \bar{g}_{3i3}, \bar{g}_{4i2}, \bar{g}_{4i3}, \bar{g}_{5i1}, \bar{g}_{6i2}, \bar{g}_{7i3}).$$

The model that specifies common values for the different estimates that pertain to the same year has the structure

$$\mathbf{E}(\bar{\mathbf{g}}_i) = \begin{bmatrix} 1 & 0 & 0 & 1 & 0 & 1 & 0 & 0 & 0 & 1 & 0 & 0 \\ 0 & 1 & 0 & 0 & 1 & 0 & 0 & 1 & 0 & 0 & 1 & 0 \\ 0 & 0 & 1 & 0 & 0 & 0 & 1 & 0 & 1 & 0 & 0 & 1 \end{bmatrix}' \begin{bmatrix} \mu_{i1} \\ \mu_{i2} \\ \mu_{i3} \end{bmatrix} \tag{50}$$

Table 9–13. Weighted least-squares estimates (and standard errors) for proportions of children with colds and Wald goodness-of-fit statistics from observational study

Area	Sex	Year 1	Year 2	Year 3	Q_W	df	Approximate p value
Area 1	Male	0.427	0.473	0.472	10.95	9	0.279
		(0.016)	(0.016)	(0.015)			
Area 1	Female	0.520	0.533	0.548	10.10	9	0.342
		(0.016)	(0.017)	(0.016)			
Area 2	Male	0.474	0.479	0.493	17.71	9	0.039
		(0.018)	(0.019)	(0.018)			
Area 2	Female	0.584	0.591	0.550	10.40	9	0.319
		(0.019)	(0.020)	(0.020)			

For each (area × sex), the weighted least-squares estimates ($\bar{\mu}_{ij}$) of the (μ_{ij}) and their estimated standard errors are shown in Table 9-13. Wald goodness-of-fit statistics are also given in the table and indicate reasonable support for use of model (50); the only noteworthy departure is the significant result ($p = 0.042$) for males in area 2, whereas the results for the other three (area × sex) combinations are clearly nonsignificant ($p > 0.150$). Thus the components of the ($\bar{\mathbf{g}}_i$) for the respective data patterns can be interpreted as representing the same population.

Hypotheses concerning the variation of the proportions (μ_{ij}) of children with colds across areas, sexes, and years can be specified through **C** matrices as in (9); results from the corresponding Wald statistics in (10) are shown in Table 9-14. They indicate that sex and area effects are significant ($p < 0.010$), but that year effects and all interactions for sex, area, and year are nonsignificant ($p > 0.150$).

Table 9–14. Results of hypothesis tests for proportions of children with colds from observational study

Source of variation[a]	Q_C	df	Approximate p value
Sex (S)	54.86	1	<0.010
Area (A)	8.38	1	<0.010
Year (Y)	2.69	2	0.261
$S \times A$	0.49	1	0.485
$S \times Y$	2.10	2	0.350
$A \times Y$	3.33	2	0.189
$S \times A \times Y$	2.45	2	0.294
Reduction to model with sex and area only	11.49	9	0.244

[a]The contrast for sex is an average over ($A \times Y$), the contrast for area is an average over ($S \times Y$), the contrasts for year are averages over ($S \times A$); the ($S \times A$) interaction is an average over Y, the ($S \times Y$) interactions are averages over A, and the ($A \times Y$) interactions are averages over S.

Thus the variation among the (μ_{ij}) can be described by a reduced model with only sex and area effects. This model has the structure

$$
\mu = \begin{bmatrix} 1 & 1 & 1 & 1 & 1 & 1 & 1 & 1 & 1 & 1 & 1 & 1 \\ 0 & 0 & 0 & 1 & 1 & 1 & 0 & 0 & 0 & 1 & 1 & 1 \\ 0 & 0 & 0 & 0 & 0 & 0 & 1 & 1 & 1 & 1 & 1 & 1 \end{bmatrix}' \begin{bmatrix} \beta_1 \\ \beta_2 \\ \beta_3 \end{bmatrix} = \mathbf{Z}\boldsymbol{\beta} \qquad (51)
$$

where $\boldsymbol{\mu} = (\mu_{11}, \mu_{12}, \mu_{13}, \mu_{21}, \ldots, \mu_{43})$; also β_1 denotes the predicted proportion of male children in area 1 with colds, β_2 is the increment for females, and β_3 is the increment for area 2. The application of weighted least-squares methods to the estimates $(\bar{\mu}_{ij})$ as the functions $\mathbf{F}$ in (17) and their corresponding covariance structure provides estimates $\mathbf{b}$ for the parameters $\boldsymbol{\beta}$ in (51); these estimates and their corresponding estimated covariance matrix are

$$
\mathbf{b} = \begin{bmatrix} 0.454 \\ 0.083 \\ 0.032 \end{bmatrix} \qquad \mathbf{V}_b = \begin{bmatrix} 80.49 & -59.00 & -54.36 \\ -59.00 & 125.25 & 3.52 \\ -54.36 & 3.52 & 128.58 \end{bmatrix} \times 10^{-6}
$$

The results from the reduced model can be interpreted as indicating that the estimated proportions of colds are higher for females than males, are higher for area 2 than area 1, and are similar across the three years.

Appendix
Computational Procedures to Obtain
the Results for the Examples

A variety of computer programs are available to perform the analyses described in this paper. Although most of the computing initially was done with the Fortran program GENCAT [Landis, et al. (1976)], the SAS (1990) procedure CATMOD (which replaces its predecessor FUNCAT) can also be used to perform many of the same analyses. CATMOD is a multi-purpose procedure which fits linear models to the functions created from response frequencies. It can be used in linear modeling, repeated measurements analyses, log-linear modeling, and logistic regression. Weighted least squares procedures are applied to estimated parameters for a variety of linear models for specified response functions, or maximum likelihood estimation is performed for the analysis of log-linear models for response probabilities. Goodness-of-fit statistics are computed, and Wald statistics are calculated for linear hypotheses concerning model parameters. Options are available for computing predicted response probabilities; both the predicted values and the estimated parameters and covariance matrix can be output to external datasets so that they can be further processed.

The clinical trial example with the proportion for excellent outcome in (18) as the response function provides a good example for the illustration of

CATMOD. The reader is assumed to have a basic understanding of the SAS system data step. If the entries of Table 9-2 correspond to a SAS dataset named SKIN with the variables D1-D4 representing the responses for 3 days, 7 days, 10 days, and 14 days respectively, and a variable named TRT taking the appropriate values "active" or "placebo," then the following SAS statements will convert the responses to the binary outcomes analyzed and put the data in the form illustrated in Table 9-4.

```
DATA TRANSFORM
    SET SKIN;
    D1 = 1*(D1 < 1); D2 = 1*(D2 < 1);
    D3 = 1*(D3 < 1); D4 = 1*(D4 < 1);
PROC FREQ DATA = TRANSFORM;
    TABLES TRT*D1*D2*D3*D4/NOPRINT OUT = EXAMPLE1;
```

The following is displayed when one uses the SAS procedure PRINT to look at the resulting dataset EXAMPLE1. There are 16 possible profiles for each treatment or 32 altogether; FREQ puts out an observation for each profile with a non-zero count; see Table 9-4.

OBS	TRT	D1	D2	D3	D4	COUNT	PERCENT
1	ACTIVE	0	0	0	0	10	13.8889
2	ACTIVE	0	0	0	1	8	11.1111
3	ACTIVE	0	0	1	0	2	2.7778
4	ACTIVE	0	0	1	1	1	1.3889
5	ACTIVE	0	1	0	0	2	2.7778
6	ACTIVE	0	1	0	1	3	4.1667
7	ACTIVE	0	1	1	1	5	6.9444
8	ACTIVE	1	0	1	0	2	2.7778
9	ACTIVE	1	1	1	1	3	4.1667
10	PLACEBO	0	0	0	0	19	26.3889
11	PLACEBO	0	0	0	1	6	8.3333
12	PLACEBO	0	0	1	0	3	4.1667
13	PLACEBO	0	0	1	1	3	4.1667
14	PLACEBO	0	1	0	0	2	2.7778
15	PLACEBO	0	1	0	1	1	1.3889
16	PLACEBO	0	1	1	1	1	1.3889
17	PLACEBO	1	0	1	0	1	1.3889

The following data step then created variables T1-T4, which take the value 'E' if the corresponding D1-D4 equals 0 and 'N' otherwise.

```
DATA EXAMPLE;
    SET EXAMPLE1;
    ARRAY D{4} D1-D4; ARRAY T{4} $ T1-T4;
    DO I = 1 TO 4;
        IF D{I} = 1 THEN T{I} = 'E';
        ELSE T{I} = 'N';
    END;
```

CATMOD is first used to model the marginal response probabilities. The input to CATMOD consists of the dataset EXA7PLE1, the observations of which contain the frequency count of those subjects who had a particular response profile for either the active or placebo treatments. When input is of this nature, CATMOD requires that a WEIGHT statement be used to identify the variable which contains the profile frequencies. The RESPONSE statement is necessary to request the response function desired to be modeled. Possible specifications are MEANS, LOGITS, MARGINALS, and JOINT, as well as more specific transformations which are to be applied to the proportion vector corresponding to each subpopulation. If no RESPONSE s5atement is used, then generalized logits are the functions modeled by default. Specifying MARGINALS indicates that the response functions are the marginal probabilities for each of the dependent variables referenced in the MODEL statement, e.g., sets of proportions like those shown in Table 9-3. CATMOD generates the appropriate A matrix internally (such as is described in Equation (24)) and applies it to the response vector to produce the appropriate functions. The following statements illustrate these and other statements required to use CATMOD to fit an identity model to the estimated marginal probabilities and perform the tests for the hypotheses specified in Table 9-5.

```
PROC CATMOD DATA = EXAMPLE;
    WEIGHT COUNT;
    POPULATION TRT;
    RESPONSE MARGINALS;
    MODEL T1*T2*T3*T4  =  ( 1 0 0 0 0 0 0 0,
                            0 1 0 0 0 0 0 0,
                            0 0 1 0 0 0 0 0,
                            0 0 0 1 0 0 0 0,
                            0 0 0 0 1 0 0 0,
                            0 0 0 0 0 1 0 0,
                            0 0 0 0 0 0 1 0,
                            0 0 0 0 0 0 0 1);
    CONSTRAST 'TREAT AVE OVER TIME'
        ALL_PARMS   1    1    1    1   -1   -1   -1   -1;
    CONTRAST 'VISIT AVE OVER TREAT'
        ALL_PARMS  -1    1    0    0   -1    1    0    0,
        ALL_PARMS  -1    0    1    0   -1    0    1    0,
        ALL_PARMS  -1    0    0    1   -1    0    0    1;
    CONTRAST 'INTERACTION'
        ALL_PARMS  -1    1    0    0    1   -1    0    0,
        ALL_PARMS  -1    0    1    0    1    0   -1    0,
        ALL_PARMS  -1    0    0    1    1    0    0   -1;
```

Variables which determine the subpopulations to be formed are listed on the POPULATION statement. The MODEL statement is used to specify the response and design effects to be used in modeling. In addition, if no POPULATION statement is included, the independent effects listed in the MODEL statement determine the subpopulation structure, subpopulation structure, SAS GLM-like syntax can be used to specify effects in the model or the X matrix itself can be input directly on the MODEL statement. This is done here in order to specify a cell-mean (identity model.) The CONTRAST statement provides a way of specifying the C matrices for the hypotheses in Table 9-5. ALL_PARMS is used to indicate that the contrasts are to be applied to the entire estimated parameter vector (versus the capacity of application to a subset of parameters corresponding to the components of a particular effect). CATMOD prints the following information for each analysis:

Response: T1*T2*T3*T4	Response Levels (R)=9
Weight Variable: COUNT	Populations (S)=2
Data Set: EXAMPLE1	Total Frequency (N)=72
	Observations (Obs)=17

In addition, CATMOD prints out the population profiles and response profiles.

Population Profiles

Sample	TRT	Sample size
1	ACTIVE	36
2	PLACEBO	36

Response Profiles

Response	T1	T2	T3	T4
1	E	E	E	E
2	E	N	E	N
3	N	E	E	E
4	N	E	N	E
5	N	E	N	N
6	N	N	E	E
7	N	N	E	N
8	N	N	N	E
9	N	N	N	N

The response functions printed below are the estimated marginal probabilities of excellent response for placebo (Sample 2) and active treatment (Sample 1) for 3 days, 7 days, 10 days, and 14 days (Function Numbers 1, 2, 3, 4). These are the same as those listed in the first row of Table 9-3. The model specification matrix X is that which was specified on the MODL statement. All this information can be suppressed from being printed by specifying the appropriate options.

Sample	Function number	Response function	Covariance matrix			
			1	2	3	4
1	1	0.1389	0.003322	0.000922	0.002465	0.000171
	2	0.3611	0.000922	0.006409	0.002551	0.002915
	3	0.3611	0.002465	0.002551	0.006409	0.001372
	4	0.5556	0.000171	0.002915	0.001372	0.006859
2	1	0.0278	0.000750	−0.000086	0.000600	−0.000236
	2	0.1111	−0.000086	0.002743	0.000086	0.000600
	3	0.2222	0.000600	0.000086	0.004801	0.001200
	4	0.3056	−0.000236	0.000600	0.001200	0.005894

Sample	Function number	Design matrix							
		1	2	3	4	5	6	7	8
1	1	1	0	0	0	0	0	0	0
	2	0	1	0	0	0	0	0	0
	3	0	0	1	0	0	0	0	0
	4	0	0	0	1	0	0	0	0
2	1	0	0	0	0	1	0	0	0
	2	0	0	0	0	0	1	0	0
	3	0	0	0	0	0	0	1	0
	4	0	0	0	0	0	0	0	1

Since the identity model was used, the parameter estimates displayed here are marginal response functions. The Chi-square printed for each parameter is a Wald statistic for the test that the parameter is zero.

Analysis of Weighted Least Squares Estimates

Effect	Parameter	Estimate	Standard error	Chi-square	Prob
MODEL	1	0.1389	0.0576	5.81	0.0160
	2	0.3611	0.0801	20.35	0.0001
	3	0.3611	0.0801	20.35	0.0001
	4	0.5556	0.0828	45.00	0.0001
	5	0.0278	0.0274	1.03	0.3105
	6	0.1111	0.0524	4.50	0.0339
	7	0.2222	0.0693	10.29	0.0013
	8	0.3056	0.0768	15.84	0.0001

The remaining output from this invocation of CATMOD is the hypothesis tests. These results are shown below and are given formally in Table 9-5.

Analysis of Contrasts

Contrast	DF	Chi-square	Prob
Treat ave over time	1	9.03	0.0027
Visit ave over treat	3	37.02	0.0001
Interaction	3	1.95	0.5835

The previously described analysis required the use of a directly input X matrix since it involved the cell mean model. It is possible to specify effects on the MODEL statement which correspond to sources of variation in the structure of the dependent variables through the use of the _RESPONSE_ keyword. The REPEATED statement can be used when there is more than one dependent variable and the _RESPONSE_ effect is being used. It allows one to specify the names and levels of a repeated measurement factor as well as to define the _ RESPONSE_ effect. Then, the specification of effects on the MODEL statement is possible to generate an appropriate X matrix. In the statements listed below, the REPEATED statement is used to name a repeated measure effect (DAY) and define the levels (4). If this value is missing, it is assumed to be equal to the number of response functions per population. The _RESPONSE_ keyword specifies effects. It is then used in the specifications of model effects on the MODEL statement.

```
PROC CATMOD DATA = EXAMPLE1;
    WEIGHT COUNT;
    POPULATION TRT;
    RESPONSE MARGINALS;
    MODEL T1*T2*T3*T4 = TRT _RESPONSE_ TRT*_RESPONSE_;
    REPEATED DAY 4 / _RESPONSE_ = DAY;
```

What follows is selected and edited output from the resulting CATMOD run. Note that the model specification matrix generated corresponds to a centerpoint parameterization with deviation from mean effects. One needs to use directly input model specification matrices if reference cell parameterization is desired. It is of interest to note that the average effects tests requested with contrast matrices for the cell mean (or identity) model are the same as those automatically generated by CATMOD for each effect in the model with centerpoint parameterization displayed in the Analysis of Variance table. Thus, if one is interested in performing tests for average effects in a cell mean model, one can use the model statement for centerpoint parameterization and obtain the test statistics for sources of variation rather than inputting an identity matrix and contrast test specifications.

Sample	Function number	Response function	Design matrix							
			1	2	3	4	5	6	7	8
1	1	0.13889	1	1	1	0	0	1	0	0
	2	0.36111	1	1	0	1	0	0	1	0
	3	0.36111	1	1	0	0	1	0	0	1
	4	0.55556	1	1	−1	−1	−1	−1	−1	−1
2	1	0.02778	1	−1	1	0	0	−1	0	0
	2	0.11111	1	−1	0	1	0	0	−1	0
	3	0.22222	1	−1	0	0	1	0	0	−1
	4	0.30556	1	−1	−1	−1	−1	1	1	1

Analysis of Variance Table

Source	DF	Chi-square	Prob
Intercept	1	561.85	0.0001
Trt	1	9.03	0.0027
Day	3	37.02	0.0001
Trt*_response_	3	1.95	0.5835
Residual	0	0.00	1.0000
Note:_response_ = day			

Analysis of Weighted Least Squares Estimates

Effect	Parameter	Estimate	Standard error	Chi-square	Prob
Intercept	1	0.7396	0.0312	561.85	0.0001
Trt	2	−0.0937	0.0312	9.03	0.0027
Day	3	0.1771	0.0317	31.26	0.0001
	4	0.0243	0.0353	0.47	0.4908
	5	−0.0312	0.0366	0.73	0.3934
Trt*_response_	6	0.0382	0.0317	1.45	0.2278
	7	−0.0313	0.0353	0.78	0.3756
	8	0.0243	0.0366	0.44	0.5068

Note:_response_ = day

The following code specifies the analysis for the model displayed in Equation (26) and leads to the results displayed in Table 9-6. Here, the goodness-of-fit statistic for the model is model is $Q(w) = 1.95$ with d.f. = 3. Immediately following is the Analysis of Contrasts table produced by the procedure.

```
PROC CATMOD DATA = EXAMPLE1;
    WEIGHT COUNT;
    POPULATION TRT;
    RESPONSE MARGINALS;
    MODEL T1*T2*T3*T4 = (1 0 0 0 0,
                         1 0 1 0 0,
                         1 0 0 1 0,
                         1 0 0 0 1,
                         1 1 0 0 0,
                         1 1 1 0 0,
                         1 1 0 1 0,
                         1 1 0 0 1);
CONTRAST 'TREATMENT EFFECT'
    ALL_PARMS 0 1 0 0 0;
CONTRAST 'VISIT EFFECTS'
    ALL_PARMS 0 0 1 0 0,
ALL_PARMS 0 0 0 1 0,
    ALL_PARMS 0 0 0 0 1;
CONTRAST 'LACK OF LINEARITY'
    ALL_PARMS 0 0 −7  4 0,
    ALL_PARMS 0 0 −11 0 4;
```

Analysis of Contrasts

Contrast	DF	Chi-square	Prob
Treatment effect	1	9.21	0.0024
Visit effects	3	35.56	0.0001
Lack of linearity	2	0.07	0.9641

The final model implied by the results of these tests is not reproduced here; however options are available in the software to produce the final model predicted proportions and their standard errors as displayed in Table 9-7.

The analysis of the mean scores in (30) is also easily accomplished with the use of the MEANS keyword on the RESPONSE statement in CATMOD. Mean scores are computed from the original SKIN dataset for each visit × treatment.

The tests for treatment effects, visit effects, and (treatment × visit) effects can be performed with CATMOD through the use of the REPEATED statement and the _RESPONSE– effect. In the statements below, CATMOD is asked to perform an analysis on the mean score for each visit. A centerpoint model is requested with effects for treatments, time, and (treatment × time) interaction. The effect for time is named 'day' with the REPEATED statement; the _ RESPONSE_ keyword is required in the MODEL specification since the effect involves dependent variables. Here, _RESPONSE_ is regarded by CATMOD as a variable with four levels corresponding to the four mean score functions for each subpopulation and thus having 3 d.f. As previously noted, the tests for the effects produced for the centerpoint parameterization are equivalent to the average effects tests for the cell mean model as described in the text. These results are illustrated below in the Analysis of Variance Table printed out by CATMOD.

```
PROC CATMOD DATA = SKIN;
    POPULATION TRT;
    RESPONSE MEANS;
    MODEL T1*T2*T3*T4 = TRT _RESPONSE_ TRT*_RESPONSE_;
    REPEATED DAY 4 / _RESPONSE_ = DAY;
```

Analysis of Variance Table

Source	DF	Chi-square	Prob
Intercept	1	347.59	0.0001
Trt	1	13.90	0.0002
Day	3	107.35	0.0001
Trt*_response_	3	3.06	0.3826
Residual	0	−0.00	1.0000
Note:_response_ = day			

The final model (26) for the mean scores (30) can be fit with CATMOD through the use of a directly input design matrix in the MODEL statement. The following is the code which can be used to replicate the analysis fo the functions (40) for the proportional odds model using the CATMOD procedure.

```
PROC CATMOD DATA = SKIN;
TITLE2 'PROPORTIONAL ODDS CREATION AND ANALYSIS';
POPULATION TRT;
RESPONSE
1  0 −1  0  0  0  0  0  0  0  0  0  0  0  0,
0  1  0 −1  0  0  0  0  0  0  0  0  0  0  0,
0  0  0  0  1  0 −1  0  0  0  0  0  0  0  0,
0  0  0  0  0  1  0 −1  0  0  0  0  0  0  0,
0  0  0  0  0  0  0  0  1  0 −1  0  0  0  0,
0  0  0  0  0  0  0  0  0  1  0 −1  0  0  0,
0  0  0  0  0  0  0  0  0  0  0  0  1  0 −1  0,
0  0  0  0  0  0  0  0  0  0  0  0  0  1  0 −1
```

LOG
1 1 0 0 0 0 0 0 0 0 0 0 0 0 0 0 0 0 0 0 0 0 0 0 0 0,
1 1 1 1 1 1 1 1 1 1 1 1 1 0 0 0 0 0 0 0 0 0 0 0 0 0,
0 0 1 1 1 1 1 1 1 1 1 1 1 1 1 1 1 1 1 1 1 1 1 1 1 1,
0 0 0 0 0 0 0 0 0 0 0 0 0 1 1 1 1 1 1 1 1 1 1 1 1 1,
1 0 1 1 1 0 0 0 0 0 0 0 0 1 1 1 0 0 0 0 0 0 0 0 0 0,
1 1 1 1 1 1 1 1 1 1 1 1 1 0 1 1 1 1 1 1 1 1 0 0 0 1,
0 1 0 0 0 1 1 1 1 1 1 1 1 0 0 0 1 1 1 1 1 1 1 1 1 1,
0 0 0 0 0 0 0 0 0 0 0 0 1 0 0 0 0 0 0 0 0 1 1 1 1 0,
1 1 1 0 0 1 1 1 0 0 0 0 0 0 0 0 1 0 0 0 0 0 0 0 0 0,
1 1 1 1 1 1 1 1 1 1 0 0 1 1 1 0 1 1 1 0 0 1 0 0 0 0,
0 0 0 1 1 0 0 0 1 1 1 1 1 1 1 1 0 1 1 1 1 1 1 1 1 1,
0 0 0 0 0 0 0 0 0 0 1 1 0 0 0 1 0 0 0 1 1 0 1 1 1 1,
1 0 1 1 0 1 0 0 1 0 1 0 0 0 0 1 1 1 0 1 0 0 1 0 0 0,
1 1 1 1 1 1 1 1 0 1 1 1 1 1 1 1 0 1 1 1 1 1 1 1 1 1,
0 1 0 0 1 0 1 1 0 1 0 1 1 1 1 0 0 0 1 0 1 1 0 1 1 1,
0 0 0 0 0 0 0 1 0 0 0 0 0 0 1 0 0 0 0 0 0 0 0 0 0 0;

The linear and log transformations on the vector of marginal proportions described in (42) are specified to CATMOD via the RESPONSE statement. Working from bottom to top (right to left in (42)), the first matrix defines the $\{f(ij0)\}$, $\{f(ij1) + f(ij2) + f(ij3)\}$, $\{f(ij0) + f(ij1)\}$, and $\{f(ij2) + f(ij3)\}$. A log transformation is then performed, followed (at top) by the leftmost matrix in (42) which forms the cumulative logits of interest. The proportional odds model of (44) can be investigated via CATMOD by directly inputting the specification matrix on the MODEL s5atement. One can proceed with this framework to compute the test statistics for effects and then fit the subsequent reduced model discussed in the text.

The analysis of rank measures of association is also possible with CATMOD, through the similar use of the RESPONSE statement to specify a series of transformations to the response vector in order to produce the functions of interest. It is tedious to do, however, and the details are not included here; see Carr, Hafner, and Koch (1989) for discussion of a more straightforward computational method.

The analysis for the observational study concerning health status for children also relies on the use fo the RESPONSE statement in order to produce the response functions of interest. The data set used by CATMOD includes the variables AREA, GENDER and YEAR1, YEAR2 and YEAR3. The YEAR* variables take on the values 'Y' 'N' and 'U', where 'Y' indicates the presence of cold symptoms for that year, 'N' indicates the absence, and 'U' represents undefined, meaning that there is no information for that year for that subject. Note that these translate fairly readily into the frequencies displayed in Table 9-12.

1 M Y Y Y 80   1 M Y Y N 46   1 M Y N Y 38   1 M Y N N 61
1 M N Y Y 57   1 M N Y N 60   1 M N N Y 59   1 M N N N 121
....

The following statements will produce the analysis for the model specified in (50), given that the data are sorted by AREA and GENDER:

```
PROC CATMOD ORDER = DATA;
BY AREA GENDER;
WEIGHT COUNT;
POPULATION·AREA GENDER;
RESPONSE
EXP
1 0 0 −1 0 0   0 0 0   0 0 0   0 0   0 0   0 0   0,
0 1 0 − 0   0 0 0   0 0 0   0 0   0 0   0 0   0,
0 0 1 −1 0 0   0 0 0   0 0 0   0 0   0 0   0 0   0,
0 0 0   0 1 0 −1 0 0   0 0 0   0 0   0 0   0 0   0,
0 0 0   0 0 1 −1 0 0   0 0 0   0 0   0 0   0 0   0,
0 0 0   0 0 0   0 1 0 −1 0 0   0 0   0 0   0 0   0,
0 0 0   0 0 0   0 0 1 −1 0 0   0 0   0 0   0 0   0,
0 0 0   0 0 0   0 0 0   0 1 0 −1 0   0 0   0 0   0,
0 0 0   0 0 0   0 0 0   0 0 1 −1 0   0 0   0 0   0,
0 0 0   0 0 0   0 1 0   0 0 0   0 1 −1 0   0 0   0,
0 0 0   0 0 0   0 0 0   0 0 0   0 0   0 1 −1 0   0,
0 0 0   0 0 0   0 0 0   0 0 0   0 0   0 0   0 1 −1

LOG
1 1 0 1 1 0 0 0 0 0 0 0 0 0 0 0 0 0 0 0 0 0 0 0 0 0,
1 1 0 0 0 0 0 0 0 1 1 0 0 0 0 0 0 0 0 0 0 0 0 0 0 0,
1 0 0 1 0 0 0 0 0 1 0 0 1 0 0 0 0 0 0 0 0 0 0 0 0 0,
1 1 0 1 1 1 1 1 1 0 0 1 0 0 0 0 0 0 0 0 0 0 0 0 0 0,
0 0 1 0 0 1 0 0 0 0 0 0 0 0 0 0 0 0 0 0 0 0 0 0 0 0,
0 0 1 0 0 0 0 0 0 0 1 0 0 0 0 0 0 0 0 0 0 0 0 0 0 0,
0 0 1 0 0 1 0 0 0 0 1 0 0 1 0 0 0 0 0 0 0 0 0 0 0 0,
0 0 0 0 0 0 1 1 0 0 0 0 0 0 0 0 0 0 0 0 0 0 0 0 0 0,
0 0 0 0 0 0 1 0 0 0 0 0 0 0 0 1 0 0 0 0 0 0 0 0 0 0,
0 0 0 0 0 0 1 1 0 0 0 0 0 0 0 1 1 0 0 0 0 0 0 0 0 0,
0 0 0 0 0 0 0 0 0 0 0 0 0 0 0 0 0 1 1 0 0 0 0 0 0 0,
0 0 0 0 0 0 0 0 0 0 0 0 0 0 0 0 0 1 0 0 1 0 0 0 0 0,
0 0 0 0 0 0 0 0 0 0 0 0 0 0 0 0 0 1 1 0 1 1 0 0 0 0,
0 0 0 0 0 0 0 0 1 0 0 0 0 0 0 0 0 0 0 0 0 0 0 0 0 0,
0 0 0 0 0 0 0 0 1 0 0 0 0 0 0 0 0 1 0 0 0 0 0 0 0 0,
0 0 0 0 0 0 0 0 0 0 0 0 0 0 0 0 0 0 0 1 0 0 0 0 0 0,
0 0 0 0 0 0 0 0 0 0 0 0 0 0 0 0 0 0 0 1 0 0 1 0 0 0,
0 0 0 0 0 0 0 0 0 0 0 0 0 0 0 0 0 0 0 0 0 0 0 1 0,
0 0 0 0 0 0 0 0 0 0 0 0 0 0 0 0 0 0 0 0 0 0 0 1 1;

MODEL YEAR1*YEAR2*YEAR3 = (1 0 0,   0 1 0,   0 0 1,
                          1 0 0,   0 1 0,   1 0 0,
                          0 0 1,   0 1 0,   0 0 1,
                          1 0 0,   0 1 0,   0 0 1);
```

In this specification, the ORDER = DATA option transforms the input ordering shown in Table 9-12 to one for which the successive response profiles for each area and gender is (YYY,YYN,YYU,YNY,YNN,YNU,...UUY,UUN). The results for this analysis are not included here.

The example concerned with estimated from a national health survey was analyzed with the GENCAT program, utilizing a capacity which allows a function vector and covariance matrix to be read directly. Other means were used to compute the covariance matrix, which involved making adjustments for the survey design. Version 6 of the SAS system also has such a capacity through the FACTORS statement.

ACKNOWLEDGMENTS

This chapter was first prepared as a paper for Workshop on Longitudinal Methods in Health Research, West Berlin, June 23–26, 1986. The research was supported in part by the U.S. Bureau of the Census through Joint Statistical Agreement JSA-84-5. The work of Julio M. Singer was also supported in part by a grant from FAPESP, Sao Paulo, Brazil. We would like to express appreciation to Bea O'Quinn, Amy Goulson, Jean Harrison, and Ann Thomas for editorial assistance.

REFERENCES

Agresti A (1984). *Analysis of Ordinal Categorical Data.* New York, Wiley.
Agresti A. (1989). "A survey of models for repeated ordered categorical response data." *Statistics in Medicine* 8:1209–1224.
Anderson JA, Pemberton JD (1985). "The grouped continuous model for multivariate ordered categorical variables and covariate adjustment." *Biometrics* 41:875–885.
Bhapkar VP (1966). "A note on the equivalence of two test criteria for hypotheses in categorical data." *Journal of the American Statistical Association* 61:228–235.
Bishop YMM, Fienberg SE, Holland PW (1975). *Discrete Multivariate Analysis: Theory and Practice.* Cambridge, Mass., MIT Press.
Cohen SB (1982). "Estimated data collection organization effect in the National Medical Care Expenditure Survey." *American Statistician* 36:337–341.
Cook NR, Ware JH (1983). "Design and analysis methods for longitudinal research." *Annual Review of Public Health* 4:1–24.
Corr GJ, Hafner KB, Koch GG (1989). "Analysis of rank measures of association for ordinal data from longitudinal studies." *Journal of the American Statistical Association* 84.
Cox DR, Oakes D (1984). *Analysis of Survival Data.* New York, Chapman and Hall.
Freeman DH Jr, Freeman JL, Brock DB, Koch GG (1976). "Strategies in the multivariate analysis of data from complex surveys. II. An application to the United States National Health Interview Survey." *International Statistical Review* 44:317–330.
Haber M (1985). "Maximum likelihood methods for linear and log-linear models in categorical data." *Computational Statistics and Data Analysis* 3:1–10.
Imrey PB, Koch GG, Stokes ME, et al. (1981, 1982). "Categorical data analysis: Some reflections on the log linear model and logistic regression." *International Statistical Review* 49:265–283 (Part I); 50:35–74 (Part II).

Kalbfleisch JD, Prentice RL (1980). *The Statistical Analysis of Failure Time Data*. New York, Wiley.

Koch GG, Amara IA, Davis GW, Gillings DB (1982). "A review of some statistical methods for covariance analysis of categorical data." *Biometrics* 38:563–595.

Koch GG, Amara IA, Singer JM (1985). "A two-stage procedure for the analysis of ordinal categorical data." In Sen PK (ed), *Biostatistics: Statistics in Biomedical, Public Health and Environmental Sciences*, New York, North Holland, pp 357–387.

Koch GG Bhapkar VP (1982). "Chi-square tests." in Johnson NL, Kotz S (eds), *Encyclopedia of Statistical Sciences* 1. New York, Wiley, pp 442–457.

Koch GG, Carr GJ, Amara IA, Stokes ME, Uryniak TJ (1990). "Categorical data analysis." In Berry DA (ed), *Statistical Methodology in the Pharmaceutical Sciences*, New York, Marcel Dekker, pp 389–473.

Koch GG, Elashoff JD, Amara IA (1986). "Repeated measurements studies, design and analysis." In Johnson NL, Kotz S (eds), *Encyclopedia of Statistical Sciences* 8, New York, Wiley, pp 46–73.

Koch GG, Freeman DH Jr, Freeman JL (1975). "Strategies in the multivariate analysis of data from complex surveys." *International Statistical Review* 43:59–78.

Koch GG, Gillings DB (1983). "Inference, design based vs. model based." In Johnson NL, Kotz S (eds), *Encyclopedia of Statistical Sciences* 4. New York, Wiley, pp 84–88.

Koch GG, Imrey PB, Reinfurt DW (1972). "Linear model analysis of categorical data with incomplete response vectors." *Biometrics* 28:663–692.

Koch GG, Imrey PB, Singer JM, Atkinson SS, Stokes ME (1985). "Analysis of categorical data." In Sabidussi G (ed), *Collection Seminaire de Mathematiques Superieures* 96. Montreal, Les Presses de L'Université de Montreal.

Koch GG, Landis JR, Freeman JL, Freeman DH Jr, Lehnen R G (1977). "A general methodology for the analysis of experiments with repeated measurement of categorical data." *Biometrics* 33:133–158.

Koch GG, Stokes ME (1982). Chi-square tests: Numerical examples. In Johnson NL, Kotz S (eds), *Encyclopedia of Statistical Sciences* 1. New York, Wiley, pp 457–472.

Kruskal WH, Wallis WA (1953). "Use of ranks in one criterion variance analysis." *Journal of the American Statistical Association* 46:583–621.

Landis JR, Koch GG (1979). "The analysis of categorical data in longitudinal studies of behavioral development." Chapter 9 in Nesselroade JR, Baltes PB (eds), *Longitudinal Research in the Study of Behavior and Development*. New York, Academic Press, pp 233–261.

Landis JR, Lepkowski JM, Eklund SA, Stehouwer SA (1982). *A Statistical Methodology for Analyzing Data from a Complex Survey: The First National Health and Nutrition Examination Survey*. Vital and Health Statistics, Series 2, No. 92 DHHS Pub. 82-1366. Public Health Service. Washington, D.C., Government Printing Office.

Landis JR, Stanish WM, Freeman JL, Koch GG (1976). "A computer program for the generalized chi-square analysis of categorical data using weighted least squares (GENCAT)." *Computer Programs in Biomedicine* 6:196–231.

Lee ET (1980). *Statistical Methods for Survival Data Analysis*. Belmont, Calif., Wadsworth.

Liang K, Zeger SL (1986). "Longitudinal data analysis using generalized linear models." *Biometrika* 73:13–22.

McCullagh P (1980). "Regression models for ordinal data" (with discussion). *Journal of the Royal Statistical Society* B 42:109–142.

McCullagh P, Nelder JA (1983). *Generalized Linear Models*. New York, Chapman and Hall.

Mann HB, Whitney DR (1947). "On a test of whether one of two random variables is stochastically larger than the other." *Annals of Mathematical Statistics* 18:50–60.

Mantel N (1963). "Chi-square tests with one degree of freedom: Extensions of the Mantel-Haenszel procedure." *Journal of the American Statistical Association* 58:690–700.

Neyman J (1949). "Contributions to the theory of the χ^2-test." In Neyman J (ed), *Proceedings of the Berkeley Symposium on Mathematical Statistics and Probability*. Berkeley, University of California Press, pp 239–273.

Ochi Y, Prentice RL (1984). "Likelihood inference in correlated probit regression." *Biometrika* 71:531–543.

SAS (1990). *SAS User's Guide: Statistics*. Cary, N.C., SAS Institute.

Semenya KA, Koch GG, Stokes ME, Forthofer RN (1983). "Linear models methods for some rank function analyses of ordinal categorical data." *Communications in Statistics—Theory and Methods* 12:1277–1298.

Singer B (1985). Longitudinal data analysis. In Johnson NL, Kotz S (eds), *Encyclopedia of Statistical Sciences* 5. New York, Wiley, pp 142–155.

Stanek EJ, Diehl SR (1988). "Growth curve models of repeated binary response." *Biometrics* 44:973–983.

Stanish WM, Gillings DB, Koch GG (1978). "An application of multivariate ratio methods for the analysis of a longitudinal clinical trial with missing data." *Biometrics* 34:305–317.

Stiratelli R, Laird N, Ware J (1984). "Random effects models for serial observations with binary responses." *Biometrics* 40:961–971.

Stram DO, Wei LJ, Ware JM (1988). "Analysis of repeated ordered categorical outcomes with possibly missing observations and time dependent coordinates." *Journal of the American Statistical Association* 83:631–637.

Walker SH, Duncan DB (1967). "Estimation of the probability of an event as a function of several independent variables." *Biometrika* 54:167–179.

Ware JH (1985). "Linear models for the analysis of longitudinal studies." *American Statistician* 39:95–101.

Woodruff RS (1971). "A simple method for approximating the variance of a complicated estimate." *Journal of the American Statistical Association* 66:411–414.

Zeger S, Liang KY (1986). "Longitudinal data analysis for discrete and continuous outcomes." *Biometrics* 42:121–130.

Zeger SL, Liang KY, Self SG (1985). "The analysis of binary longitudinal data with time independent covariates." *Biometrika* 72:31–38.

III
Special Problems in the Modeling of Longitudinal Observations

10

Nonrandom Attrition in the Framingham Heart Study
Application: Age Trends in Blood Pressure

MANNING FEINLEIB AND JOAN PINSKY

In epidemiology, longitudinal studies have been used primarily to relate suspected causes of a disease subsequent incidence of or death from the disease. This usually involves ascertaining exposure status or measuring characteristics (so-called risk factors) for each individual in the study sample and relating this information to the subsequent occurrence of disease or death in these same individuals. Such studies have also been called *cohort, prospective,* or *follow-up studies.* In the social sciences, longitudinal studies have been concerned primarily with measurement of changes within each individual for a set of characteristics measured on two or more occasions. Studies involving multiple measurements of the same variables have also been called *panel surveys, growth studies,* and *tracking studies.* Some studies, such as the Framingham Heart Study, have collected both types of data and permit both types of analyses.

Longitudinal studies have often been called "natural experiments" because they proceed in the same temporal direction as a true experiment involving intentional manipulation of the putative causal factor (from cause to effect), but do not involve control by the investigator of which persons in the sample are exposed to the causal factor. Often in these "natural experiments" there is attrition from the study group for reasons that are also beyond the control of the investigator. This lack of control at both the initial and end phases of a study make longitudinal studies subject to biases that can seriously interfere with the investigator's ability to draw valid conclusions from the data that are available.

This chapter provides an illustration of the extent of attrition in a long-term epidemiologic study in relation to a key variable of interest. Although the degree of differential attrition observed in this example may not occur in studies of shorter duration or for variables that do not bear as strong a relation to the endpoints of interest, the specter of such attrition bias should lead to more careful examination of longitudinal data and caution in their interpretation.

The variable used in this example is systolic blood pressure (SBP), which is now well known to be related to the risk of development of myocardial infarction and stroke (Kannel, 1974; Kannel, Dawber & McGee, 1980). However, for certain investigations performed with the Framingham data, as well as in other studies, the analysts were not concerned with the risk factor–disease relationship but with the natural history or "trajectory" of level of systolic blood pressure as the individuals in the study grew older. A number of questions were addressed:

1. On the average, across individuals, does SBP tend to increase with age (Clarke, Woolson, & Lauer, 1986; Feinleib, Halperin, & Garrison, 1969; Miall & Lovell, 1967; Miall & Oldham, 1958; Pickering, 1968)?
2. Can the regression curve of blood pressure on age be adequately fitted with a linear relation, or is a higher degree polynomial or some other model needed Feinleib et al., 1969; Miall & Oldham, 1958)?
3. If the average "trajectory" of SBP with age can be described by a straight line, how does the slope of this line (the rate of increase) depend on the "initial" level of blood pressure (Blomqvist, 1977; Feinleib et al., 1969; Miall & Lovell, 1967; Rosner, Hennekens, Kass, & Miall, 1977; Svardsudd, Wedel, & Wilhelmsen 1980; Wu, Wang, & Feinleib, 1980)?
4. Does the rate of increase in blood pressure depend on other covariables such as gender, family history of hypertension or cardiovascular disease, degree of obesity, amount of salt intake, level of physical fitness, and measures of psychosocial "stress" (Clarke et al., 1986; Feinleib et al., 1979; Havlik et al., 1980; Lauer, Anderson, Beaglehole, & Burns, 1984; Miall, Bell, & Lovell, 1968; Sparrow, Garvey, Rosner, & Thomas, 1982)?
5. Can distinct subgroups of the population be identified that differ so much in their rates of increase of SBP that one can classify individuals into "hypertension prone" and "nonhypertension prone" strata (Pickering, 1968; Platt, 1959)?

If answers could be found to these questions, it was felt that it might be possible to clarify further the risk relationship between SBP and clinical endpoints (Hofman, Feinleib, Garrison, & Van Laar, 1983). Since it is widely believed that hypertension is an insidious chronic condition that may have precursors in childhood and show premonitory signs of development in early adulthood, early detection might be possible and effective treatment might ameliorate, if not totally prevent, clinical sequelaw.

Although some progress has been made in answering these questions, it has been quite limited (Clarke et al., 1986; Hofman et al., 1983; Svardsudd et al., 1980). This has been due partly to a scarcity of adequate data bases and partly to the complexity of formulating adequate models. But also, we believe, it may have been due to an almost subliminal realization that there were inherent biases in available data that were of sufficient magnitude to make most analyses virtually meaningless. Key among these suspected biases was that of differential attrition on the basis of level of blood pressure. This is the theme of the example we wish to illustrate here.

METHODS

The material to be presented was drawn from the rich data base of the Framingham Heart Study. This is a general-population longitudinal study initiated in 1948 to study the precursors of cardiovascular diseases. The respondent sample of 5209 men and women aged 28 through 62 at entry have been followed for more than thirty years by means of biennial medical examinations and surveillance for disease endpoints. Detailed descriptions of the sample and methods used have been presented elsewhere (Dawber, 1980; Dawber, Kannel, & Lyell, 1963; Feinleib, 1985). This report uses information collected through the twelfth biennial examination, which is equivalent to twenty-two years of follow-up. Depending on the date of first examination of the individual, this constituted calendar years 1971 to 1973. For those individuals who were not examined at the twenty-two year follow-up, vital status was determined through several surveillance methods (Dawber, 1980; Feinleib, 1985). Vital status shown in this report was that which was known through 1981.

Blood pressure was measured three times during each examination—first by a nurse shortly after the participant entered the examination area and then twice by the examining physician, once at the beginning and once at the end of his or her examination. All measurements were done on the left arm with the subject seated, using standard mercury sphygmomanometers with cuffs of the appropriate size. An effort was made to record all measurements to the nearest 2 mm Hg. Both systolic and fifth-phase diastolic pressures were measured, but only the means of the two SBP measurements recorded by the physician are used in the present analysis.

RESULTS

The vital status after twenty-two years of follow-up for the 2336 men and 2873 women are shown by age in Table 10-1. (The majority of participants came in for their twelfth biennial examination—59.0% of the men and 65.5% of the women. This represents 81.1% of the men and 79.1% of the women not known to be dead.) Among men, attrition due to death was considerably greater than among women in each age group, amounting to a 60-percent excell overall. As would naturally be expected, attrition in the older age groups due to deaths was about fourfold greater than among the younger cohorts for both men and women. Likewise, attrition due to nonparticipation in the twelfth examination among those not known to be dead increased with age, being about twice as great among the oldest group compared with the youngest. However, the participation rate (pe) for surviving men was actually slightly better than for surviving women for each age group.

The status of the cohort at twenty-two years by initial level of systolic blood pressure is displayed Tables 10-2 and 10-3. Attrition due to three causes is examined: (1) attrition due to death (2) attrition due to nonparticipation at the twelfth examination of those not known to be dead, and (3) attrition due to

Table 10-1. Number of participants and status at twenty-two-year follow-up examination, by sex and age at Examination 1, Framingham Heart Sstudy

	Age at Examination 1							
	Men				Women			
Status at 22-year follow-up	29–39	40–49	50–62	Total	28–39	40–49	50–62	Total
Examined	641	469	269	1378	808	653	422	1883
Dead	87	195	355	637	82	140	269	491
Not known dead, not examined	107	115	99	321	152	169	178	499
Total	835	779	722	2336	1042	962	869	2873
				Percent				
Examined	76.77	60.21	37.12	58.99	77.54	67.88	48.56	65.54
Dead	10.42	25.03	49.17	27.27	7.87	14.55	30.96	17.09
Not known dead, not examined	12.81	14.76	13.71	13.74	14.59	17.57	20.48	17.37
Not examined, of those not known to be dead	14.30	19.69	26.98	18.89	15.83	20.56	29.67	20.95

intentional manipulation of the study variable beyond the control of the investigators as manifested by self-reported treatment with antihypertensive medications at the time of examination ("Treated for HBP" and "Treated (as % of examined)" in tables).

The association between casual systolic blood pressure measured at a single point in time and cumulative mortality over the next twenty-two years is shown in Figure 10-1 for men and in Figure 10-2 for women. The previously well-documented positive relation between blood pressure and risk of death is clearly evident. The possibility of a quadratic U-shaped relation, which is suggested by the data for women, has not been adequately investigated. It is not the intent of the present report to examine this possibility, but rather to highlight the differential attrition due to death across the blood pressure range.

Of those participants in the Framingham Heart Study who were not known to be dead at the twenty-two-year follow-up, 80 percent returned for their twelfth biennial examination. Many of those who did not attend the twelfth examination were (or will be) examined at a later examination cycle and thus were (will be) ascertained to be alive at their twenty-two-year follow-up anniversary, while others were (or will be) determined through various surveillance activities to have died after the twenty-two-year follow-up. A few will be found to have died prior to the twenty-two-year follow-up. In surprisingly few cases (about 2%) of the original cohort), vital status will be indeterminable.

The proportion of those not known to be dead who did not return for the twelfth examination are shown by SBP level at the first examination in Figure 10-3 for men and in Figure 10-4 for women. There is a positive association

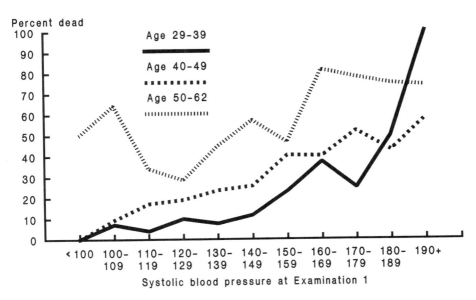

Figure 10-1. Proportion of men known to be dead at twenty-two-year follow-up by age and systolic blood pressure at Examination 1.

Table 10–2. Status of Framingham Heart Study Male Cohort at twenty-two-year follow-up, by age and systolic blood pressure at entry into the Study (Examination 1)

Age at Examination 1 and status at 22-year follow-up	Systolic blood pressure at Examination 1											
	<100	100–	110–	120–	130–	140–	150–	160–	170–	180–	190+	Total
Ages 29–39 at Examination 1												
Total number	3	41	145	229	221	110	56	16	8	4	2	835
Examined	3	33	119	172	184	81	35	7	5	2	0	641
Dead	0	3	6	23	17	13	13	6	2	2	2	87
Lost	0	5	20	34	20	16	8	3	1	0	0	107
Treated for HBP[a]	0	2	6	9	30	19	11	4	2	2	0	85
Dead (as % of total)	0.0	7.3	4.1	10.0	7.7	11.8	23.2	37.5	25.0	50.0	100.0	10.4
Lost (as % of not dead)	0.0	13.2	14.4	16.5	9.8	16.5	18.6	30.0	16.7	0.0	0.0	14.3
Treated (as % of examined)[a]	0.0	6.1	5.0	5.2	16.3	23.5	31.4	57.1	40.0	100.0	0.0	13.3
Examined (as % of total)	100.0	80.5	82.1	75.1	83.3	73.6	62.5	43.8	62.5	50.0	0.0	76.8
Examined, not treated[b] (as % of total)	100.0	75.6	77.9	71.2	69.7	56.4	42.9	18.8	37.5	0.0	0.0	66.6
Age 40–49 at Examination 1												
Total number	3	21	116	167	211	132	57	30	23	7	12	779
Examined	1	13	80	109	135	76	30	12	7	2	4	469
Dead	0	2	20	32	50	34	23	12	12	3	7	195
Lost	2	6	16	26	26	22	4	6	4	2	1	115
Treated for HBP[a]	0	0	3	9	23	19	13	3	4	1	3	78
Dead (as % of total)	0.0	9.5	17.2	19.2	23.7	25.8	40.4	40.0	52.2	42.9	58.3	25.0
Lost (as % of not dead)	66.7	31.6	16.7	19.3	16.1	22.4	11.8	33.3	36.4	50.0	20.0	19.7
Treated (as % of examined)[a]	0.0	0.0	3.8	8.3	17.0	25.0	43.3	25.0	57.1	50.0	75.0	16.6
Examined, (as % of total)	33.3	61.9	69.0	65.3	64.0	57.6	52.6	40.0	30.4	28.6	33.3	60.2
Examined, not treated[b] (as % of total)	33.3	61.9	66.4	59.9	53.1	43.2	29.8	30.0	13.0	14.3	8.3	50.2

Age 50–62 at Examination 1

Total number	2	14	73	150	145	129	81	49	32	20	27	722
Examined	1	5	42	79	60	38	28	7	2	2	4	268
Dead	1	9	25	43	65	74	38	40	25	15	20	355
Lost	0	0	6	28	20	17	15	2	5	3	3	99
Treated for HBP[a]	0	0	3	11	7	11	11	2	1	2	3	51
Dead (as % of total)	50.0	64.3	34.2	28.7	44.8	57.4	46.9	81.6	78.1	75.0	74.1	49.2
Lost (as % of not dead)	0.0	0.0	12.5	26.2	25.0	30.9	34.9	22.2	71.4	60.0	42.9	27.0
Treated (as % of examined)[a]	0.0	0.0	7.1	13.9	11.7	28.9	39.3	28.6	50.0	100.0	75.0	19.0
Examined (as % of total)	50.0	35.7	57.5	52.7	41.4	29.5	34.6	14.3	6.3	10.0	14.8	37.1
Examined, not treated[b] (as % of total)	50.0	35.7	53.4	45.3	36.6	20.9	21.0	10.2	3.1	0.0	3.7	30.1

All ages

Total number	8	76	334	546	577	371	194	95	63	31	41	2336
Examined	5	51	241	360	379	195	93	26	14	6	8	1378
Dead	1	14	51	98	132	121	74	58	39	20	29	637
Lost	2	11	42	88	66	55	27	11	10	5	4	321
Treated for HBP[a]	0	2	12	29	60	49	35	9	7	5	6	214
Dead (as % of total)	12.5	18.4	15.3	17.9	22.9	32.6	38.1	61.1	61.9	64.5	70.7	27.3
Lost (as % of not dead)	28.6	17.7	14.8	19.6	14.8	22.0	22.5	29.7	41.7	45.5	33.3	18.9
Treated (as % of examined)[a]	0.0	3.9	5.0	8.1	15.8	25.1	37.6	34.6	50.0	83.3	75.0	15.5
Examined (as % of total)	62.5	67.1	72.2	65.9	65.7	52.6	47.9	27.4	22.2	19.4	19.5	59.0
Examined, not treated[b] (as % of total)	62.5	64.5	68.6	60.6	55.3	39.4	29.9	17.9	11.1	3.2	4.9	49.8

[a]Self-reported treatment with antihypertensive medication at twenty-two-year follow-up.
[b]Not receiving treatment at twenty-two-year follow-up.

Table 10-3. Status of Framingham Heart Study female cohort at twenty-two-year follow-up, by age and systolic blood pressure at entry into the study (Examination 1)

Age at Examination 1 and status at 22-year follow-up	Systolic blood pressure at Examination 1											
	<100	100–	110–	120–	130–	140–	150–	160–	170–	180–	190+	Total
Age 28–39 at Examination 1												
Total number	19	124	323	315	4	76	25	10	3	1	2	1042
Examined	15	104	264	252	98	52	15	6	1	0	1	808
Dead	2	7	19	21	13	11	3	3	1	1	1	82
Lost	2	13	40	42	33	13	7	1	1	0	0	152
Treated for HBP[a]	0	3	18	33	29	22	10	4	1	0	1	121
Dead (as % of total)	10.5	5.6	5.9	6.7	9.0	14.5	12.0	30.0	33.3	100.0	50.0	7.9
Lost (as % of not dead)	11.8	11.1	13.2	14.3	25.2	20.0	31.8	14.3	50.0	0.0	0.0	15.8
Treated (as % of examined)[a]	0.0	2.9	6.8	13.1	29.6	42.3	66.7	66.7	100.0	0.0	100.0	15.0
Examined (as % of total)	78.9	83.9	81.7	80.0	68.1	68.4	60.0	60.0	33.3	0.0	50.0	77.5
Examined, not treated[b] (as % of total)	78.9	81.5	76.2	69.5	47.9	39.5	20.0	20.0	0.0	0.0	0.0	65.9
Age 40–49 at Examination 1												
Total number	13	51	172	205	207	119	81	48	35	15	16	962
Examined	7	34	122	157	147	81	47	23	20	6	9	653
Dead	4	7	15	15	31	20	16	12	8	6	6	140
Lost	2	10	35	33	29	18	18	13	7	3	1	169
Treated for HBP[a]	0	2	9	32	36	35	24	14	14	5	8	179
Dead (as % of total)	30.8	13.7	8.7	7.3	15.0	16.8	19.8	25.0	22.9	40.0	37.5	14.6
Lost (as % of not dead)	22.2	22.7	22.3	17.4	16.5	18.2	27.7	36.1	25.9	33.3	10.0	20.6
Treated (as % of examined)[a]	0.0	5.9	7.4	20.4	24.5	43.2	51.1	60.9	70.0	83.3	88.9	27.4
Examined (as % of total)	53.8	66.7	70.9	76.6	71.0	68.1	58.0	47.9	57.1	40.0	56.3	67.9
Examined, not treated[b] (as % of total)	53.8	62.7	65.7	61.0	53.6	38.7	28.4	18.8	17.1	6.7	6.3	49.3

Total number	4	15	54	113	163	144	118	79	64	38	77	869
Examined	2	8	38	74	90	66	49	42	23	9	21	422
Dead	2	5	10	20	43	38	38	24	31	18	40	269
Lost	0	2	6	19	30	40	31	13	10	11	16	178
Treated for HBP[a]	0	0	3	6	18	23	25	22	16	7	16	136
Dead (as % of total)	50.0	33.3	18.5	17.7	26.4	26.4	32.2	30.4	48.4	47.4	51.9	31.0
Lost (as % of not dead)	0.0	20.0	13.6	20.4	25.0	37.7	38.8	23.6	30.3	55.0	43.2	29.7
Treated (as % of examined)[a]	0.0	0.0	7.9	8.1	20.0	34.8	51.0	52.4	69.6	77.8	76.2	32.2
Examined (as % of total)	50.0	53.3	70.4	65.5	55.2	45.8	41.5	53.2	35.9	23.7	27.3	48.6
Examined, not treated[b] (as % of total)	50.0	53.3	64.8	60.2	44.2	29.9	20.3	25.3	10.9	5.3	6.5	32.9
All ages												
Total number	36	190	549	633	514	339	224	137	102	54	95	2873
Examined	24	146	424	483	335	199	111	71	44	15	31	1883
Dead	8	19	44	56	87	69	57	39	40	25	47	491
Lost	4	25	81	94	92	71	56	27	18	14	17	499
Treated for HBP[a]	0	5	30	71	83	80	59	40	31	12	25	436
Dead (as % of total)	22.2	10.0	8.0	8.8	16.9	20.4	25.4	28.5	30.2	46.3	49.5	17.1
Lost (as % of not dead)	14.3	14.6	16.0	16.3	21.5	26.3	33.5	27.6	29.0	48.3	35.4	20.9
Treated (as % of examined)[a]	0.0	3.4	7.1	14.7	24.8	40.2	53.2	56.3	70.5	80.0	80.6	23.2
Examined (as % of total)	66.7	76.8	77.2	76.3	65.2	58.7	49.6	51.8	43.1	27.8	32.6	65.5
Examined, not treated[b] (as % of total)	66.7	74.2	71.8	65.1	49.0	35.1	23.2	22.6	12.7	5.6	6.3	50.4

[a]Self-reported treatment with antihypertensive medication at twenty-two-year follow-up.
[b]Not receiving treatment at twenty-two-year follow-up.

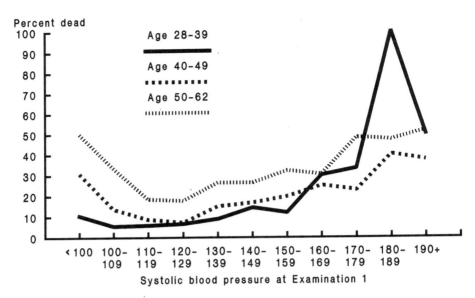

Figure 10-2. Proportion of women known to be dead at twenty-two-year follow-up by age and systolic blood pressure at Examination 1.

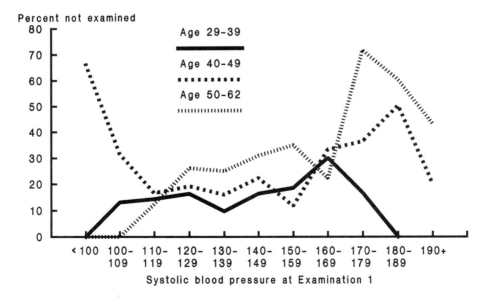

Figure 10-3. Proportion of men not examined at Examination 12 of those not known to be dead at twenty-two-year follow-up.

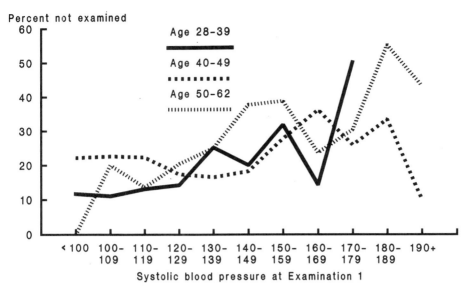

Figure 10-4.   Proportion of women not examined at Examination 12 of those not known to be dead at twenty-two-year follow-up.

between SBP at the initial examination and failure to attend the twelfth examination for most of the age-sex groups, with some departures from this trend appearing for the sparse extreme groups.

The third type of attrition considered here is that produced by intentional manipulation of the study variable outside of the study protocol and the control of the investigators. In the Framingham Heart Study—an observational cohort study without treatment component—this type of attrition in the present context is produced by treatment by the participants' own physicians. Of the 3261 participants who took the twelfth biennial examination, 650 reported that they were currently being treated with antihypertensive medications, 15.5 percent of the men and 23.2 percent of the women. Since such treatment is offered practically only because of the presence of elevated blood pressures observed by the patient's physician, and since subsequent clinically elevated blood pressure correlates highly with the casual blood pressure measured at the first Framingham examination, a strong positive relation between treatment and initial SBP would be expected. That this is indeed the case is shown in Tables 10-2 and 10-3 ("Treated (as % of examined)") and in Figures 10-5 and 10-6.

The net result of these three forms of attrition for studies of the natural history of SBP in untreated adults followed for twenty-two years in the Framingham Heart Study is that only 50.1 percent of the originally examined cohort were available (1164 men and 1447 women of the 5209 total examined initially). The proportions available differed markedly by sex, age, and particularly initial SBP as shown in Tables 10-2 and 10-3 ("Examined, not treated")

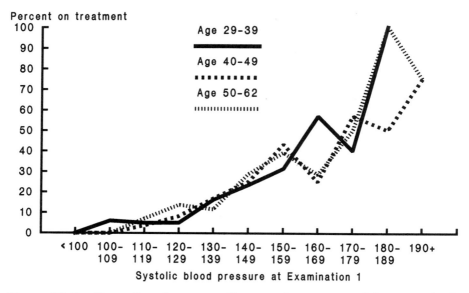

Figure 10–5. Proportion of men on antihypertensive treatment of those examined at twenty-two-year follow-up.

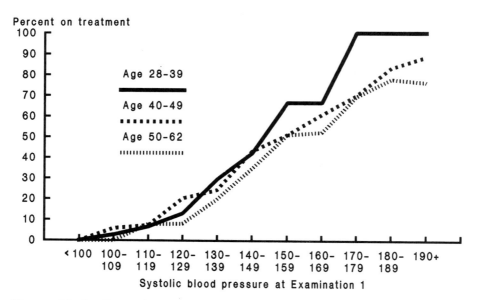

Figure 10–6. Proportion of women on antihypertensive treatment of those examined at twenty-two-year follow-up.

and in Figures 10-7 and 10-8. Among men, age at entry was an important covariable for determining who would be available for natural history studies of SBP. Age at entry was not as important for women. However, for all sex and age groups, initial level of SBP was of paramount importance. Whereas in every age-sex group more than half of the entrants with initial SBP of 110–119 nm Hg were available twenty-two years after entry, less than 10 percent those with SBP over 190 mm Hg were available.

DISCUSSION

The general trends discussed in this chapter seem almost trivially self-evident. It is well established that elevated blood pressure levels are associated with fatal conditions such as myocardial infarctions and strokes and, thus, with total mortality. To the extent that nonfatal infracts and strokes might be related to chronic disability or institutionalization, high blood pressure would also affect the ability of surviving subjects to return for clinical examination. And since blood pressure measurements are rather highly correlated over time within individuals (r is approximately .6 for measurements taken two to ten years apart), antihypertensive treatment by a physician should be correlated with blood pressure measures taken years earlier. All of this is confirmed by the present data.

What is not so self-evident is the magnitude of these effects and how they may impact on one's ability to assess the validity of certain hypotheses regarding the long-term behavior of blood pressure levels. It is the great magnitude of the differential attrition between higher compared with lower initial levels of blood pressure that these data highlight. This severe censoring of the duration of follow-up has not been well addressed in previous analyses.

For example, early studies of the relation of blood pressure with age were based on cross-sectional samples (Miall & Oldham, 1958). Little explicit attention was paid to the selective biases inherent in survival to the older ages and how this might be related to blood pressure at younger ages. Later studies using longitudinal data also largely ignored the biases demonstrated here and analyzed data as if the surviving subjects were representative of all of the initial participants (Miall & Lovell, 1967). Unfortunately, few efforts seem to have been made until quite recently (Rosner et al., 1985) to take into account explicitly the effect of the differential attrition in the models that have been suggested for analyzing longitudinal trends in blood pressure.

Without belaboring the point further, it would seem essential that models for the longitudinal behavior of variables that might be associated with the types of attrition demonstrated here should take into account simultaneously both the patterns of observed measurements and the risk of attrition. That is, the models should incorporate the risk relations examined in cohort studies with the repeated measurement relations usually examined in tracking or growth studies.

Although such composite models are apt to be more complex than usual growth models, their information content would be commensurately richer. The

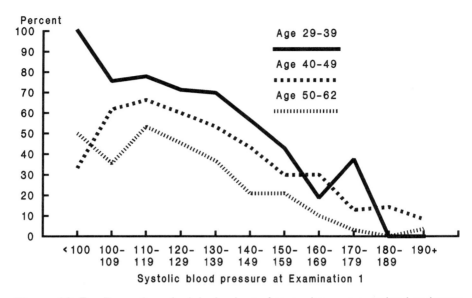

Figure 10–7. Proportion of original cohort of men who were examined and were not being treated for hypertension at twenty-two-year follow-up.

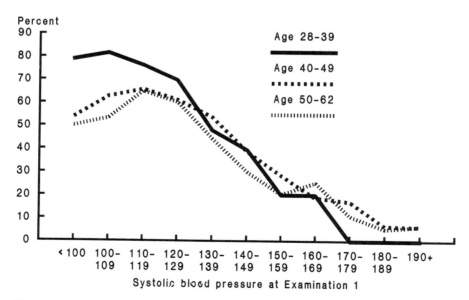

Figure 10–8. Proportion of original cohort of women who were examined and were not being treated for hypertension at twenty-two-year follow-up.

development of such models to account for these combined effects are challenges facing future investigators of longitudinal phenomena. Meanwhile, epidemiologists who examine longitudinal data should try to be more explicit about the possible presence of differential attrition and how it might limit the generalizability of their conclusions.

REFERENCES

Blomqvist N (1977). "On the relation between change and initial value." *Journal of the American Statistical Association* 72:746–749.

Clarke WR, Woolson RF, Lauer RM (1986). "Changes in ponderosity and blood pressure in childhood: The Muscatine Study." *American Journal of Epidemiology* 124:195–206.

Dawber TR (1980). *The Framingham Study.* Cambridge, Mass., Harvard University Press.

Dawber TR, Kannel WB, Lyell LP (1963). "An approach to longitudinal studies in a community. The Framingham Study." *Annals of the New York Academic of Sciences* 107:539–556.

Feinleib M (1985). "The Framingham Study: Sample selection, follow-up, and methods of analysis." *National Cancer Institute Monograph* 67:59–64.

Feinleib M, Garrison RJ, Stallones L, Kannel WB, Castelli WP, McNamara PM (1979). "A comparison of blood pressure, total cholesterol and cigarette smoking in parents in 1950 and their children in 1970." *American Journal of Epidemiology* 110:291–302.

Feinleib M, Halperin M, Garrison RJ (1969). "Relationship between blood pressure and age: Regression analysis of longitudinal data." Paper presented at the 97th Annual Meeting of the American Public Health Association, Philadelphia.

Havlik RJ, Garrison RJ, Feinleib M, Padgett S, Castelli WP, McNamara PM (1980). "Evidence for additional blood pressure correlates in adults 20–56 years old." *Circulation* 61:710–715.

Hofman A, Feinleib M, Garrison RJ, van Laar A (1983). "Does change in blood pressure predict heart disease?" *British Medical Journal* 287:267–269.

Kannel WB (1974). "Role of blood pressure in cardiovascular morbidity and mortality." *Progress in Cardiovasculat Disease*, 17:5–24.

Kannel WB, Dawber TR, McGee DL (1980). "Perspectives on systolic hypertension. The Framingham Study." *Circulation* 61:1179–1182.

Lauer RM, Anderson AR, Beaglehole R, Burns TL (1984). "Factors relating to tracking of blood pressure in children. U.S. National Center for Health Statistics Health Examination Surveys Cycles II and III." *Hypersion* 6:307–314.

Miall WE, Bell RA, Lovell HG (1968). "Relation between change in blood pressure and weight." *British Journal of Preventive and Social Medicine* 22:73–80.

Miall WE, Lovell HG (1967). "Relation between change in blood pressure and age." *British Medical Journal;* 2:660–664.

Miall WE, Oldham PD (1958). "Factors influencing arterial blood pressure in the general population." *Clinical Science* 17:409–444.

Pickering G (1968). *High Blood Pressure.* New York, Grune & Stratton.

Platt R (1959). "The nature of essential hypertension." *Lancet* 2:55–57.

Rosner B, Hennekens CH, Kass EH, Miall WE (1977). "Age-specific correlation analysis of longitudinal blood pressure data." *American Journal of Epidemiology* 106:306–313.

Rosner B, Muñoz A, Tager I, Speizer F, Weiss S (1985). "The use of an autoregressive model for the analysis of longitudinal data in epidemiologic studies." *Statistics in Medicine* 4:457–467.

Sparrow D, Garvey AJ, Rosner B, Thomas HE Jr (1982). "Factors in predicting blood pressure change." *Circulation* 65:789–794.

Svardsudd K, Wedel H, Wilhelmsen L (1980). "Factors associated with the initial blood pressure level and with subsequent blood pressure increase in a longitudinal population study." *European Heart Journal*, 1:345–354.

Wu M, Ware JH, Feinleib M (1980). "On the relation between blood pressure change and initial value." *Journal of Chronic Diseases*, 33:637–644.

11

Missing Data in Longitudinal Studies
Application: Height and Blood Pressure in Adolescents

ROBERT WOOLSON, WILLIAM CLARKE,
AND JAMES LEEPER

Longitudinal studies are rarely complete due to patient attrition, mistimed visits, premature study termination, and other factors. When the data are missing at random, a number of standard approaches may be implemented to handle the incomplete response vectors. In this chapter we review selected methods for the handling of randomly missing longitudinal data and describe the limitations and strengths of the approaches. More problematic is the case of nonrandomly missing data, in which case the techniques for inclusion of the incomplete response vectors are less well studied. We also discuss this problem of handling nonrandomly missing data and delineate some difficulties inherent in modeling nonrandomly incomplete longitudinal data.

To limit the discussion to a focused set of problems, we restrict consideration to the problem of the analysis of a single continuous variable that is scheduled to be measured at a set of (at most) p specified times. This eliminates the case where measures are taken at arbitrary times, but does not eliminate the case where it is planned to measure each person at most $t(t < p)$ times. We also restrict attention to the case where the major missing data question is one of item, rather than unit, nonresponse; specifically, we are concerned with the treatment of incomplete response vectors rather than with the problem of dealing with individuals for whom the entire data vector is missing.

Following the review of missing data techniques, we discuss a two-stage estimation procedure for the estimation of growth norms. We then discuss a specific problem associated with the analysis of the Muscatine Study of Coronary Risk Factors in Children. This well-known epidemiologic study consists of a series of six biennial surveys of the school-aged children in Muscatine, Iowa. The goals of this study are multifaceted and include questions regarding the establishment of age- and sex-specific norms of blood pressure, body size, serum lipids, and a number of other factors. For purposes of this analysis we examine the data by age at last birthday (5, 6,..., 18 years). Accordingly, there are fourteen ($p = 14$) ages of measurement. One question is to estimate mean values and changes in body size and blood pressure measurements for each age and sex. It may be noted that while there are fourteen ages of measurement possible, each child could only be measured for at most six of the ages, since only six biennial surveys have been conducted. Thus, an individual who was age 6 in 1971 (the year of the first biennial survey) was eligible for measurement at age 8 (the next biennial survey) and at ages 10, 12, 14, and 16. By design, this individual has data missing for the remaining eight ages, and may also be missing data for at least one of the six eligible ages. Naturally, for a group as large as the Muscatine school population there is a large amount of "missing" data in the sense that an individual may provide data for only one of the fourteen ages, two of the fourteen ages, and so on up to at most six of the fourteen ages. Furthermore, the missing data may be viewed as partly due to the design, and partly missing at random. The latter is assumed for school screens missed because of illness or other absence. Obviously, a more thorough analysis of the data would examine the specific reasons for the incomplete data and give consideration to modeling such nonresponse.

If there is interest in estimating norms and changes in norms at each age for each sex, then an analysis of the Muscatine data should take into account the various incomplete data configurations, in order to utilize fully the longitudinal information available in the sample. A naive, but not necessarily efficient, analysis would disregard the longitudinal aspects of the data and consider a response for each child at each age as an independent observation regardless of whether there are additional observations for this child or not. This approach may yield unbiased estimates of age norms and growth rates, but the variances (and covariances) of the estimates would not be correct, since correlated data are treated as independent observations in the analysis. We describe a two-stage procedure for the estimation of norms and growth rates and append an SAS (Sall, 1982) program for the implementation of this approach. This approach is based on earlier work of Kleinbaum (1970, 1973), Woolson, Leeper, and Clarke (1978), and Fairclough and Helms (1983) and relies heavily on the concept of seemingly unrelated regression estimation described and studied by Zellner (1962, 1963), Williams (1967), and Revankar (1974, 1976). While this two-stage approach provides a method for estimation of age-sex-specific norms and growth rates, it is not intended to be viewed as a recommendation for all missing data estimation problems for longitudinal studies. It is an approach that has worked well for the Muscatine data, perhaps due to the large number of children and number of observations per child. We begin with a presentation of the underlying statistical model to establish notation and fix ideas.

THE STATISTICAL MODEL

As just stated, it is assumed that the data are to be obtained from an experiment or observational study in which a fixed number of distinct ages (times), p, are possible for observation. It is assumed that the response to be measured is a continuous one and that the data may be incomplete in the sense that individual i has measurements at $p_i(\leqslant p)$ of the possible ages. For individual i, we place these observations in a vector: y_i, $p_i \times 1$ and it is assumed that y_i conforms to the model

$$y_i = T_i\beta + e_i \qquad (1)$$

for $i = 1, \ldots, N$ and T_i is a $(p_i \times v)$ known model matrix, β is a $(v \times 1)$ vector of unknown parameters, and e_i is a $(p_i \times 1)$ error vector distributed $N(0, \Sigma_i)$, where Σ_i is a $(p_i \times p_i)$ positive definite covariance matrix assumed to be a submatrix of a $(p \times p)$ matrix Σ, the covariance matrix for the entire array of p ages.

Naturally, models other than the multivariate normal may be assumed or the y_i may be discrete (or categorical) variables. These situations, while of general interest, will not be discussed here.

The major question to be addressed for data conforming to model (1) is to draw an inference on β; that is, estimate β and test hypotheses regarding β. To study β it is necessary to estimate Σ, and perhaps model Σ as a function of fewer parameters than the $(p(p + 1))/2$ distinct parameters represented in Σ itself. If this is possible, then the efficiency in estimating β may be increased. On the other hand, an incorrect model for Σ may translate into improper variability estimates for the resulting estimator of β. Nevertheless, when the total sample size is small relative to p and the data are incomplete, modeling Σ becomes an attractive alternative to leaving Σ unstructured, since the number of parmeters in Σ to be estimated will be large and the sample size too small to provide stable estimators for all parameters. There are several simple examples of modeling Σ in terms of fewer parameters. For example, if the repeated observations on a child are independent with equal variance, then $\Sigma = \sigma^2 I$, I is the identity matrix, and Σ can be modeled as one parameter, σ^2. The usual mixed model would represent Σ as $\sigma_1^2 I + \sigma_2^2 1$, where 1 is a $(p \times p)$ matrix of ones, and therefore Σ would be modeled with two parameters, σ_1^2 and σ_2^2. Other structures can be set for Σ either by modeling e_i or writing Σ in some structural model form. Laird and Ware (1982, 1984), Cook (1983), and Ware (1984, 1985) have studied the longitudinal data problem by writing a model for e_i thereby inducing a structure for Σ. These works have primarily employed the EM algorithm (Dempster, Rubin, & Tsutakawa, 1977; Orchard & Woodbury, 1972) as a device to provide maximum likelihood estimators for the resulting parameter of Σ and β. Helms (1984) has modeled Σ as

$$\sum_{i=1}^{r} \alpha_i W_i$$

where W_i are known matrices and $\alpha_1, \ldots, \alpha_r$ are unknown parameters. Estimation of the α's in this linear covariance model is followed by estimation of β. Finally, LaVange and Helms (1983) have modeled the Σ matrix in the classic time series form by considering various autoregressive covariance structures. All of these workers have focused on the problem of analyzing randomly missing longitudinal data. Although the individual approaches to parameter estimation may differ in some fundamental ways, the incompleteness in the data is assumed to be at random. In the next section we give an overview of various major methods that have been proposed for randomly missing longitudinal data.

TREATMENT OF RANDOMLY MISSING LONGITUDINAL DATA

There has been a proliferation of literature in recent years regarding the statistical analysis of (randomly) incomplete longitudinal data. In spite of the number of papers, essentially two general approaches have been proposed for dealing with this problem.

One is a generalized least-squares estimation and the use of Wald's (1943) test statistic. This approach was initially proposed for this problem by Kleinbaum (1970, 1973). The outcome of this approach is an estimator of β, its estimated variance–covariance matrix, and test statistics to test $H_0: C\beta = 0$, where C is a known matrix of full row rank. In addition to Kleinbaum (1970), this approach has been studied by Schwertman (1974), Schwertman and Allen (1973, 1979), Leeper (1977). Leeper and Woolson (1982), and others. Fairclough and Helms (1983) have described a series of SAS macros written for estimation and hypothesis testing in this generalized linear model. Their approach consists of three steps: (1) An estimator of Σ is produced by utilizing the pairwise complete data. (2) This estimate is used to estimate β by using the step 1 estimator of Σ as the covariance matrix in a generalized least-squares estimation of β. Since the pairwise complete estimator of Σ is a consistent estimator of Σ, this sample covariance–generalized least-squares estimator of β is asymptotically unbiased and efficient as an estimator of β. As this estimator of β is also asymptotically normal, tests of $H_0: C\beta = 0$ can be produced by constructing appropriate quadratic forms in $C\hat{\beta}$ (where $\hat{\beta}$ is the estimator of β). (3) Test statistics are produced. These statistics are asymptotically chi square (Kleinbaum, 1973).

One of the difficulties with this approach is that the estimator of Σ may not be positive definite. This was originally noted by Kleinbaum (1970), and Schwertman and Allen (1979) suggested a "smoothing procedure" that produces a positive semidefinite estimator of Σ. The finite sample properties of the test statistics, when the smoothed estimator is used, have been studied only for certain restricted problems. When the response variables are highly correlated with incomplete data vectors, indefinite estimation of Σ can be common (Fairclough & Helms, 1983; Leeper & Woolson, 1983). Since the effect of the smoothing procedure on the parameter estimates is not well understood, this approach should be avoided in these cases. Nevertheless, for large data sets with numerous patterns of missing data, this generalized least-squares approach is attractive, since statistical packages sufficiently general to handle matrix operations and linear models can be adapted for the analysis, as illustrated by the software developed by Fairclough and Helms (1983). We analyze the Muscatine data and write a program that illustrates the utility of the approach to compute these estimators. To conclude our discussion of this approach, it should also be noted that this approach generally leaves Σ unstructured and does not model it as a function of fewer parameters. Such modeling can be undertaken, then coupled with the foregoing generalized least-squares estimation of β (Helms, 1984; LaVange & Helms, 1983).

The second approach to inference with randomly incomplete longitudinal data is based on consideration of the likelihood function. This approach addresses the estimation of β and Σ through maximum likelihood. Likelihood-based analysis for incomplete data has been a topic of considerable interest in the literature (see Beale & Little, 1975; Hocking, 1958; Little, 1979; Rubin, 1974, 1976a, 1976b; and Szatrowski, 1983, and for an account of the general development in this area.) Little and Schluchter (1985) developed incomplete data algorithms for maximum likelihood estimators for mixed continuous and discrete data. Their paper is a very general approach to problems of random incomplete data, and makes use of the EM algorithm.

At this point it is convenient to discuss the EM algorithm due to its fundamental role in likelihood analysis of incomplete data. The EM algorithm was initially introduced into the statistical literature by Orchard and Woodbury (1972), and was more thoroughly developed and extended by Dempster, Laird, and Rubin (1977). For the general multivariate incomplete data problem, Beale and Little (1975) have programmed the algorithm. This algorithm forms the basis for likelihood-based estimation in the presence of incomplete data. This algorithm may be described in a variety of ways, but in its simplest form it may be described as an iterative procedure consisting of two steps at each iteration: an expectation (E) step and a maximization (M) step. One version of the general E step consists of estimation of the posterior expectation of the sufficient statistics for the complete data given the observed (incomplete) data. The M step uses the estimated complete data along with the observed data and considers the estimated data as if they are the real data to find maximum likelihood estimates of the population parameters (β and Σ). These steps are iterated until convergence is reached (Dempster et al., 1977, 1981). The 1977 paper of Dempster and colleagues, and the discussion to it, enumerate several advantages and disadvantages of this algorithm compared with other competitive maximum likelihood estimation procedures such as Newton–Raphson and Fisher scoring algorithms. Some advantages are

1. The convergence of the algorithm is usually guaranteed.
2. Computations in the algorithm are quite simple.
3. The algorithm is easily programmed.
4. Estimates of the missing values are provided.
5. The algorithm has wide applicability.
6. The estimated covariance matrix is positive definite at each iteration provided the initial estimate provided by the user is also positive definite.

The algorithm has several disadvantages, including

1. The rate of convergence can be slow (in terms of the required number of iterations).
2. Results can be sensitive to starting values.
3. Convergence may be to a local, instead of a global, maximum.

Meneses (1984) has performed a limited study of the role of starting values in the EM algorithm and has reported that generalizations about the effect of starting values are premature for the incomplete, one-sample multivariate normal problem. He noted that further study is warranted to better understand the roles patterns of missing data and the underlying covariance structure have on the algorithm. This problem is more complex for incomplete longitudinal data. The difficulty of the EM algorithm (and its possible sensitivity to starting values) was further detailed by Bentler and Tanaka (1983), who critiqued its application to a problem in factor analysis. Different starting values led to three essentially different solutions. Two of the solutions had indefinite Hessian matrices with one of the two matrices being very close to singular. The third solution yielded a proper negative definite Hessian; it is the solution achieved by classical factor analysis. These findings prompted Bentler and Tanaka (1983) to remind readers of the limitations of the EM algorithm:

1. It has slow convergence.
2. The convergence rate may go to zero when improper solutions are required.
3. It may converge to a saddle point.
4. It does not yield standard error estimators.
5. The second-order sufficiency condition for a maximum is not directly evaluated by the algorithm.

These authors conjectured that the algorithm may not iterate effectively when it encounters an ill-conditioned Hessian matrix. They favored, as discussants of the original Dempster et al. 1977 paper did, modification of the algorithm by use of Newton–Raphson or Fisher scoring. Most important, they advised against the uncritical application of the algorithm, especially without further computations of the score (gradient) vector and the Hessian matrix to evaluate the condition for attainment of a local maximum.

For the longitudinal data problem, Fairclough and Helms (1985) reported slow convergence of the EM algorithm, especially when Σ is estimated by a near singular matrix. To deal with these problems for the analysis of incomplete longitudinal data, Jennrich and Schluchter (1985) have written programs implementing three general algorithms: Fisher scoring, Newton–Raphson, and the EM algorithm. Their basic approach to the EM algorithm is to specify the complete data by considering the p vectors $\mathbf{y}_1^*, \ldots, \mathbf{y}_N^*$ that contain the observed vectors $\mathbf{y}_1, \ldots, \mathbf{y}_N$ as subvectors. Each $\mathbf{y}_i^*$ is distributed as $N(T_i^* \beta, \Sigma)$ where T_i^* contains the T_i as submatrices. They performed the E and the M steps with regard to the complete data (y_i^*) given the incomplete data, and iterated to a solution. They included several special provisions in their EM algorithm including a "scoring step" for the covariance matrix when Σ is assumed to be structured. These various steps are intended to improve the convergence rate of the algorithm and to identify problems such as a singular estimate of Σ. They noted that the amount of computation required by the EM algorithm increases linearly with N for a fixed p, v, and number of covariance parameters to be estimated. They also noted that one cost savings device is to group the subjects according to pattern of missing data, prior to initiating the algorithm. The major problems encountered with their EM algorithm occur when there are a small number, possibly zero, of complete cases.

To conclude this discussion of the EM algorithm, it should be noted that there are a number of EM algorithms that could be used to maximize the likelihood function, but only two are in general use for the analysis of incomplete longitudinal data. The one used by Jennrich and Schluchter (1985) uses the vector $\mathbf{y}_i^*$ as the complete data. In contrast to this approach, Laird and Ware (1982), Fairclough and Helms (1985), and others have modeled the complete data as the $\mathbf{y}_i$ and $\mathbf{b}_i$, where the $\mathbf{b}_i$ are the unobserved vectors in a random coefficients model. In this instance the $\mathbf{b}_i$ represent the random vectors used to model Σ in a structured form. As stated by Laird and Ware (1982), this use of the EM algorithm is fundamentally different from the usual approach based on $\mathbf{y}_i^*$ and $\mathbf{y}_i$, since they treat no data missing but treat the $\mathbf{b}_i$ as unobservable vectors. This approach has been used extensively by Cook (1983), Laird and Ware (1982), and others and is advantageous for those problems in which the number of observation times is not fixed in advance and the covariance matrix can be assumed to be of a specific form. As noted by Jennrich and Schluchter (1985), the approach of using $\mathbf{y}_i^*$ as the complete data is useful because it facilitates the handling of arbitrary structures for Σ. Nevertheless it should be noted that Cook (1983) has produced a FORTRAN computer program for the class of random-effects model; Cook and Ware (1983), however, have noted that special programs or tailormade modifications are still required for incomplete longitudinal data analysis. Berk (1984a, 1984b) provided examples of modifications of widely available general statistical software for the analysis of incomplete longitudinal data. This work and that of Fairclough and Helms (1983), Jennrich and Schluchter (1985), and Cook (1983) are promising, since taken together they represent a set of algorithms with broad applicability for the analysis of randomly incomplete longitudinal data. They also show that much remains to be done by way of producing a single set of programs for the treatment of randomly missing longitudinal data.

TREATMENT OF NONRANDOMLY MISSING DATA

Efficient and unbiased estimation of parameters in a univariate or multivariate regression model will generally depend on the mechanism generating the incomplete data. Rubin (1974, 1976a, 1976b, 1978) has provided a discussion of the general incomplete data problem and has examined the various interpretations of the likelihood function depending on the incomplete data assumptions (1976a). When data are missing at random, the observed sample of data may be viewed as a random subsample of the unobserved, complete data; this simplifies the problem of missing data analysis, since the mechanism for incompleteness is assumed to be random. When randomness cannot be assumed, it may be feasible to model the missing data by assuming a relationship among the probability that the response variable is incomplete, the response variable, and the regression variables to be used in the analysis. Note that we are implicitly assuming here that there is one response variable, and that it is either missing or not missing for each individual. We also assume the regression variables are known for all individuals in the sample. Naturally, there are many variations of missing data possible, but we restrict attention in this section to the case where only the univariate response variable can be incomplete. Accordingly, we are not discussing longitudinal data in this section, but single univariate response data. Little work has been done on the problem of nonrandomly missing longitudinal data by way of formal modeling of the incompleteness, although models do exist for handling special types of incompleteness such as censoring or truncation of data beyond a certain time period.

Models for a univariate incomplete response variable arise by consideration of the probability of being missing in a probit or logistic model and modeling of the observed respondents in a multiple regression model. For univariate response data, Tobin (1958) proposed a model for the analysis of a limited dependent variable, a response variable that has a lower limit. This model is a combination of a probit model and the multiple linear regression model. The model is dichotomous for the response, and it is a multiple linear regression model for the respondents. Tobin (1958) developed the likelihood equation and estimators for this problem. Heckman (1974, 1976) generalized this approach and presented a unified treatment of statistical models for truncation, sample selection (i.e., incomplete data), and limited dependent variables. He also provided generalized least-squares estimators of the parameters and empirically demonstrated that these estimators are close to the maximum likelihood estimators. As Heckman (1976) noted, this problem extends quite easily to the case of multivariate response, although the missing data patterns must surely be restricted to a few, because it would be unreasonable to expect the analyst to be able to assume a different model for each pattern of missing data.

To our knowledge, these types of models have not been applied to incomplete longitudinal data in a systematic way. It would appear that one approach would be to apply them for problems involving nonrandom attrition or serial dropouts from a long-term study. Attempts to apply these models to the most general incomplete longitudinal data problem are likely to be complex, since it would be necessary to model each incomplete response and the longitudinal correlation between incomplete and/or complete responses at different time points. This would necessitate the specification of a covariance structure for the incomplete/complete data.

The area of modeling of nonrandomly incomplete longitudinal data is richly deserving of further study. The availability of a general procedure for the handling of nonrandomly missing longitudinal data would greatly facilitate incomplete longitudinal data analysis.

A TWO-STAGE GENERALIZED LEAST-SQUARES ESTIMATION PROCEDURE

As has been discussed in the previous two sections, there are a number of estimation procedures and approaches for the treatment of incomplete longitudinal data. We have found the procedures of Kleinbaum (1970, 1973) quite useful for certain questions in the analysis of the Muscatine study. This project will be briefly described in the next section, but may be characterized as a longitudinal study with fourteen ages of measurement and no person having measurements at more than six ages. In addition, there are a very large number of individuals in the study $(10,000+)$ and numerous missing data patterns. In this section we describe a general two-stage procedure we have used and programmed for selected questions in this study. The methods are based on the work of Zellner (1962, 1963), Kleinbaum (1973), Fairclough and Helms (1982), and Leeper and Woolson (1982).

To outline the procedure, we assume, as before, that there are p ages for which data have been collected. Some individuals have been measured at one age only, others at two ages, and so on. The number of times measured and the ages at measurement uniquely determine a data pattern for each child. For convenience we assume that there are s such distinct patterns of data. In addition, for persons in pattern k, it is assumed that they have data at exactly p_k of the p ages $(p_k \leqslant p)$.

If we order the p ages from 1 to p, the ages at which data are available for those in pattern k will be denoted by a $(p_k \times p)$ indicator matrix $K^{(k)}$ in which each row has one 1 and $p - 1$ 0's. As an example, if a pattern is characterized by individuals having data at ages 1, 2, and 4, then the K matrix is

$$\begin{bmatrix} 1 & 0 & 0 & 0 & 0 & \cdots & 0 \\ 0 & 1 & 0 & 0 & 0 & \cdots & 0 \\ 0 & 0 & 0 & 1 & 0 & \cdots & 0 \end{bmatrix}$$

At this point it will be necessary to complicate slightly the notation previously given in the second section. This is due to the need to identify the data for each age. We denote the response variable, for example systolic blood pressure, by $y_{ij}^{(k)}$ for the ith child at age j in pattern k. Note that $y_{ij}^{(k)}$ is unknown if the child was not measured at age j. For simplicity we assume that the "complete data" (with * for missing y's) are placed into an $(N \times p)$ array Y where the first n_1 rows correspond to missing data pattern 1, the next n_2 to missing pattern 2, and so on. Further, we let $Y = [Y_1, \ldots, Y_p]$ where Y_j is the array of data (complete and incomplete) at age j. Let X_j denote the model matrix corresponding to Y_j where rows of X_j are assumed to be zeros for the unobserved (missing) individuals at that age. The two-stage estimation procedure follows the lines of Zellner (1962, 1963), where we first estimate Σ from residuals determined by performing an ordinary least-squares regression analysis of $\dot{Y}_j$ or $\dot{X}_j$, where $\dot{Y}_j$ and $\dot{X}_j$ are the corresponding observed parts of Y_j and X_j. This is done for each of the p ages. If the data are missing at random we have the model

$$\dot{Y}_j = \dot{X}_j \beta_j + \dot{e}_j \quad \text{for } j = 1, 2, \ldots, p \tag{2}$$

The ordinary least-squares estimator of β_j is

$$\hat{\beta}_j = (\dot{X}_j' \dot{X}_j)^{-1} \dot{X}_j' \dot{Y}_j \quad \text{for } j = 1, \ldots, p \tag{3}$$

Residuals from (3) are

$$r_j = Y_j - X_j \hat{\beta}_j \quad \text{for } j = 1, \ldots, p$$

where it is understood that the residuals are undefined for the incomplete components of $\mathbf{Y}_j$. An estimator of Σ is $S = (s_{jj'})$ where

$$s_{jj'} = \frac{\mathbf{r}_j' \mathbf{r}_j'}{N_{jj'} - 1} \tag{4}$$

and $N_{jj'}$ is the number of individuals with observations at both ages j and j'. Also it is assumed that $\mathbf{r}_j' \mathbf{r}_{j'}$ is computed over only those individuals with data at both ages j and j'.

Expression (4) is but one estimator of Σ and is analogous to the "restricted" estimator discussed by Revankar (1976) for complete data. It should be noted that while Σ is positive definite, it does not follow that S is. For the second stage of the estimation we require that $K^{(k)} S K^{(k)'}$ be positive semidefinite for $k = 1, \ldots, s$. If positive definiteness is not attained for all of these matrices, one alternative path to follow is to estimate $K^{(k)} \Sigma K^{(k)'}$ from each of the patterns of missing data. In particular, an estimator of $K^{(k)} \Sigma K^{(k)'}$ could be obtained by first performing an OLS regression of $\mathbf{y}_j^{(k)}$ on $X_j^{(k)}$ resulting in an estimator $\hat{\boldsymbol{\beta}}_j^{(k)}$ for $\boldsymbol{\beta}_j$. Then residuals can be computed by $\mathbf{r}_j^{(k)} = (\mathbf{y}_j^{(k)} - X_j^{(k)} \hat{\boldsymbol{\beta}}_j^{(k)})$. Following this, an estimator $S^{(k)} = (s_{jj'}^{(k)})$ for $K^{(k)} \Sigma K^{(k)'}$ can be computed. In particular

$$s_{jj'}^{(k)} = \frac{\mathbf{r}_j^{(k)'} r_{j'}^{(k)}}{(n_k - I)} \quad \text{for } j, j' = 1, \ldots, p \tag{5}$$

where $\mathbf{r}_j^{(k)}$ are the residuals for the kth missing data pattern.

Hence at least two procedures can be employed to generate an estimator of $K^{(k)} \Sigma K^{(k)'}$.

The estimator for $\boldsymbol{\beta}$ that we propose is a generalized least-squares estimator and is a natural extension of the usual two-stage estimator of Zellner (1962, 1963). To define this estimator it is useful to first define the vector $\mathbf{z}^{(k)}$ as the column-concatenation of the $n_k p_k$ vector in missing data pattern k. The vector of y's for the first child is stacked in column form on top of that for the second child, and so forth. Hence, $\mathbf{z}^{(k)}$ is a vector of length $n_k p_k$. Let $A^{(k)}$ be the model matrix corresponding to $\mathbf{z}^{(k)}$ so that $E(\mathbf{z}^{(k)}) = A^{(k)} \boldsymbol{\beta}$ and

$$E[(\mathbf{z}^{(k)} - A^{(k)} \boldsymbol{\beta})(\mathbf{z}^{(k)} - A^{(k)} \boldsymbol{\beta})'] = K^{(k)} \Sigma K^{(k)'} \quad \otimes I \quad \text{for } k = 1, \ldots, s$$

where $\otimes$ is the right-Kronecker product. Since the s groups of data corresponding to the patterns are independent of one another, it follows that the weighted least-squares estimator of $\boldsymbol{\beta}$ is:

$$\tilde{\boldsymbol{\beta}} = \left(\sum_{k=1}^{s} [A^{(k)'} (K^{(k)} \Sigma K^{(k)'} \otimes I)^{-1} A^{(k)}] \right)^{-1} \sum_{k=1}^{s} A^{(k)'} (K^{(k)} \Sigma K^{(k)'} \otimes I)^{-1} \mathbf{z}^{(k)}$$

Since Σ, and therefore $K^{(k)} \Sigma K^{(k)'}$, is unknown, we propose estimating $\boldsymbol{\beta}$ by $\hat{\boldsymbol{\beta}}$ where $\hat{\boldsymbol{\beta}}$ is $\tilde{\boldsymbol{\beta}}$ with $K^{(k)} \Sigma K^{(k)'}$ estimated by $\hat{\Sigma}^{(k)}$, one of the estimators described earlier.

The estimator of $\boldsymbol{\beta}$ which we propose is

$$\hat{\boldsymbol{\beta}} = \left\{ \sum_{k=1}^{s} [A^{(k)'} (\hat{\Sigma}^{(k)} \otimes I)^{-1} A^{(k)}] \right\}^{-1} \sum_{k=1}^{s} A^{(k)'} (\hat{\Sigma}^{(k)} \otimes I)^{-1} \mathbf{z}^{(k)} \tag{6}$$

where $\hat{\Sigma}^{(k)}$ is a consistent estimator of $K^{(k)} \Sigma K^{(k)'}$.

If $\hat{\Sigma}^{(k)}$ is consistent as an estimator of $K^{(k)}\Sigma K^{(k)'}$, it follows that $\hat{\beta}$ is a consistent estimator of β. In addition, if the rows of the original Y matrix arise from a multivariate normal distribution, then $z^{(k)}$ is multivariate normal and $\hat{\beta}$ is multivariate normal. Accordingly, $\hat{\beta}$ is asymptotically multivariate normal. In particular, $\hat{\beta}$ is approximately normal with a mean vector of β and a covariance matrix estimated by

$$\left[\sum_{k=1}^{s} A^{(k)'} (\hat{\Sigma}^{(k)} \otimes I)^{-1} A^{(k)} \right]^{-1} \tag{7}$$

Linear functions of β, say $C\beta$, can be estimated by $C\hat{\beta}$ and would have a covariance matrix estimated by

$$C \left[\sum_{k=1}^{s} A^{(k)'} (\hat{\Sigma}^{(k)} \otimes I)^{-1} A^{(k)} \right]^{-1} C'$$

It may be of interest to model the components of β as a function of age, and C can be chosen to do this. For example, one can model the response variable as linear function of age and test the hypothesis that this model is adequate. In general, to test hypotheses of the form $H_0 : C\beta = 0$ the statistic

$$(C\hat{\beta})' \left\{ C \left[\sum_{k=1}^{s} A^{(k)'} (\hat{\Sigma}^{(k)} \times I)^{-1} A^{(k)} \right]^{-1} C' \right\}^{-1} (C\hat{\beta}) \tag{8}$$

may be compared to a chi-square statistic with c degrees of freedom, where c is the row rank of C.

APPLICATION OF TWO-STAGE PROCEDURE TO THE MUSCATINE DATA

These data come from the Muscatine Coronary Risk Factor study, a longitudinal study of coronary risk factors in school children. This study began in 1971; between 1971 and 1981 six biennial cross-sectional school screens were completed. An additional survey was conducted in 1974. Only children who were enrolled in school during the year of a survey were eligible to participate; about 70 percent of those eligible actually participated. School leavers were no longer eligible, and two new classes became eligible for each survey; there were many patterns of participation over the eleven years of the study.

Height, systolic blood pressure, and other variables were measured on each participant in a survey. For this illustration we simply analyze the height (cm) and systolic blood pressure (mm Hg) as a function of age. We restrict attention to the girls.

Over 4500 girls are included in this analysis. Some have participated in only one survey, whereas others have participated in all six surveys. The distribution of children by the number of surveys in which they participated is presented in

Table 11-1. Number of individuals sampled by frequency of sampling

Number of times sampled	Number of individuals	Number of samples
1	2,095	2,095
2	1,078	2,156
3	618	1,854
4	411	1,644
5	366	1,830
6	116	696
Total	4,684	10,275

Table 11-1. As stated earlier, there are a number of reasons why children have participated in fewer than six survey years. Some children did not reach school age until 1981 and were eligible for only one survey year. Others graduated and were no longer eligible. For the fourteen ages considered, over 400 different patterns of incomplete data are represented in the data set.

By way of summary statistics, Table 11-2 exhibits the age-survey-year-specific mean and standard errors for the height and systolic blood pressure. The final column is a summary collapsed across all survey years; approximately 500 observations are in this summary ("All") for ages 5, 15, 16, 17, and 18, while there are over 1000 for each of the ages 6 through 14. The overall cross-sectional summary fails to take into account the correlation between repeated observations on the same child; therefore, the variance–covariance matrix is not estimated properly with such a cross-sectional analysis.

If there is interest in estimation of the age-specific means and growth rates, then the two-stage procedure of the previous section may be applied. In the appendix we outline an SAS program that was prepared for this specific application. This program generates the two-stage estimator and the estimated variance–covariance matrix. In Table 11-3 these estimators and their standard errors are displayed along with the overall cross-sectional and 1981-only data estimators. The lower standard errors for the two-stage estimator are a reflection of the utilization of the correlation between repeated observations on the same child. In addition to the estimated means, we also estimated the two-year growth rates (displayed at the ending age in Table 11-3) and their standard errors for each of the three analyses. Here the two-stage estimators have considerably lower standard errors compared with the other two procedures for height, and have slightly lower standard errors for systolic blood pressure. The ability of the two-stage procedure to use the correlation between repeated observations is a distinct advantage over the cross-sectional analyses of the data. Also shown in the table (last column) are the correlation estimates between repeated observations separated by two years. This summary illustrates the magnitude of the correlation between the repeated values and reinforces the need to take it into account in the analyses.

Mean systolic blood pressure by age and survey year, girls only

	1971		1973		1974		1975		1977		1979		1981		All	
Age	Mean	SE	Mean	SE	Mean	SE	Mean	SE	Mean	SE	Mean	SE	Mean	SE	Mean	SE
Height (cm)																
5	126.55	9.65	106.50	8.90	112.81	0.53	111.90	0.66	113.48	0.61	112.69	0.59	113.36	0.58	112.90	0.27
6	119.45	0.47	119.73	0.57	118.52	0.44	116.61	0.40	116.74	0.39	117.04	0.40	116.82	0.37	117.56	0.16
7	123.96	0.41	123.67	0.38	121.78	0.67	123.81	0.47	122.82	0.43	123.94	0.46	122.95	0.46	123.44	0.17
8	129.96	0.32	130.18	0.43	124.57	1.79	128.44	0.44	128.48	0.41	129.06	0.41	129.34	0.45	129.32	0.16
9	135.32	0.34	135.01	0.42	—	—	135.00	0.42	135.34	0.46	135.25	0.48	135.38	0.43	135.22	0.17
10	140.79	0.46	141.08	0.46	—	—	141.72	0.48	140.64	0.48	141.02	0.47	141.14	0.47	141.06	0.19
11	147.72	0.45	148.45	0.50	—	—	147.15	0.48	146.85	0.49	148.49	0.55	148.16	0.59	147.78	0.21
12	154.51	0.50	153.57	0.51	—	—	154.45	0.45	155.28	0.47	152.93	0.57	154.07	0.49	154.19	0.20
13	158.47	0.51	159.02	0.43	—	—	158.68	0.47	158.09	0.49	158.64	0.46	159.23	0.48	158.68	0.19
14	161.41	0.40	161.77	0.45	—	—	161.31	0.45	160.99	0.43	161.91	0.53	161.15	0.52	161.42	0.19
15	162.09	0.47	163.12	0.53	—	—	163.14	0.42	162.30	0.49	162.95	0.51	161.70	0.54	162.58	0.20
16	162.78	0.52	163.33	0.60	—	—	163.93	0.51	163.53	0.54	163.60	0.45	163.34	0.61	163.43	0.22
17	164.11	0.54	162.71	0.72	—	—	164.17	0.64	164.48	0.52	163.31	0.56	163.12	0.71	163.76	0.25
18	162.98	0.79	162.62	1.50	—	—	163.27	1.04	163.94	0.80	164.37	0.71	164.28	1.05	163.75	0.37
Systolic blood pressure (mm Hg)																
5	107.50	0.50	93.00	3.00	91.40	1.25	91.43	1.35	96.39	1.05	96.11	1.13	96.27	1.17	94.30	0.55
6	99.92	0.86	100.51	1.14	93.64	0.93	95.61	0.81	96.97	0.62	94.56	0.76	98.28	0.65	96.76	0.31
7	100.83	0.75	101.12	0.70	96.33	1.43	98.77	0.90	98.32	0.68	95.95	0.82	98.77	0.86	98.96	0.32
8	104.56	0.61	103.11	0.87	91.33	10.73	97.85	0.89	100.01	0.71	96.19	0.61	98.46	0.75	100.52	0.31
9	107.24	0.68	105.64	0.88	—	—	101.71	0.76	102.47	0.84	99.30	0.77	101.41	0.70	103.45	0.33
10	109.49	0.81	108.95	0.79	—	—	102.49	0.81	103.23	0.79	102.15	0.73	100.93	0.65	104.86	0.33
11	114.53	0.85	110.55	0.89	—	—	106.93	0.88	107.54	0.81	107.09	0.88	104.78	0.78	108.87	0.36
12	117.81	1.00	110.89	0.92	—	—	110.07	0.81	108.27	0.76	107.02	0.99	108.51	0.81	110.56	0.37
13	119.68	0.97	115.25	0.82	—	—	112.99	0.99	112.86	0.83	109.61	0.83	111.33	0.91	113.86	0.38
14	120.14	1.00	116.62	0.89	—	—	113.35	0.88	112.99	0.73	110.08	0.84	108.53	0.80	113.98	0.38
15	117.29	1.00	116.27	0.93	—	—	113.73	0.85	114.96	0.79	113.16	0.93	109.06	1.00	114.18	0.38
16	116.05	1.06	114.05	1.24	—	—	114.18	0.86	114.71	0.81	113.23	0.96	111.58	1.06	114.01	0.41
17	116.41	1.20	115.84	1.74	—	—	114.33	1.17	115.70	1.00	113.21	0.93	112.91	1.23	114.71	0.48
18	122.06	2.17	115.20	3.15	—	—	108.88	1.65	114.78	1.32	112.80	1.21	112.62	1.85	114.38	0.73

Table 11–3. Summary statistics for three analyses: Age-specific means, standard errors, and two-year differences by height and systolic blood pressure, girls only

| | 1981 cross-sectional survey | | | | All cross-sectional surveys | | | | Two-stage estimates | | | | Stage I |
| | | | Two-year differences | | | | Two-year differences | | | | Two-year differences | | Two-year correlations |
Age	Mean	SE	Mean	SE	Mean	SE	Mean	SE	Mean	SE	Mean	SE	
Height (cm)													
5	113.36	0.58			112.90	0.27			111.36	0.10			
6	116.82	0.37			117.56	0.16			117.03	0.11			
7	122.95	0.46	9.59	0.74	123.44	0.17	10.54	0.32	123.35	0.10	11.99	0.05	0.87
8	129.34	0.45	12.52	0.58	129.32	0.16	11.76	0.23	129.43	0.11	12.40	0.11	0.88
9	135.38	0.43	12.43	0.63	135.22	0.17	11.78	0.24	135.26	0.12	11.91	0.10	0.92
10	141.14	0.47	11.80	0.65	141.06	0.19	11.74	0.25	140.56	0.14	11.13	0.12	0.91
11	148.16	0.59	12.78	0.73	147.78	0.21	12.56	0.27	148.32	0.16	13.06	0.13	0.90
12	154.07	0.49	12.93	0.68	154.19	0.20	13.13	0.28	153.20	0.14	12.64	0.10	0.91
13	159.23	0.48	11.07	0.76	158.68	0.19	10.90	0.28	158.93	0.15	10.61	0.15	0.86
14	161.15	0.52	7.08	0.71	161.42	0.19	7.23	0.28	161.60	0.13	8.40	0.13	0.82
15	161.70	0.54	2.47	0.72	162.58	0.20	3.90	0.28	162.58	0.19	3.65	0.14	0.89
16	163.34	0.61	2.19	0.80	163.43	0.22	2.01	0.29	163.39	0.17	1.79	0.11	0.95
17	163.12	0.71	1.42	0.89	163.76	0.25	1.18	0.32	163.44	0.27	0.86	0.32	0.96
18	164.28	1.05	0.94	1.21	163.75	0.37	0.32	0.43	164.20	0.45	0.81	0.50	0.99

Systolic blood pressure (mm Hg)

5	96.27	1.17			94.30	0.55			95.33	0.55			
6	98.28	0.65			96.76	0.31			97.65	0.31			
7	98.77	0.86	2.50	1.45	98.96	0.32	4.66	0.64	99.52	0.32	4.19	0.60	0.42
8	98.46	0.75	0.18	0.99	100.52	0.31	3.76	0.44	101.22	0.32	3.57	0.42	0.38
9	101.41	0.70	2.64	1.11	103.45	0.33	4.49	0.46	103.98	0.34	4.46	0.42	0.41
10	100.93	0.65	2.47	0.99	104.86	0.33	4.34	0.45	105.20	0.35	3.97	0.42	0.73
11	104.78	0.78	3.37	1.05	108.87	0.36	5.42	0.49	108.71	0.38	4.73	0.45	0.73
12	108.51	0.81	7.58	1.04	110.56	0.37	5.70	0.50	110.78	0.38	5.58	0.45	0.41
13	111.33	0.91	6.55	1.20	113.86	0.38	4.99	0.52	113.55	0.38	4.84	0.46	0.48
14	108.53	0.80	0.02	1.14	113.98	0.38	3.42	0.53	113.69	0.38	2.92	0.47	0.43
15	109.06	1.00	−2.27	1.35	114.18	0.38	0.32	0.54	113.85	0.41	0.30	0.49	0.46
16	111.58	1.06	3.05	1.33	114.01	0.41	0.03	0.56	113.83	0.42	0.14	0.48	0.46
17	112.91	1.23	3.85	1.59	114.71	0.48	0.53	0.61	114.50	0.51	0.65	0.59	0.43
18	112.62	1.85	1.04	2.13	114.38	0.73	0.37	0.84	114.34	0.73	0.51	0.76	0.54

DISCUSSION

Longitudinal data are rarely complete, particularly if long follow-up intervals are involved. Accordingly, statistical procedures for the estimation of mean values and other parameters should be sufficiently flexible to accommodate incomplete data. In this chapter we have reviewed selected approaches that have been applied to the analysis of incomplete longitudinal data. Our review emphasizes the area of randomly incomplete longitudinal data, since the majority of the existing statistical literature focuses on this topic. Maximum likelihood and generalized least-squares estimation procedures have been well studied in an asymptotic sense for incomplete longitudinal data; much work, however, remains to be done in understanding these procedures for finite samples. Computer programs are available for general randomly incomplete longitudinal data; however, such software is more "demonstration" than "production" software. At this point most problems require special programming to adapt the software for a particular application.

The two-stage example is but one illustration of an adaption we have used for the Muscatine study. It is essentially an application of the general Kleinbaum (1970, 1973) methodology. It is easy to implement on the standard statistical packages that provide matrix procedures (appendix), although the procedure does involve a large amount of computational effort. In addition, numerical problems may be encountered in the estimation of β if the estimators of $\Sigma^{(k)}$ are not positive semidefinite. In this case a smoothed estimator of $\Sigma^{(k)}$ can be obtained by using the procedure described in Schwertman and Allen (1973) and in Leeper and Woolson (1982). This procedure ensures a positive semidefinite estimator of $\Sigma^{(k)}$. In this case the inverse of $\hat{\Sigma}^{(k)}$, which is used in (6) and (7), is replaced by its generalized inverse. For large data sets, the two-stage generalized least-squares procedure may be useful. In addition, it is useful in this case due to the large number of patterns of incomplete data. While the two-stage procedure described has desirable large sample properties, further study of its small sample properties is warranted.

There has been considerably less work done on the problem of nonrandomly missing longitudinal data. This area is a likely future area of further research, and the methods of Heckman (1974, 1976) may be especially useful in its further study. Little and Rubin (1986) have provided detailed treatment of general problems regarding missing data; this publication may be consulted for more discussion of nonresponse problems.

Appendix
SAS Computer Methods for Two-Stage
Estimation Procedure

This appendix briefly describes an SAS MATRIX procedure program to compute the two-stage estimates for the parameter matrix and its variance–covariance matrix. The procedure was used for each sex and for height and systolic blood pressure separately.

Various SAS programs had already prepared the data sets that are required as input to this procedure. The programs necessary for this first phase of the analysis depend heavily on the source and form of the original data and are only outlined here.

STAGE I

An SAS data set was prepared with all observations on the dependent variable (height or systolic blood pressure) for each subject. This data set had one 14×1 vector (one element for each of the possible ages 5 to 18 years) for each subject. This vector contained the observed value of the dependent variable for each age at which the child had been measured and the missing attribute for all other ages. These vectors of observations were used to calculate the 14×14 covariance matrix for all possible pairs of ages, and this matrix was saved on an SAS data set. Impossible age pairs were given the missing attribute in this covariance matrix.

A second file was created that had one observation for each observed age profile. This data file contained for each profile a 14×1 vector of 0's and 1's describing the profile, a unique profile identification number, and a count of the number of observations for the profile. (The profile ID was created from the profile by converting the pattern of 14 0's and 1's into the decimal equivalent of the binary number.) The profile ID number was also merged onto a file containing one record for each observation on a child. The resulting file was sorted in profile ID order.

At the end of Stage I we had the following:

1. The 14×14 covariance matrix computed from the residuals (called SSET in the Stage II program).
2. A profile data set (called PSET in the Stage II program) that had one record for each unique profile. This file contained a 1×14 vector that described the profile, the unique profile ID, and a count of the number of observations for the profile. This set was sorted in profile ID order.
3. A data file (called ZSET in the Stage II program) containing one record for each measurement on each child. This file contained the profile ID for

that child and the 14×1 observation for that child. This set was sorted first by profile ID and then subject ID.

4. A fourth data file (called ASET in the Stage II program) contained the child's ID, the profile ID for that child, andthe $1 \times q$ vector for the design matrix A for that observation. This file was created in a separate data step in SAS and its contents depended on the model being used. This file was also sorted by profile ID, then subject ID, so that the observations would correspond appropriately in ZSET and ASET.

STAGE II

A listing of an SAS MATRIX procedure program to compute the second-stage estimates and their covariance matrix using equations (6) and (7) follows. Two features of this procedure are important. First, because the submatrices of the Stage-I covariance matrix would not need to be positive definite, we smoothed the estimates (Schwertman and Allen, 1979) and used generalized inverses in subsequent analyses. Second, some of the matrices described in the theoretical portion of this chapter were very large for the data we were analyzing and quickly exceeded the core capacity of the machine we were using. It was necessary to include coding that would avoid creating very large matrices.

The procedure first computes the eigenvalues and eigenvectors for the covariance matrix. The smoothed generalized inverse is computed by deleting the nonpositive eigenvalues and summing the inner product of the eigenvectors, divided by the corresponding eigenvalues. In equation (8) the Kroneker product term has dimension $n_k p_k \times n_k p_k$, which became very large for our data. Creation of these large matrices was avoided by using the coding detailed in the procedure.

PROC MATRIX DUMP:
*

   THIS PROCEDURE WILL COMPUTE STAGE II ESTIMATES FOR BETA MATRIX AND OUTPUT ESTIMATED;
   BETA MATRIX
   COVARIANCE OF BETA MATRIX
INPUT TO THIS ROUTINE MUST INCLUDE THE FOLLOWING FOUR DATA SETS:
   1. THE COVARIANCE MATRIX (CALLED SSET).
   2. A FILE WITH ONE RECORD PER SAMPLING PROFILE CONTAINING A UNIQUE PROFILE ID, THE PROFILE WITH 1'S FOR SAMPLED AGES AND 0 FOR NONSAMPLED AGES, AND ACOUNT OF THE NUMBER OF OBSERVATIONS FOR THE PROFILE (CALLED PSET).
   3. A DATA FILE CONTAINING TNE RESIDUAL FOR EACH MEASUREMENT ON EACH CHILD (CALLED ZSET).

4. A FILE CONTAINING THE DESIGN MATRIX FOR EACH OBSERVATION
   (CALLED ASET).

THE EQUATIONS USED IN THE COMPUTATIONS ARE DESCRIBED IN THE
BODY OF THE PAPER.

```
;
*  SET UP DIMENSION OF THE BETA MATRIX;
Q = 20;
*
   GET STAGE I SIGMA MATRIX;
FETCH SIGMA DATA-SSET;
*
   GET P MATRIX
   THIS MATRIX CONTAINS PROFILES FOR S DIFFERENT PATTERNS;
FETCH P DATA = PSET;
   S = NROW(P);
*  CREATE MATRICES TO HOLD SUMS OF C(K) AND F(K) MATRICES;
   SC = J(Q,Q,0);
   SF = J(Q,1,0);


*

   COMPUTE C(K) AND F(K) FOR EACH PATTERN;
DO K = 1 TO S;
   NK = NUMBER OF SUBJECTS IN THIS PATTERN
   PK = NUMBER OF AGES IN THIS PATTERN
   NPK = NUMBER OF OBSERVATIONS FOR THIS PATTERN;
   PP = P(K,1:14);
   NK = P(K,15);
   PK = PP(1,+);
   NPK = NK*PK;
*  GET DESIGN MATRIX A(K) AND DATA MATRIX Z(K) FOR THIS PROFILE
   ;
FETCH ZK NPK DATA = ZSET;
FETCH AK NPK DATA = ASET;
*  PICK OFF APPROPRIATE ROWS AND COLUMNS OF SIGMA
   FOR THIS PATTERN;
   T = J(PK,14,0);
   KI = 0;
   DO IX = 1 TO 14 WHILE (KI < PK);
     IF PP(1,IX) = 1 THEN DO;
       KI = KI + 1;
       T(KI,IX) = 1;
     END;
   END;
   TSTP = T * SIGMA * T';
*  IN ORDER TO SAVE CORE, HANDLE PK = 1 AS SEPARATE CASE;
```

```
IF PK = 1 THEN DO;
  VAR = TSTP(1,1);
    CK = (AK' * AK) #/VAR;
    FK = (AK' * ZK) #/VAR;
END;


*   COMPUTE CONTRIBUTION FOR PK > 2 ;
ELSE DO;
*   GET EIGEN VALUES AND EIGEN VECTORS FOR SUBMATRIX;
    EIGEN EVAL EVEC TSTP;
*   CALCULATE GENERALIZED INVERSE FOR THIS SUBMATRIX;
WK = J(PK,PK,0);
  DO IX = 1 TO PK;
    L = EVAL(IX,1);
    IF I < = 0 THEN GO TO DONE INV;
    EP = EVEC(,IX);
    WK = WK + ((EP * EP') #/L);
  END;


*   COMPUTE CONTRIBUTIONS TO COVARIANCE AND BETA FROM THIS
PATTERN;
*   CREATE AW MATRIX
    AW = A' * (W * I)
    TO AVOID EXTREMELY LARGE REGION REQUIREMENT
    ;
DONE INV:     AW = J(Q,NPK,0);
  DO JJ = 1 TO Q;
    IND = 0;
    DO LL = 1 TO PK;
      DO IS = 1 TO NK;
        IND = IND + 1;
        IM = IS;
        DO M = 1 TO PK;
          AW(JJ,IND) = AW(JJ,IND) + WK(M,LL)*AK(IM,JJ);
          IM = IM + NK;
        END;
      END;
    END;
  END;
END;
  CK = AW * AK;
  FK = AW * ZK;
END;   *  END OF DO GROUP FOR PK > 2;
*  ACCUMULATE CONTRIBUTIONS THIS PATTERN ;
    SC = SC + CK;
    SF = SF + FK;
```

ENDK: END;
* ALL PATTERNS HAVE BEEN PROCESSED, COMPUT VARIANCE-
COVARIANCE MATRIX AND STAGE II ESTIMATE OF BETA;
VARCOV = INV(SC);
BHAT = VARCOV * SF;

* OUTPUT RESULTS TO PERMANENT SAS DATA SETS THEN
  PRINT RESULTS

;
OUTPUT VARCOV DATA = SAVE.FHGTCOV;
OUTPUT BHAT DATA = SAVE.FHGTBHAT;
PRINT BHAT;
PRINT VARCOV;
PRINT NSMTH;
STOP;

ACKNOWLEDGMENT

This research supported in part by grant No. MH46011-01 from the National Institute of Mental Health.

REFERENCES

Beale EML, Little RJA (1975). "Missing values in multivariate analysis." *Journal of the Royal Statistical Society B* 37:129–146.
Bentler PM, Tanaka JS (1983). "Problem with EM algorithms for ML factor analysis." *Psychometrika* 48:247–251.
Berk KN (1984a). "Computing for unbalanced repeated measures for experiments." In *Proceedings of the Eleventh Annual SUGI Conference* Cary, N.C., SAS Institute.
Berk KN (1984b). *Computing for Incomplete Repeated Measures*. BMDP Technical Report, no. 81.
Cook NR (1983). "Modeling and estimation in unbalanced repeated measures designs." Paper presented at the Joint Statistical Meetings, Toronto, Canada.
Cook NR, Ware JH (1983). "Design and analysis methods for longitudinal research." *Annual Review of Public Health* 4:1–23.
Davis CS, Wei LJ (1988). "Nonparametric methods for analyzing incomplete nondecreasing repeated measurements." *Biometrics* 44:1005–1018.
Dempster AP, Laird NM, Rubin DB (1977). "Maximum likelihood from incomplete data via the EM algorithm" (with discussion). *Journal of the Royal Statistical Society B* 39:1–38.
Dempster AP, Rubin DB, Tsutakawa RK (1981). "Estimation in covariance components model." *Journal of the American Statistical Association* 76:341–353.
Fairclough DL, Helms RW (1983). "PROC MATRIX macros for generalized incomplete (GIM) and multiple design (MDM) multivariate models." In *Proceedings of the Eighth Annual SAS Users Group International Conference*, pp 883–888.
Fairclough DL, Helms RW (1985). "A sensitivity analysis of maximum likelihood

estimators in a mixed model for analysis of incomplete and mistimed longitudinal data." Paper presented at the Interface Symposium, Lexington, Ky.

Geisser S, Greenhouse SW (1958). "An extension of Box's results on the use of the F distribution in multivariate analysis." *Annals of Mathematical Statistics* 29:885–891.

Hartley HO (1958). "Maximum likelihood estimation from incomplete data." *Biometrics* 14:174–194.

Heckman JD (1974). "Shadow prices, market wages and labor supply." *Econometrica* 42:679–694.

Heckman JD (1976). "The common structure of statistical models of truncation, sample selection and limited dependent variables and a simple estimator for such models." *Annals of Economic and Social Measurement* 5:475–492.

Helms RW (1984). "Linear models with linear covariance structure for incomplete data." Paper presented at the annual meeting of the American Statistical Association, Philadelphia.

Hocking RR, Smith WB (1968). "Estimation of parameters in the multivariate normal distribution with missing observations." *Journal of the American Statistical Association* 63:159–173.

Jennrich RI, Schluchter MB (1985). "Incomplete repeated measures models with structured covariance matrices." Paper presented at the annual meeting of the American Statistical Association, Las Vegas.

Kleinbaum DG (1970). "Estimation and hypothesis testing for generalized multivariate linear models." PhD diss. University of North Carolina, Chapel Hill.

Kleinbaum DG (1973). "A generalization of the growth curve model which allows missing data." *Journal of Multivariate Analysis* 3:117–124.

Laird NM (1988). "Missing data in longitudinal studies." *Statistics in Medicine* 7:305–315.

Laird NM, Ware JH (1982). "Random-effects models for longitudinal data." *Biometrics* 38:963–974.

Laird NM, Ware JH (1984). "Random effects models for serial categorical response." Paper presented at the annual meeting of the American Statistical Association, Philadelphia.

LaVange LM, Helms RW (1983). "The analysis of incomplete longitudinal data with time series covariance structures." Paper presented at the Joint Statistical Meetings, Toronto.

Leeper JD (1977). "A linear model approach to the analysis of incomplete longitudinal data." PhD diss. University of Iowa.

Leeper JD, Woolson RF (1982). "Testing hypothesis for the growth curve model when the data are incomplete." *Journal of Statistical Computation and Simulation* 15:97–106.

Little RJA (1979). "Maximum likelihood inference for multiple regression with missing values: A simulation study." *Journal of the Royal Statistical Society B* 41:76–87.

Little RJA, Rubin DB (1986). *The Analysis of Incomplete Data* New York, Wiley.

Little RJA, Schluchter MD (1985). "Maximum likelihood estimation for mixed continuous and categorical data with missing values." *Biometrika* 72:497–512.

Meneses J (1984). "A note on the initial estimates for the EM algorithm." In *Proceedings of the Statistical Computing Section, American Statistical Association.*

Orchard T, Woodbury MA (1972). "A missing information principle: Theory and applications." In *Proceedings of the 6th Berkeley Symposium on Methods in Statistics and Probability,* pp 697–715.

Potthoff RF, Roy SN (1964). "A generalized multivariate analysis of variance model useful especially for growth curve problems." *Biometrika* 51:313–326.

Rao CR (1965). "The theory of least squares when the parameters are stochastic and its application to the analysis of growth curves." *Biometrika* 52:447–458.

Rao CR (1973). *Linear Statistical Inference and Its Application* (2nd ed). New York, Wiley.

Rao MN, Rao CR (1966). "Linked cross-sectional study for determining norms and growth rates—a pilot survey on Indian school-going boys." *Sankhya B* 28:237–258.

Revankar NS (1974). "Some finite sample results in the context of two seemingly unrelated regression equations." *Journal of the American Statistical Association* 69:187–190.

Revankar NS (1976). "Use of restricted residuals in SUR systems: Some finite sample results." *Journal of the American Statistical Association* 71:183–188.

Rubin DB (1974). "Characterizing the estimation of parameters in incomplete data problems." *Journal of the American Statistical Association* 69:467–474.

Rubin DB (1976a). "Inference and missing data." *Biometrika* 63:581–592.

Rubin DB (1976b). "Comparing regressions when some predictor values are missing." *Technometrics* 18:201–205.

Rubin DB (1978). "Multiple imputations in sample surveys—a phenomenological Bayesian approach to nonresponse" (with discussion and reply). In *Imputation and Editing of Faulty or Missing Survey Data*. Washington, D.C., Social Security Administration and Bureau of the Census, pp 1–9.

Sall J (1982). *SAS User's Guide, Statistics*. Cary, N.C., SAS Institute.

Schluchter MD, Jackson KL (1989). "Log-linear analysis of censored survival data with partially observed covariates." *Journal of the American Statistical Association* 84:42–52.

Schwertman NC (1974). The analysis and testing of hypotheses using growth curve data with missing observations." PhD diss., University of Kentucky.

Schwertman NC, Allen DM (1973). *The smoothing of an indefinite matrix with applications to growth curve analysis with missing observations*. Technical Report, no. 56, University of Kentucky Department of Statistics, Lexington.

Schwertman NC, Allen, DM (1979). "Smoothing an indefinite variance–covariance matrix." *Journal of Statistical Computation and Simulation* 9:183–194.

Schwertman NC, Flynn W, Stein S, Schenk KL (1985). "A Monte Carlo study of alternative procedures for testing the hypothesis of parallelism for complete and incomplete growth curve data." *Journal of Statistical Computation and Simulation* 21:1–37.

Srivastava JN, McDonald LL (1974). "Analysis of growth curves under the hierarchical models." *Sankhya A* 36:251–260.

Szatrowski TH (1983). "Missing data in the one-population multivariate normal patterned mean and covariance matrix testing and estimation problem." *Annals of Statistics* 11:947–958.

Timm NH (1980). "Multivariate analysis of variance of repeated measurements." In Krishnaiah PR (ed), *Handbook of Statistics, Analysis of Variance* New York, North-Holland, vol. 1, pp 41–87.

Tobin J (1958). "Estimation of relationships for limited dependent variables." *Econometrica* 26:24–36.

Wald A (1943). "Tests of statistical hypothesis concerning several parameters when the number of observations is large." *Transactions of the American Mathematics Society* 54:426–482.

Ware JH (1984). "Linear models for the analysis of longitudinal studies." Paper presented at the annual meeting of the American Statistical Association, Philadelphia.

Ware JH (1985). "Linear models for analysis of longitudinal studies." *American Statistician* 39:95–101.

Williams JS (1967). "The variance of weighted regression estimates." *Journal of the American Statistical Association* 62:1290–1301.

Woolson RF, Leeper JD, Clarke WR (1978). "Analysis of incomplete data from longitudinal and mixed longitudinal studies." *Journal of the Royal Statistical Society A* 141 (Part 2):242–252.

Zellner A (1962). "An efficient method of estimating seemingly unrelated regressions and tests of aggregation bias." *Journal of the American Statistical Association* 57:348–368.

Zellner A (1963). "Estimators of seemingly unrelated regression equations: Some exact finite sample results." *Journal of the American Statistical Association* 58:977–992.

12

Models for the Longitudinal Analysis of Cohort and Case-Control Studies with Inaccurately Measured Exposures

Application: Dietary Ratio of Polyunsaturated to Saturated Fats and Subsequent Risk of Coronary Heart Disease

DAVID CLAYTON

RELATIVE-RISK REGRESSION IN EPIDEMIOLOGY

Recent years have seen statistical methods in epidemiology develop toward a unified approach based on the proportional hazards regression model introduced by Cox (1972). This provides a general approach for modeling time-to-failure data; it derives its name from its simplest form in which, although the hazard or risk of failure may vary over time, the *ratio* of hazards for two populations characterized by different covariates is assumed to be constant. The model may, however, be extended to include covariates that vary over time and covariates whose effects on risk vary over time in some parametrically described manner. In such cases the model no longer predicts proportional hazards. For this reason it is becoming customary to refer to this model as the *relative risk regression model*.

In the setting of chronic disease epidemiology, the failure-time of interest is the age at which individuals succumb to the disease under study. Normally this will be taken as the age at first clinical diagnosis of the disease (incidence). Sometimes, however, this information is lacking and it is necessary to use age at mortality ascribed to the studied disease as a surrogate for incidence. In these circumstances, the hazard function of failure-time theory is interpretable as an age-specific incidence (mortality) rate. Thus let $\lambda(t; X(t))$ represent the probability of disease incidence per unit time for persons of age t characterized by a covariate history $X(t)$. The relative risk regression model may be written

$$\lambda[t \mid X(t)] = \lambda_0(t)\theta[X(t); \beta] \tag{1}$$

That is, the conditional age-specific rates are expressed as the product of a baseline incidence curve, $\lambda_0(t)$, and a *relative risk* function, $\theta[X(t); \beta]$. The relative risk function could have any known parametric form, but two are of particular interest (Thomas, 1981). The log-linear relative risk regression model has

$$\log \theta[X(t); \beta] = x^*(t)\beta \tag{2}$$

while the linear relative risk regression model has

$$\theta[X(t); \beta] = 1 + x^*(t)\beta \tag{3}$$

The notation $x^*(t)$ is due to Prentice (1982) and denotes any known function of the covariate history, $X(t)$, and of t, age itself. Since relative risks must be positive, the linear form (3) is rather less generally useful, being restricted to positive-valued functions $x^*(t)$ with positive-valued coefficients β. Nevertheless, this form has sometimes been found preferable to the log-linear form (2) for the relative risk of certain cancers when $x^*(t)$ represents the cumulative lifetime dose of a carcinogen.

This framework encompasses most of modern statistical methodology in epidemiology. For cohort studies it is usual to model the baseline incidence curve, $\lambda_0(t)$, by a step function based on five- or ten-year age-groups. This leads to the "subject-years method" recently reviewed by Berry (1983). In the special case of comparison of a single study cohort to a reference set of population rates, it justifies the long-established standardized mortality ratio (Breslow, 1978). The analysis of case-control studies follows from the idea of "partial likelihood" (Cox, 1972, 1975). This eliminates the baseline incidence curve from the argument and concentrates on the *risk sets* of individuals in a study cohort who are both observed and free of disease at the ages at which disease incidence occurred. Partial likelihood is constructed by taking a product over all such ages of the probability that the disease occurred in the individual as observed, rather than in any other member of the corresponding risk set. The analysis of the epidemiologic case-control study reproduces this argument with the trivial modification that the risk set is sampled rather than identified exhaustively (Prentice & Breslow, 1978). In the case of the log-linear model (2), the method of maximum partial likelihood then leads to the *conditional* logistic regression analysis used for matched case-control sets (Breslow & Day, 1980, Chap. 7; Smith, et al., 1981). Grouping such sets into a relatively few strata allows a simplified analysis via conventional, or unconditional, logistic regression analysis (Anderson, 1970; Breslow & Day, 1980, Chap. 6). Similarly, the use of logistic regression analysis for cohort study data, frequently encountered in coronary epidemiology, may be thought of as an approximation to an analysis by relative risk regression/partial likelihood methods, although difficulties are encountered for studies involving long and/or variable follow-up times (Clayton, 1982). It should be stressed that, in principle, these methods are not restricted to specific choices of parametric form for the relative risk function (e.g. (2) or (3)) although, in practice, availability of software often limits the choice.

Despite the power and elegance of this approach, problems remain, and many of these may be traced to the fact that (1) is a *regression* model. In particular, it ignores the fact that the covariate history, $X(t)$, provides at best an inaccurate measurement of the true disease determinants, which we shall denote by $\xi(t)$ and refer to as *exposures*. Of course if the motivation for the model is to provide an actuarial prediction, then it is correct to ignore such measurement errors—if an important variable in the etiology of the disease is badly measured then it may legitimately become a much less imporant predictor. Epidemiologists are, however, not actuaries and they are rarely primarily concerned with prediction. They are concerned with *explanation* and must beware of apparent downgrading of the importance of etiologic factors. Two examples illustrate this problem.

Example 1:   This concerns the controversial finding of a relationship between cigarette smoking and the incidence of cancer of the cervix (Harris et al., 1980). It is likely that the main causal agent in cancer of the cervix is infectious and is transmitted by sexual contact. It would also seem that there is an association between cigarette smoking and those aspects of sexual behavior that lead to increased risk of disease: When one adjusts for the confounding effects of such variables as lifetime number of sexual partners and age at first intercourse in a regression analysis, the relative risk associated with smoking is reduced. However, this risk remains appreciable and statistically significant. Since we cannot measure the true etiologic factor directly, it remains possible that the remaining association is attributable to *residual confounding*, that is, the risk would disappear completely if we could measure the confounding variable accurately enough.

Example 2:   This is the interpretation of Keys' invaluable studies of coronary disease in seven countries (Keys, 1970, 1980). The seemingly paradoxical finding is that, while a relative risk regression equation based on known coronary risk factors (serum cholesterol, blood pressure, smoking, and the rest) was extremely good at predicting the eventual *order* of the geographically dispersed study cohorts in disease incidence, the *extent* of the relative risks was consistently and seriously underestimated. This led Keys to speculate that "some unidentified variable or variables, *unrelated to those considered here*, contributed to increase the risk of the Americans and the northern Europeans or to protect the southern Europeans and the Japanese" (Keys, 1980, my italics). This has been a common interpretation put on these findings, but if these hypothetical variables are indeed unrelated to the known coronary risk factors, why is the rank order of incidence rates predicted so well? We must at least consider the possibility that the known risk factors do measure the important disease determinants, but measure them imperfectly.

For problems such as this, statistical analysis based on regression must be treated with some caution and, when the data allow, should be supplemented by further analysis that takes account of the inaccuracy of measurement of exposures. This chapter reviews progress in such methods and identifies priorities for further work.

ERRORS OF MEASUREMENT

Several authors have considered the problem of errors of measurement of exposure variables in epidemiology. Prentice (1982) considered the case where the measurement error structure is entirely *known* (or at least assumed) in the formal framework set out in the last section; this paper will be reviewed in detail in the section "Two Relative Risk Regressions." Michalek and Tripathi (1980) also considered the case of known measurement errors in the closely related logistic regression and normal discrimination models. Other papers have concentrated on the incorporation of data from either test−retest reliability studies or validity studies into the inference concerning the relationship between disease incidence and underlying exposure. Two such papers appeared together in the section of the *Journal of Chronic Diseases* devoted to "Variance and Dissent." In the first, Marshall and Graham (1984) appealed for a greater use of dual response in epidemiologic studies. Two imperfect measurements, they argued, are better than one—hardly a statement liable to give rise to variance and dissent! The controversy, such as it was, concerned the analysis of studies incorporating dual response.

Marshall and Graham proposed simple and readily communicable methods, which in effect simply continue to use the regression model (1) through (3). For continuous measurements they advocated entering the mean of the dual measurements into the regression; for dichotomous responses they suggested the use of the four-level factor formed by crossing the two two-level factors. Although this strategy has the (important) virtue of simplicity, it has a number of disadvantages. It leaves unresolved the problem of what to do when replicate measurements are available on only some of the study subjects, or when there is a varying degree of replication throughout the study. Elsewhere (Calyton, 1985) it has been pointed out that this is more likely to be a realistic possibility in the design of etiologic studies. For example, in case-control studies, repeated measurements might prove feasible only in controls. Clayton (1985) also attempted to assess the relative merits of different repeated measurement strategies. Just as seriously, it would appear that the strategy is not as successful as might be hoped.

Kaldor and Clayton (1985) addressed the problem of residual confounding arising as a result of errors of measurement of a dichotomous confounder. They considered the case of a confounder C associated with a sixfold increase in risk of disease and present in 40 percent of subjects classified as exposed to some influence of interest E, but only in 10 percent of subjects not so exposed. In these circumstances, the *confounding risk ratio* (Breslow & Day, 1980, Chap. 3; Miettinen, 1972) is 2, so that if, holding C constant, there is *no* increased risk associated with exposure to E, *marginally* E will carry an apparent relative risk of 2. Figure 12-1 shows relative likelihood curves for the relative risk of the exposure of interest from case-control studies (with 200 cases and 200 controls). The curve labeled "C" is that expected from the confounded study in which the confounder is not measured. The curve labeled "1" is the likelihood curve expected when an attempt is made to allow for the confounding by including an

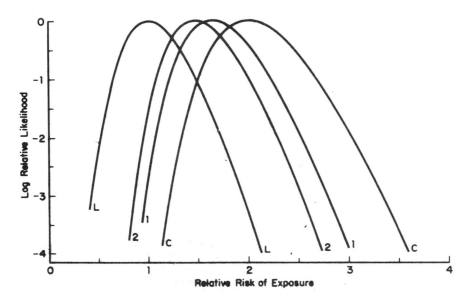

Figure 12–1. Likelihood functions for a relative risk in the presence of confounding.

imperfect measurement of the confounder in a logistic regression equation. In this case the probabilities of both false-positive and false-negative errors are taken to be a fairly modest 0.2, but it can be seen that there is considerable residual confounding. The curve labeled "2" is that expected if dual measurements were taken and simply included in the logistic regression as two variables; the improvement is, perhaps, disappointing. The curve labeled "L" is that which is achieved when the errors of measurement of the confounder are explicitly modeled using the latent class method (described in the section 7). Using this method, the effect of E is estimated correctly.

The existence of alternative methods of analyzing dual response data was pointed out by Walter (1984) in response to Marshall and Graham's paper. These methods have been the subject of several papers in the biostatistical literature (Chen, 1979; Clayton, 1985; Elton & Duffy, 1983; Hui & Walter, 1980; Kaldor & Clayton, 1985; McClish & Quade, 1985). All of these papers suggest using the method of maximum likelihood to fit the extended model that both relates underlying "true" exposures to disease and models the errors of measurement of exposures. The last-mentioned paper pointed out that all this work represents an application of *latent class (structure) analysis* (Goodman, 1974, 1978) and Kaldor and Clayton pointed out a connection with factor analysis models for categorical data (Bartholomew, 1980, 1984). There is also a strong connection with the problem of incompletely measured exposures, for example the right-censored measurements that arise in the analysis of family history data in epidemiologic studies (Clayton, 1978) and the ordinal exposure measurements considered by Cuzick (1985).

These connections will be explored more fully in the section "A General Model" after the work of Prentice (1982) has been discussed. This work is helpful in clarifying the role of *time* in the problem and therefore in elucidating differences in approach to inference from cohort and case-control studies. Before we embark on this discussion, however, it is helpful to digress to remind ourselves of well-known results for conventional least-squares linear regression analysis.

ARE THERE TWO REGRESSIONS?

This section takes its name from the classic paper of Berkson (1950) to which reference will be made later in the section. It concerns the relationship between the regression equation relating a response Y to true values ξ, of independent or exogenous variables and the *induced* regression relationship between Y and imperfect measures X of ξ. The topic has been fully reviewed by Cochran (1968). First assume that the relationship between Y and ξ is indeed a linear regression, that is,

$$E(Y \mid \xi) = \alpha + \xi\beta \qquad (4)$$

We next make the assumption that X, the erroneous measurement of ξ, is related to Y only via ξ, that is, that given the true values ξ, the measured values X cannot improve prediction of Y. In terms of conditional probability distributions $f(Y \mid .)$, this condition may be formally expressed as

$$f(Y \mid \xi, X) = f(Y \mid \xi) \qquad (5)$$

This latter assumption is necessary for any quantitative inference. To put it in an epidemiologic context, note that a good example of an error of measurement that violates (5) is *recall bias* in case-control studies. Here the measurement error depends on the outcome variable, Y, disease status.

With these two assumptions some elementary algebra shows that the induced regression relationship between Y and the imperfect measurements X is

$$E(Y \mid X) = \alpha + \bar{\xi}(X)\beta \qquad (6)$$

where

$$\bar{\xi}(X) = E(\xi \mid X) \qquad (7)$$

Now in general $\bar{\xi}(X) \neq X$, so that replacing the ξ's by inaccurate measurements will give a biased estimate of the underlying regression model (4). In fact, (7) may be regarded as a *Bayes estimate* of ξ using a squared error loss function; usually such estimates behave in such a way that, relative to the X's, they are pulled in toward the center of the distribution. Thus the slope of the regression line of Y on X will be closer to zero than β of (4).

The functional form of $\bar{\xi}(X)$ and hence of the induced regression model (6) depends on assumptions concerning the distribution of ξ in the population studied and about the distribution of errors in their measurement. Berkson pointed out that, in certain circumstances, $\bar{\xi}(X) = X$ so that the induced regression of Y on X is identical to the underlying regression of Y on ξ. This arises in an experimental context in which the experimenter aims to deliver exposure X but, owing to imperfect technique, actually delivers exposure ξ. Thus we might assume

$$\xi = X + \varepsilon \tag{8}$$

where ε is random measurement error, uncorrelated with X and with zero expectation. In these circumstances the measurement errors in X cause little difficulty, save for some lack of precision of the experiment. This is, however, an unrealistic model for measurement error in epidemiologic inquiries, which are for the most part observational studies rather than experiments. For an observational study, usually a more realistic additive error model than (8) is

$$X = \xi + \varepsilon \tag{9}$$

The measurement error is now uncorrelated with ξ.

With the model (9), to derive an expression for the Bayes estimate of ξ, (7), we must know (or assume) the population distribution of true exposures as well as the distribution of measurement errors. The simplest case arises when both of these are normal distributions. If true exposures ξ are distributed normally with mean μ and variance σ^2, and measurement errors ε are normally distributed with zero mean and variance τ^2, then it may be shown that

$$\bar{\xi}(X) = E(\xi \mid X) = cX + (1 - c)\mu \tag{10}$$

where

$$c = \frac{\sigma^2}{\sigma^2 + \tau^2} \tag{11}$$

Equation (10) defines the James–Stein estimate of a normal mean (James & Stein, 1961) and "shrinks" X toward μ using the shrinkage factor c ($\leqslant 1$). By substituting (10) into (6) it is clear that, with these assumptions, the induced regression of Y on X is linear but with slope $c\beta$ rather than β. It should be noted that the linearity of this regression depends on the assumption that the error variance is constant for all ξ. If instead we assume that, conditional on ξ, ε is normal with standard deviation proportional to ξ (i.e., with constant coefficient of variation), then large observed X's are shrunk more than small ones. Thus the induced regression becomes nonlinear—quadratic, in fact, it is therefore possible that the regression relationship of Y on X may mislead us not only as to the extent of the underlying relationship between Y and ξ, but also as to its form.

Similar considerations arise in more general linear model situations where the exposure variables are discrete. In this case, however, there is no assumption analogous to Berkson's formulation in which the two regressions are identical.

Bayes estimates such as the James–Stein estimate are known to outperform more conventional "best" estimates such as maximum likelihood estimates in situations in which a large number of parameters are to be estimated simultaneously (Efron & Morris, 1973; Maritz, 1970; Morris, 1983). Likewise, naive use of maximum likelihood or similar methods in problems involving large numbers of subsidiary or "nuisance" parameters is known in certain cases to lead to inconsistent estimators of parameters of interest. The problem considered here is just such a problem; we observe N pairs $[(Y_i, X_i), i = 1, \ldots, N]$ but have N unknown parameters in the shape of the true exposures (ξ_i) in addition to the parameters of interest, namely α and β. The discussion shows that should we estimate the (ξ_i) by the naive best estimates, that is (X_i), then we obtain inconsistent estimates of α and β. The problem is avoided if we can instead replace (ξ_i) by Bayes estimates, $[\bar{\xi}(X_i)]$. Unfortunately these estimates depend on further unknown parameters of the true exposure distribution and the measurement error distribution. These must, in turn, be estimated from the data. We must therefore adopt an empirical Bayes argument.

This section has served to introduce some important conceptual points in a familiar and straightforward statistical problem, namely normal-theory linear regression. In the next section we show how Prentice (1982) demonstrated that very similar results hold for relative risk regression.

TWO RELATIVE-RISK REGRESSIONS

We now return to the work of Prentice (1982), which derives results similar to those of the last section in the case of the relative risk regression model we discussed in the first section. We now denote the true exposure history of an individual at age t by $\xi(t)$ and let $X(t)$ represent inaccurate or incomplete measure(s) of that exposure history. Our interest as epidemiologists is in the relationship between disease risk and true exposure, and this may be expressed with little loss of generality as a relative risk model,

$$\lambda[t \mid \xi(t)] = \lambda_0(t)\theta[\xi(t); \beta] \tag{12}$$

Again it is necessary to assume that, given the *true* exposure history $\xi(t)$, the inaccurate measurements $X(t)$ are uninformative concerning disease outcome. In the last section this assumption was represented by equation (5); for relative risk regression it may be written

$$\lambda[t \mid \xi(t), X(t)] = \lambda[t \mid \xi(t)] \tag{13}$$

With these assumptions, Prentice showed that the *induced* relationship between disease risk and measured exposure, $X(t)$, may also be written as a relative risk regression model:

$$\lambda[t \mid X(t)] = \lambda_0(t)\bar{\theta}[X(t); \beta] \tag{14}$$

where

$$\bar{\theta}[X(t); \beta] = E\{\theta[\xi(t); \beta] \mid X(t), T \geq t\} \tag{15}$$

That is, leaving some notation undefined for the present, the relative risk function in the induced relative risk regression is a Bayes estimate of the true relative risk function. In general, therefore, owing to the shrinkage of Bayes estimators, true relative risks will be understated in the observed relationship between disease and measured exposure. This is a well-known (although often forgotten) fact, but the beauty of Prentice's result is that it is given a general quantitative expression.

Before continuing the discussion, we must clarify the notation of (15) and discuss the important problems of truncation and censoring arising in epidemiologic cohort and case-control studies. The notation $T \geqslant t$ in the conditional expectation, (15), means that the expectation is conditional on the individual not having succumbed to the disease under study before attaining age t. Formally, T represents the age of onset of the studied disease. This condition enters into the expectation because of the definition of an age-specific incidence rate—the probability per unit time of first occurrence of the disease in individuals free of disease until a given age. This theoretical incidence rate could only be measured in an idealized epidemiologic cohort study in which all individuals entered the study cohort at birth and in which the sole reason for termination of follow-up was occurrence of the study disease (Mantel, 1973). Real cohort studies differ from this ideal in that individuals enter the study at some age, say E, in general greater than zero. Thus had they already succumbed to disease, they would not have been included in the study cohort. This is termed *truncation* and its implication is that real epidemiologic studies measure incidence rates in survivor populations. It is necessary for us to assume that this fact will not materially bias our conclusions. Likewise, in real studies, there are many reasons for termination of follow-up other than occurrence of the single disease under study. These are collectively termed *censoring* and have the implication that real studies measure incidence rates in individuals whose follow-up has not been censored. Again we must assume that this will not affect our conclusions. Writing C for the age at which follow-up would be censored were disease occurrence not to intervene, we can express these assumptions more formally as follows

$$\lambda[t \mid \xi(t), T > E, C > t] = \lambda[t \mid \xi(t)] \tag{16}$$

which merely states that the incidence rates we can observe in real studies are the same as the ideal theoretical incidence rates. These considerations lead us to replace the conditioning on $T \geqslant t$ in (14) and (15) by $(T \geqslant t, T > E, C > t)$, the condition that the individual be free of disease *and under study* at age t. For brevity we will write this condition as $R(t)$.

Prentice suggested that, given the "posterior" distribution of true exposure history $\xi(t)$, given $X(t)$ (measurement) and $R(t)$ (being under study at t), then the expectation (15) is in principle a known function of β so that we may simply use partial likelihood methods to fit the induced relative risk regression (14), thus obtaining point and interval estimates for β. He discussed the case of a time-independent exposure ξ, measured by a simple continuous variable X, assuming the posterior distribution of ξ given X to be normal. This arises in both of the error models (8) and (9) discussed in the last section. Under the "experimental" model (8), using either the log-linear (2) or linear (3) relative risk models, the induced regression is identical to the underlying relative risk model for true exposure. Under the "observational" model (9), however, the coefficients are attenuated although the form of the relative risk function is unchanged. This follows from the following relationships: for the log-linear model,

$$E[\theta(\xi; \beta) | X, R(t)] = E[\exp(\xi\beta) | X, R(t)] = \exp(X\beta c) \tag{17}$$

and, for the linear model,

$$E[\theta(\xi; \beta) | X, R(t)] = E[(1 + \xi\beta) | X, R(t)] = 1 + X\beta c' \tag{18}$$

The "shrinkage factors," c and c', are functions of the parameters of the (normal) distributions of true exposures and measurement errors, respectively. For the log-linear model, the shrinkage c is identical to that for simple linear regression, (11), where σ^2 and τ^2 refer to the variance of ξ and ε for subjects under study at age t. For the linear relative risk model the shrinkage c' is more pronounced:

$$c' = \frac{c}{[1 + (1 - c)\mu]} \tag{19}$$

where c is again given by (11).

Prentice considered as an example the estimation of the dose-response relationship between radiation exposure and thyroid cancer in the Hiroshima atomic bomb survivors. Perhaps surprisingly, in this very nonexperimental situation, he concentrated most of his attention on Berkson's experimental error model and the preceding discussion suggests that no bias would result from ignoring measurement errors in that case. On closer consideration, this may indeed be the more appropriate error model, since X represents a *theoretical* radiation dose determined from the individual's location at the time of the blast. Even if this is so, however, Prentice showed that inference concerning the form of the relative risk dose-response curve is sensitive to assumptions concerning the variance of measurement error. If, for example, we adopt the constant coefficient of variation model ($E(\xi | X) = X$, $\mathrm{var}(\xi | X) = kX^2$), then an underlying log-linear model induces a log-quadratic relationship between relative risk and X. The importance of this issue lies in the problem of low-dose extrapolation.

There are several problems with the analysis proposed by Prentice. First, the normality assumptions are not generally admissible, since the distribution of ξ will not remain invariant over age. Even without allowing censoring to depend on ξ, the fact that disease risk depends on ξ means that an initially normal distribution of ξ will not remain normal. Other distributions do maintain the same distributional form, although their location changes in line with early removal of high risk individuals (Hougaard, 1984a, 1984b). For most applications in epidemiology, however, this effect will be small enough to ignore. The problem of the relationship between censoring and exposure may be more serious; it will be discussed in more detail later. The second problem has already been alluded to in the section "Are There Two Regressions?"; that is, the joint distribution of (ξ, X) is never known in practice so that the Bayes estimates required cannot be calculated. By validity or test–retest reliability substudies, evidence may be collected to *estimate* this distribution so that empirical Bayes estimates can be used instead. This, however, brings new problems, since there must be some effect of errors of estimation of the parameters of the assumed distribution of (ξ, X). Before we consider this problem, the next section considers an example using a heuristic empirical Bayes approach. This serves to clarify the problem in which ξ and X are both continuous variables.

AN EXAMPLE: DIET AND HEART

Perhaps, of all the exposures with which modern epidemiology is concerned, the most problematic for measurement is diet. Coronary epidemiology has long been concerned with this variable, and increasingly cancer epidemiologists are turning their attention to dietary influences on colorectal cancer, stomach cancer, bladder cancer, breast cancer, and others. The fundamental difficulty is that, while great diversity of diet exists *between* communities, there has been little diversity *within* communities (although perhaps this is changing). Further, the problems encountered in measuring the diets of free-living subjects are extremely serious. Thus dietary hypotheses are strongly indicated by "ecological" studies of geographically dispersed communities, quite often supported by the results of migrant studies, but they prove remarkably difficult to verify by traditional cohort or case-control methods.

The data reported in this section are taken from a serendipitous study reported by Morris, Marr, and Clayton (1977). In pilot studies whose aim was to develop and validate questionnaire methods for use in large-scale cohort studies of coronary heart disease, 337 men completed at least one one-week full weighed dietary survey. Seventy-six men completed two such surveys separated by approximately six months. Although these studies were abandoned, being regarded as having failed (!), these men were part of a larger study cohort whose mortality and morbidity experience was followed up. By December 1984, forty-six of the men had died of ischemic heart disease (IHD) and there had been fifty-eight incident cases. There is some reason to doubt the completeness of morbidity follow-up, and here we shall concentrate on the mortality data (although the incidence data yield very similar results). These data are listed in the appendix, together with the dietary data concerning P/S ratio—the ratio of polyunsaturated to saturated fat intake. This is one of the best indices for "explaining" between-community differences in IHD incidence and mortality.

Here we let X represent the measured P/S ratio (the first measurement if there are two) and we let ξ represent the true value, which will be assumed to be invariant within an individual. Figure 12-2 shows graphically the relevant information for a partial likelihood analysis of the relative risk regression of IHD against measured P/S ratio, X. The points represent the deaths from IHD and plot X (ordinate) against age at death (abscissa). At each age at which an IHD death occurred, a vertical bar is also plotted, and this represents the mean plus or minus one standard deviation of X for the set comprising those members of the study cohort who were alive and under study at that age. This set was termed by Cox (1972) the *risk set* corresponding to the observed death. Closer examination shows that the distribution of measured P/S ratio in risk sets is reasonably normal. Without knowledge of the measurement error introduced by the one-week weighted survey method, one would have no option but to limit inference to the predictive model, relating imperfect measurement to disease

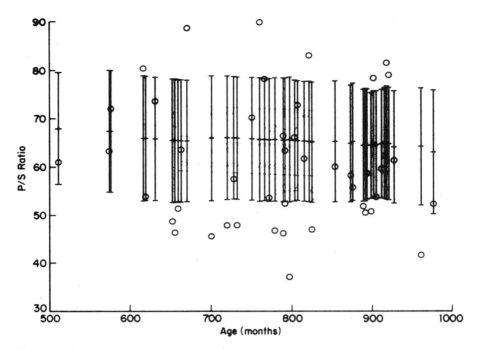

Figure 12–2. P/S ratio (polyunsaturated to saturated fat intake) in cases (ischemic heart disease deaths) and in their corresponding risk sets.

risk. Here, however, the repeated measurement on seventy-six individuals allows further progress.

In this case it is clearly the observational errors model (9) that is the more appropriate, and it seems reasonable to assume normal distributions both for true exposure within risk sets and for measurement error. In particular, let the distribution of ξ within the ith risk set be $N(\mu_i, \sigma_1^2)$ and let the measurement error ε be $N(0, \tau^2)$. Thus X will be distributed in the ith risk set as $N(\mu_i, \sigma_1^2 + \tau^2)$. We may estimate τ^2 by half the variance of the seventy-six *differences* between first- and second-week survey results, and hence obtain unbiased estimates of σ_1^2 by subtraction of our estimate of τ^2 from the conventional variance estimates of X. Finally we can estimate the shrinkage factor for each risk set, c_i, by substituting these estimates into (9).

The results of the last section show that, if the relative risk of mortality from IHD as a function of the true P/S ratio ξ is log linear, that is, $\exp(\xi\beta)$, then it is also a log-linear function of the measured P/S ratio X, that is, $\exp(Xc_i\beta)$. Thus we can estimate the parameter of the underlying model by fitting a log-linear relative risk regression model using the product Xc_i (or more precisely, $X\hat{c}_i$) as covariate. Prentice proposed that this may be carried out by using conventional maximum partial likelihood methods. Thus if $x_{(i)}$ is the value of X observed in the ith case, and R_i is the "risk set" of individuals under study at the age t_i at which the disease occurred in that case (so that the notation $j \in R_i$ means that person j belongs to that set), then the contribution of this case/risk-set to the partial likelihood is the probability that the disease attacked the observed case rather than another member of the risk set. This is simply the value of the relative risk function for the case divided by the sum of relative risks over the entire risk set, here given by

$$\frac{\exp(x_{(i)}\hat{c}_i\beta)}{\sum_{j \in R_i} \exp(x_j \hat{c}_i \beta \Omega}$$ (20)

The partial likelihood is the product of the terms (20) for all observed cases, and β may be estimated by the familiar method of maximum likelihood, even though partial likelihood is not truly a likelihood in the strict sense of the word.

The assumptions just made, however, allow an even easier method of estimation of the regression parameters in this case. From the assumption of normal distributions for both true exposures, ξ, and measurement errors, ε, in each risk set, it follows that measured exposures X are distributed normally with, in the ith risk set, mean μ_i and variance $\sigma_1^2 + \tau^2$. It may be easily shown that it follows from the log-linear assumption for the relative risk function that X should also be distributed normally in the disease case with variance equal to its variance in the corresponding risk set, but with mean shifted in location by δ_i, which is related to β by

$$\delta_i = \beta \sigma_1^2$$ (21)

Thus, using the same argument by which Truett, Cornfield, and Kannel (1967) derived the logistic model for probability of disease occurrence from multivariate normal discriminant analysis, each case and its risk set allows calculation of an estimate of β,

$$\beta_i = \frac{[x_{(i)} - \bar{x}_i]}{\hat{\sigma}_1^2}$$ (22)

where $\bar{x}_i$ is the mean of X in the ith risk set and $\hat{\sigma}_1^2$ is an estimate of σ_1^2. A final estimate is the weighted mean of these with weights inversely proportional to their variances which, assuming the risk sets to be large, are given by

$$\text{var } \hat{\beta}_i = \frac{(\sigma_i^2 + \tau_i^2)}{\sigma_i^4}$$ (23)

so that

$$\hat{\beta} = \frac{\sum_i \hat{c}_i [x_{(i)} - \bar{x}_i]}{\sum_i \hat{c}_i \hat{\sigma}_i^2}$$ (24)

This argument may readily be generalized to the multivariate case where ξ is a vector of true exposures; σ_i^2 is replaced by Σ_i, the variance–covariance matrix of true exposures; and τ^2 is replaced by T, the variance–covariance matrix of measurement errors (which will generally be assumed to be diagonal).

In the case of a time scale coarsely granulated so that many cases occur in the same epoch and of no measurement errors for X, these two methods of analysis become equivalent to logistic regression analysis and Fisher discriminant analysis, respectively. These approaches have been compared by Halperin, Blackwelder, and Verter (1971) who concluded that, when the distribution of exposure variables deviates from multivariate normality, the estimates of β obtained by the discriminant analysis argument may be markedly biased but that, nevertheless, this method may be useful in determining which variables are likely to be of importance. A theoretical comparison of logistic regression and normal discriminant analysis in the presence of errors of measurement was reported by Michalek and Tripathi (1980), who showed that errors of measurement of exposures leads to similar loss of performance of both methods (as would be expected from the present discussion). They also considered the problem, not addressed here, of misclassification of disease status so that some individuals classed as cases are, in reality, free of disease and that other members of risk sets classed as healthy are not. Since this cross-contamination causes deviation from normal assumptions, such errors of diagnosis seem more serious for normal discrimination than for logistic regression.

In the example considered here, the two procedures yield very similar estimates (Table 12-1). Either method leads to an estimated coefficient around 50 percent larger than is obtained by ignoring errors of measurement. It should also be stressed that test–retest reliability studies must be expected to yield *conservative* estimates of the error variance, τ^2, so that even the corrected estimates will be attenuated to some degree. Also it should be stressed that the standard errors obtained for the corrected estimates are conservative since they ignore the fact that the shrinkage factors, c_i, are not known constants but depend on estimates of variance components. This general problem will be discussed in more detail later. The specific problem of correction of normal discriminant coefficients by allowing for a diagonal variance component due to errors of measurement is nearly the same as the problem looked at by Goldstein (1979). Goldstein considered multiple linear regression in a multivariate normal context with errors in measurement of exogenous variables. He explicitly dealt with the consequences for the precision of the estimates of regression coefficient of the errors attending the estimation of the measurement error component from a test–retest reliability study. These results could readily be adapted to the discriminant analysis solution to the relative risk regression problem.

It might be considered that the preceding analyses underutilize the data in that, for the seventy-six subjects in whom duplicate measurements were

Table 12–1.   Estimates (and standard errors) of β

Method of analysis	Measurement error assumption			
	$\tau^2 = 0.0$		$\tau^2 = 55.0$[a]	
Maximum partial likelihood	-0.0349	(0.0134)	-0.0550	(0.0209)
Normal theory discriminant function	-0.0310	(0.0119)	-0.0486	(0.0185)

[a]Estimated from the repeated measurements.

available, only the first measurement has been used for estimation of the relative risk regression. The second measurement is used only to estimate the factors c_i used to correct the bias. This omission is deliberate and raises a further problem that has very general implications. If the duplicate measurements are true replicates (that is, if they are exchangeable), the argument developed above may be simply modified to incorporate the extra data. It is necessary to consider the induced relative risk regression, which uses the mean of the replicate measures within each subject as covariate. To obtain the correct regression coefficient for the underlying relative risk regression, each of these means must be shrunk toward the estimated true mean exposure for the appropriate risk set. The amount of shrinkage will no longer be constant, however; measured exposure based on one replicate measurement will be shrunk more than measured exposure based on two, so that subjects with more replicate measurements will have rather more weight in the analysis. Instead of (11), the shrinkage factor for an observed exposure based on k replicate measurements is of the form

$$c = \frac{\sigma^2}{(\sigma^2 + \tau^2/k)} \tag{25}$$

Unfortunately this would not seem to be the most appropriate analysis here, since there is evidence that the two measurements cannot be regarded as true replicates—there is a systematic tendency for the second measurement to be less than the first. With only six months separating measurements, it is unlikely that this reflects genuine change in dietary habits and we would suspect some methodologic bias. For example dietary survey methods tend to find some "learning" effect as subjects become accustomed to the detailed record keeping these methods necessitate (Marr, 1971). There are also seasonal fluctuations in diet. The model presented above makes no provision for such influences. Clearly there is a need for greater elaboration in the process of modeling the relationship between true exposure and measured exposure than has been considered so far. This is particularly the case for analyzing cohort studies, such as the Framingham study, which incorporate longitudinal measurement of changes in X variables over the follow-up period in subsamples or in the entire study cohort. In some cases it might well be that underlying trends in exposure variables may be important in determining relative risk. For example, in the trial of the drug clofibrate, which lowers serum cholesterol level, for the primary prevention of myocardial infarction the investigators attempted to identify a relationship between the extent of cholesterol change and subsequent risk of heart attack (Report from the Committee of Principal Investigators, 1978).

DICHOTOMOUS VARIABLES

In this section the discussion is broadened to include discrete variables, and some further problems are highlighted. Several main themes should, by now, have emerged:

1. "Causal" risk models in epidemiology are *latent variable* models, the latent variables being the hypothetically causal exposures.

2. Simply replacing such exposures by inaccurate measurements, although adequate for building predictive models, is incorrect for drawing inferences about the underlying causal model. The unknown values of the latent variable comprise, in effect, a large number of nuisance parameters, and their replacement by naive "good" estimates leads to inconsistent estimates of the parameters of interest.
3. On the other hand, replacement of these unknown values of the latent variable by empirical Bayes estimates leads to consistent estimates of the parameters of the causal model.
4. Unfortunately, the construction of these estimates involves further extraneous parameters, notably parameters describing the distributions of true exposures and of their measurement errors.
5. Finally, these distributions may themselves be complicated and might necessitate further statistical models, possibly involving other covariates.

Although the discussion so far has been concerned largely with true exposures ξ and measurements X, which are both continuous variables, these are not necessary assumptions. This case was considered first in order to explore the link with discriminant analysis, which was important in the early development of multifactor risk scores. In general, however, we must recognize that many measurements in epidemiology are discrete in nature. It is also possible that some underlying exposure variables are discrete, even dichotomous. In the next section a general framework is suggested. Before we discuss this, some further insights into the general problem may be gained from consideration of another "polar" simple case: that in which both ξ and X are dichotomous. This is the case considered in the papers of Marshall and Graham (1984), Hui and Walter (1980), Walter (1984), Clayton (1985), and Kaldor and Clayton (1985). All of these papers deal with an unstratified case-control study, but may be equally thought of as dealing with one stratum of an age-matched study. As we have seen, this is closely related to the idea of "partial likelihood," the comparison of each case with its risk set. Thus a more general representation of the problem than all the papers just referenced requires simply a subscripted notation in which subscript i indicates the ith case/risk-set comparison.

Let π_i represent the proportion of truly exposed ($\xi = 1$) individuals in the population studied at age t_i, and denote the corresponding probabilities of false-positive and false-negative misclassification by, respectively,

$$\Pr(X = 1 \mid \xi = 0) = \gamma_i \qquad \Pr(X = 0 \mid \xi = 1) = \gamma_{2i} \qquad (26)$$

Then, if the relative risk function is 1 for unexposed individuals and $\theta(t)$ for truly exposed individuals of age t, the relative risks for *measured* exposure X are given by the Bayes estimates:

$$E[\theta \mid X = 0, R(t_i)] = \frac{[\pi_i \gamma_{2i} \theta(t_i) + (1 - \pi_i)(1 - \gamma_{i1})]}{[\pi_i \gamma_{2i} + (1 - \pi_i)(1 - \gamma_{i1})]}$$

$$E[\theta \mid X = 1, R(t_i)] = \frac{[\pi_i(1 - \gamma_{2i})\theta(t_i) + (1 - \pi_i)\gamma_{1i}]}{[\pi_i(1 - \gamma_{2i}) + (1 - \pi_i)\gamma_{1i}]} \qquad (27)$$

Given known π_i, γ_{i1}, and γ_{2i}, the relative risk function (27) is a known function of the underlying relative risk function, $\theta(t)$. Thus the underlying model could be fitted by partial likelihood methods.

These results generalize readily to the case of dual response and multiple response. If the responses are assumed to be exchangeable, then X may represent the number of positive responses and, conditional on ξ, is binomially distributed. If not, then further parameters are needed for the error probabilities associated with measurements X_1, X_2, and so on. In either case, extended versions of the expressions (27) may be obtained using elementary probability theory. Again, if all the parameters, π, γ_1, and γ_2 are known, partial likelihood can be used to estimate the underlying relative risk function. However, the existence of some multiple response data in the study also allows estimation of these parameters when they are not known. This in turn has consequences for the precision of the estimate of the true relative risk equation. An added complication is that, since disease outcome is related to ξ, disease outcome provides information concerning ξ and is therefore in principle relevant to the estimation of misclassification error probabilities. Separating out the two estimation problems is thus not likely to be optimal. Instead we should attempt to estimate simultaneously all the unknowns from the total information contributed by the study. The next section outlines some approaches to this, but first the special case considered in this section raises some general issues concerning the specification of models.

First, although we might be prepared to assume that the error probabilities γ_1 and γ_2 are constant across risk sets, we would not in general wish to make the same assumption about the proportions exposed, π_i. As noted earlier, this assumption would not be justified, first because of selective removal of exposed individuals from a study population by the action of the disease studied and second and more importantly because of the nature of the censoring and truncating mechanisms involved. For example, an age-matched case-control study might recruit cases over a relatively short period of time. Each case is then compared with controls of the same age, and these are regarded as being a sample of the healthy members of the risk set in the population from which the cases arose. Because of the study design, however, each of these risk sets is a different birth cohort, and we would certainly be rash to assume that different birth cohorts have identical distributions of exposure. Technically speaking, it cannot in general be assumed that censoring is independent of exposure.

These $\{\pi_i\}$ represent further nuisance parameters and are potentially very numerous—one for each risk set. In the absence of measurement errors, there are established ways of avoiding these becoming troublesome; partial likelihood and conditional logistic regression circumvent the problem by arguing conditionally on the distribution of exposure in each risk set. However, when true exposures are not observed, this option is no longer open to us. Another approach would be to estimate the $\{\pi_i\}$ by maximum likelihood, but even when true exposures are observed, this is known to be hazardous. For example, in the case of the 1 : 1 matched case-control study, this analysis leads to estimates of the relative risk of exposure that tend to the square of the correct value (Andersen,

1973). Pike, Hill, and Smith (1979) showed this bias still to be appreciable in studies that match each case with, for example, ten controls.

The general problem of uncertainty concerning the distribution of true exposures in relative risk regression when only flawed measurements are available, remains unresolved and presents a considerable theoretical challenge. The next section sets out the whole problem in some generality and identifies special cases in which some progress has been made or seems imminent.

A GENERAL MODEL

The last two sections have demonstrated the style of model that needs to be set up to deal with the problems considered in this chapter. This section sets out a more general description of this model, which turns out to have important links with other problems that might have seemed, at the outset, to be unrelated. The general model has three submodels, as follows:

1. *Submodel I* (the "disease model"). This model relates risk of incidence of, or mortality from, a disease to certain exposure variables. Exposures may be either *correctly observed* (these shall be denoted by Z) or *latent variables* ξ measured by flawed indicators X. The variables Z, ξ, and X may all be dependent on age t (or on other time scales). There would seem to be no doubt as to the choice of the relative risk regression model, introduced by Cox and since extended by others, for this model. In the notations introduced earlier, this can be written

$$\lambda[t \mid X(t), \xi(t), Z(t)] = \lambda[t \mid \xi(t), Z(t)]$$

$$= \lambda_0(t)\theta[\xi(t), Z(t)] \tag{28}$$

2. *Submodel II* (the "measurement model"). This model relates the measurements X to the true underlying exposures ξ. The measurements may also depend on age t and on further extraneous covariates Z. For example, the dietary measurements discussed in the section "An Example: Diet and Heart" might be related to the season of dietary survey as well as to any persistent level of intake that might be related to the incidence of chronic disease. Here the model choice is much more diverse, reflecting the range of measurements encountered. A wide family is the generalized linear models of Nelder and Wedderburn (1972), which includes multiple regression with normal errors, and logit and probit regression models for dichotomous measurements. This family can be extended to include the ordered categorical measurements that often are encountered in epidemiology (McCullagh, 1980; McCullagh & Nelder, 1984). A further interesting possibility for ordered or partially ordered categorical measurements is the "stereotype regression" model introduced by Anderson (1984), which bears the same relationship to k-group multivariate normal discriminant analysis as logistic regression bears to two-group discriminant analysis. An interesting further problem that may be viewed within this framework is the analysis of family history data in which the latent variable ξ (family proneness or "frailty") is measured by right-censored ages at disease onset of other family members (Clayton, 1978). In this case the natural choice for the measurement model is

another relative risk regression model. The system is then symmetric and may be viewed as a multivariate generalization of the proportional hazards model (Clayton & Cuzick, 1985).

3. *Submodel III* (the "exposure model"). This model specifies the distribution of latent exposures ξ in the healthy population. This distribution will, in general, depend on further known covariates Z and, as discussed in the last section, will also depend on age, first as a result of relationship between the censoring/truncation implicit in the study design and exposures, and second as a result of the action of the disease studied. Again there is some diversity among possible choices for this model. In particular, one must decide whether the latent exposure is discrete or continuous. If the former, the number of discrete states must be chosen and, if the latter, further distributional assumptions may be necessary. In the section "An Example: Diet and Heart" a continuous normal model was assumed for the latent exposure, while in the section "Dichotomous Variables" a two-point distribution was assumed. Much work in survival models involving latent "frailties," which are simply multiplicative effects of latent exposures on hazard, have assumed gamma-distributed frailties (e.g., Clayton & Cuzick, 1985). This choice follows from the analytical convenience of the gamma distribution as a mixing distribution for an exponential survival-time distribution. This and other models for the distribution of frailty has been reviewed by Hougaard (1984a), who has also recently proposed the use of the positive stable distributions (Hougaard, 1984b). Finally, Aitkin (1985) has made the interesting suggestion that latent frailty distributions (and by implication the distribution of latent exposures) may be modeled nonparametrically in the same way as Laird (1978) has considered nonparametric estimation of a mixing distribution. In such cases the distribution of the latent variable may be estimated by nonparametric maximum likelihood, and Laird showed that the estimated distribution has its support concentrated on relatively few distinct values. The algorithms for fitting nonparametric maximum likelihood estimates of the distribution of a continuous latent variable mirror those for fitting a discrete latent variable distribution, with the additional requirement that the algorithm detect coalescence of adjacent support points. This suggestion would free us from detailed decisions about the true exposure distribution, which would be modeled to the level of complexity that the data would support. In relation to the discussion of the sections "Are There Two Regressions?" and "Two Relative Risk Regressions," this suggestion leads to the estimation of effects of latent exposures by distribution-free empirical Bayes estimates in the spirit of those suggested by Robbins (1956). For an example of the use of such methods in the analysis of educational data, see Aitkin, Anderson, and Hinde (1981).

The preceding discussion sets out a framework and indicates the diversity of analyses that might be required in the analysis of real epidemiologic studies using causal models. Figure 12-3 represents this model diagrammatically using the extended LISREL-style diagram suggested by Palmgren and Ekholm (1986). Observed random variables (age at event, T, and erroneously measured exposures, X) are represented by a square and latent random variables (true exposures, ξ) by a triangle. Fixed explanatory variables (accurately measured

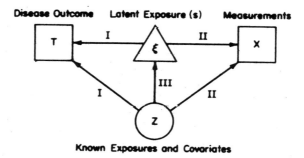

Figure 12–3. The general model; the labels I, II, and III denote the submodels (see text).

exposures and covariates of other models, Z) are represented by a circle. The arrows represent the relationships specified by the three submodels just discussed.

As indicated in earlier sections, the search for a general solution to the problem of inference in this general class of models faces daunting difficulties. Some progress has, however, been made in special cases. Most of this work has already been referenced, but it is helpful to look again at these seemingly diverse pieces of work within the general framework set out in this section.

Only one paper attacks the problem of inference from prospective data in the full relative risk regression disease model. This is the work of Clayton and Cuzick, outlined previously. In effect they advocated an iterative method in which the unknown family frailties are replaced by empirical Bayes estimates derived from a gamma "prior" population frailty distribution and the likelihood of the observed family histories conditional on frailty. Clayton and Cuzick justified this work rather heuristically in terms of marginal likelihood arguments. Gill (1985) gave a similarly heuristic justification in terms of nonparametric maximum likelihood estimation of the baseline hazard functions $\lambda_0(t)$. This method remains hard to justify rigorously despite two notable practical limitations: (1) the problem of truncated observation times is not dealt with and (2) the method implicitly assumes that the frailty distribution varies with age only as a result of action of the disease under study (that is, it assumes censoring to be independent of ξ).

An interesting related paper by Cuzick (1985) considered the $1:M$ matched case-control study in which exposure is incompletely measured to the extent that the data consist only of the positions of each case in the ranking of each set of $(M + 1)$ subjects by exposures.

The remaining work considers case-control analyses based on a coarse granulation of the age scale, so that the difficulties of large numbers of nuisance parameters can be avoided by analyzing in large strata. (In fact, all of these papers consider only a single stratum, but the extension of their results to several strata is trivial.) It is probably necessary also to assume that the disease is rare, so that there is a negligibly small probability of a control selected for one case also turning up as a case or as a control at a later age. While the factorization on which partial likelihood is based renders it nonproblematic in the simple relative risk regression case, it cannot be assumed that this property is maintained in the more complicated models considered here. With these assumptions, the disease model within each stratum may be treated as an unconditional logistic regression of the (binary) disease status Y (taking values 0 and 1 for control and case, respectively), against the exposure variables.

When the measured exposures X are categorical variables and any repeated measurements are available for *all* individuals in the study, the data may be presented as simple contingency tables. Conventional analyses of the categorical regression model for Y on X may be viewed as a special case of the log-linear model (see, for example, Breslow & Day, 1980). If, however, we assume a causal model in which there is one or more discrete-valued latent exposures, and adopt logistic regression for the disease submodel and a log-linear model for the measurement submodel, then we arrive at the model considered in its simplest form by Hui and Walter (1980). Clayton (1985) pointed out that this is an example of the "latent class" model proposed by Goodman (1978) and Kaldor and Clayton (1985) set out a more general description. Elton and Duffy (1983) described inference with the same model when the case-control study is supplemented by a validity substudy. Chen (1979), and more recently McClish and Quade (1985), described a similar analysis of disease prevalence from repeated measures in the presence of measurement errors. The general use of such models for the analysis of problems involving categorical data with errors of observation has been reviewed by Palmgren and Ekholm (1986), who also discuss computational details of maximum likelihood estimation.

Assuming the latent exposures are continuous leads to a discrete factor analysis model (Bartholomew, 1980). Several authors have proposed multivariate probit models in which observation of an underlying multivariate normal model is restricted to whether or not the hypothetical response variables exceed unknown "cut-points" or thresholds. The most general of these formulations is due to Muthén (1979), who accorded this treatment to the LISREL (linear structural relationships) model (Jöreskog, 1973, 1977). This was an attractive choice for the measurement submodel, since ordered categorical measurements could be accommodated by invoking multiple cut-points (following McCullagh, 1980). An extended model of this form that allows for continuous, dichotomous, or ordered categorical responses is described by Muthén (1984). However, a probit model for the relationship between disease status and exposure variables is not in accord with the mainstream methods of modern quantitative epidemiology, which, as we have seen, hinge around relative risk regression; the probit model is not expressible in terms of a simple or natural relative-risk model. However, Muthén's model can be modified to become a hybrid logit/probit model by making a multivariate normal assumption for the distribution of latent exposures *conditional on disease status*. In this way the relationship between disease status and latent exposures would be represented by a normal discriminant model, leading to a logistic risk-exposure relationship as described by Truett, Cornfield, and Kannel (1967), while that between disease and fixed explanatory variables would continue to be represented by a logistic regression model free of the normality assumption. This is the model adopted for the analysis in the section "An Example: Diet and Heart" save that, in that case, there was no discretization of the dietary measurement by cut-points.

This model seems tractable (although some numerical integration of multivariate normal densities is involved) and would be generally useful in epidemiology, but further discussion is beyond our scope here. A further possibility is to assume multivariate normality for the continuous latent variables conditional on both disease stuatus Y and the measurements X. This model predicts not only a logistic regression relationship between latent exposures and disease status, but also a logistic relationship between latent exposures and dichotomous indicators of exposure. Ordered categorical measurements could be related to latent exposures via the stereotype regression model of Anderson (1984). This model could be termed the *latent discriminant model* and is much more tractable, since it avoids the numerical integration problems. It does not seem to have been proposed before and is worthy of further investigation.

Bartholomew (1980) argued that the choice of distribution of latent variables is arbitrary since it requires only a monotone transformation to meet any assumption. He therefore suggested a uniform distribution of the latent variable, and considered both logit and probit response models. However, a monotone transformation of a variable so as to make it uniformly distributed on (0, 1) must also modify the form of its relationship to response, and it is by no means clear that the logit and probit models are realistic in this case. Taken together, the disease model and the exposure models specify relative risk as a function of the centile points of the distribution of latent exposure, and it is this relationship that must be plausibly modeled.

In view of these ambiguities, my preference would be to model the distribution of continuous latent variables nonparametrically. This effectively removes any distinction between discrete and continuous latent variable models; both reduce to latent class models. Some difficulties remain, however, particularly when there are fixed exposure variables in addition to the latent ones.

Computational methods for the models discussed in this section are, as yet, in their infancy. The next section discusses some general principles.

DISCUSSION: FITTING THE MODEL

This chapter has set recent developments in the use of latent variable models for improved estimates of underlying causal relationships from data marred by errors of measurement against the modern unified approach to the analysis of cohort and case-control studies, within the general theory of relative risk regression. Considerable theoretical difficulties present themselves, but there would seem to be some hope of progress. The implementation of existing knowledge is hindered, to some extent, by lack of computer software, but the case-control studies matched in large strata may be analyzed using latent class models. In reviewing these models, Clogg (1981) offered a computer program, and other authors have indicated that general purpose software such as GLIM (Baker & Nelder, 1978) may be used.

In using programs such as GLIM to fit models such as are indicated in Figure 12-1, considerable use has been made of the EM algorithm (Dempster, Laird, & Rubin, 1978). Writing the data concerning age of disease onset in a study, including censoring information as t and x, z, and ξ for the corresponding data concerning flawed measurements, known covariates, and latent exposures, respectively, the total likelihood may be written as

$$L(\beta, \lambda_0, \gamma, \delta; t, x, z)$$

$$= \int_\xi \phi_i(t \mid \xi, z; \beta, \lambda_0)\phi_2(x \mid \xi, z; \gamma)\phi_3(\xi \mid z; \delta)\,d\xi \qquad (29)$$

where ϕ_1, ϕ_2, and ϕ_3 are conditional densities derived from the disease, measurement, and exposure submodels, respectively. The parameters of these models are β, γ, and δ, respectively, and the disease model also involves the unknown baseline age-specific risk function, $\lambda_0(t)$. The EM algorithm follows largely from the fact that the score vector computed by differentiating the logarithm of (29) with respect to β, γ, and δ has components

$$\frac{\partial l}{\partial \beta} = E\left[\frac{\partial}{\partial \beta} \log \phi_1(t \mid \xi, z; \beta, \lambda_0)\right]$$

$$\frac{\partial l}{\partial \gamma} = E\left[\frac{\partial}{\partial \gamma} \log \phi_2(x \mid \xi, z; \gamma)\right]$$

$$\frac{\partial l}{\partial \delta} = E\left[\frac{\partial}{\partial \delta} \log \phi_3(\xi \mid z; \delta)\right] \qquad (30)$$

where the expectations are taken over the *posterior* distribution of ξ given (t, x, z). Each step of the algorithm consists of solving the equations formed by setting (30), evaluated using the current parameter estimates, to zero, thus yielding a new set of parameter estimates. For certain important models these expectations are, at least approximately, linear in ξ so that the evaluation of (30) is equivalent to the replacement of the unobserved values of latent variables by empirical Bayes estimates. In other cases, (30) involves replacing simple functions of latent variables by empirical Bayes estimates. Thus computer programs such as GLIM, which have extensive macro facilities and maximize likelihoods for individual component submodels in a single command, may be adapted to fit the composite model using the EM iteration.

This algorithm can, however, be very slow in converging, and better ones have been proposed. Palmgren and Ekholm (1986) discussed iteratively re-weighted least-squares methods for fitting latent class models, and Ekholm and Palmgren (1982) described their implementation using the GLIM program. An alternative is use of a quasi-Newton method such as the Fletcher–Powell–Davidon algorithm (Fletcher & Powell, 1963) for solution of the nonlinear set of equations (30). This algorithm, and its later refinements, carries out steps of a Newton–Raphson algorithm, but rather than computing the second derivatives of the log-likelihood (which may be intractable), it uses an approximation to the inverse of the second derivative matrix based on previous values of the vector of first derivatives at earlier stages in the iteration. In general, this method performs much better than the EM algorithm. The EM algorithm can, however, be useful as a way of getting the iteration started.

Much remains to be done. In particular, further work is necessary to validate and extend nonparametric exposure models. The parametric exposure models discussed in the previous section also require some evaluation. The analysis presented in the section "An Example: Diet and Heart" makes clear that the conditional normality assumption has two roles: (1) to allow a parametric empirical Bayes estimation of the true exposures and (2) to allow a one-step normal discriminant solution rather than the iterative logistic regression calculations. My experience is that empirical Bayes estimates are not greatly influenced by the precise choice of parametric form for the underlying distribution, while general experience indicates that the normal discriminant solution may be seriously affected by deviation from normality. This suggests that it might be possible to discover a compromise method similar to our use of partial likelihood in Table 12-1—to use the normality assumption for empirical Bayes estimation of exposures but not for estimation of the disease/exposure relationship. Again, the formal details remain to be worked out.

For the present, available software limits us to the analysis of simple discrete problems by latent class analysis and to rather heuristic analyses of continuous exposures such as has been presented in the section just mentioned. Nevertheless, experience with these methods has been promising and suggests that they might offer an opportunity to extend the methodology of quantitative epidemiology.

Appendix
Diet and Heart Data

The following data give (1) age at entry to study (months), (2) age at study termination (months), (3) reason for study termination (1 = IHD death, 0 = other reason), (4) ratio of polyunsaturated to saturated fat uptake (P/S ratio), and (5) month of survey. The last two fields are repeated in some individuals.

595	839	0	74.83	8	727	970	0	73.75	9
606	846	0	41.75	12	527	778	1	46.69	12
705	902	0	65.17	9	669	892	0	68.90	5
705	897	0	60.99	11	752	959	1	41.72	5
713	944	0	61.22	9	717	788	0	78.79	2
612	849	0	50.71	3	731	884	0	77.84	2
542	855	0	57.31	11	731	816	0	73.29	2
605	840	0	80.81	5	710	959	0	77.56	2
805	1057	0	58.80	2	731	989	0	55.82	6
722	925	1	61.30	7	761	818	0	67.72	1
726	899	0	53.17	10	780	934	0	53.07	12
719	964	0	85.79	7	786	1086	0	73.63	12

775	938	0	56.75	12	693	956	0	75.11	1
566	871	0	49.50	7	688	905	0	64.83	11
583	888	0	75.58	7	726	987	0	76.46	3
566	618	0	83.95	8	693	962	0	75.41	7
576	761	0	62.46	6	692	963	0	64.69	5
563	790	0	51.22	7	706	872	0	56.43	5
582	796	1	36.99	8	584	893	0	56.55	3
702	915	0	63.58	5	601	914	0	61.05	2
721	1028	0	53.27	5	610	763	0	77.63	5
718	914	1	62.22	4	594	816	0	82.67	6
745	939	0	66.20	1	592	796	0	68.60	2
773	918	1	79.10	12	712	977	0	68.38	11
423	729	0	85.30	6	690	876	0	88.35	8
569	875	0	59.02	6	673	942	0	57.65	7
554	860	0	72.16	6	734	866	0	42.45	7
692	953	0	67.02	3	737	823	1	46.91	7
468	756	0	92.01	12	480	775	0	76.65	5
736	959	0	75.51	5	550	787	0	63.64	3
581	870	0	56.52	11	732	941	0	54.77	7
546	834	0	56.52	12	725	789	1	66.39	5
536	712	0	74.20	11	545	851	0	62.87	6
704	895	0	80.68	7	522	574	1	63.17	10
522	808	0	71.25	2	535	837	0	84.04	10
680	888	1	51.82	4	517	819	0	56.23	10
448	671	0	70.53	5	481	778	0	41.64	3
457	742	0	71.52	3	481	780	0	70.20	1
739	971	0	55.37	8	570	872	0	66.55	10
707	885	0	73.83	8	571	873	0	56.79	10
554	618	1	53.74	3	553	855	0	66.03	10
543	719	1	47.79	3	582	799	0	64.15	11
547	779	0	81.68	11	570	871	0	67.80	11
568	805	0	56.96	3	364	653	0	74.53	11
589	808	0	46.00	9	439	729	0	60.75	10
560	872	1	58.19	11	445	737	0	53.72	8
543	816	0	73.43	11	374	664	0	63.58	10
606	943	0	80.16	11	573	862	0	57.79	11
534	871	0	65.25	11	736	755	0	64.73	6
620	957	0	82.62	11	595	884	0	53.72	11
608	945	0	51.82	11	731	922	0	54.14	6
656	965	0	69.23	1	523	813	0	67.68	10
591	928	0	80.25	11	543	831	0	53.00	12
554	891	0	107.11	11	412	700	0	59.28	12
546	575	1	72.00	12	361	651	0	75.65	10
649	806	1	72.83	1	578	866	0	88.28	12
558	894	0	58.65	12	568	855	0	98.73	1
618	748	0	69.34	12	458	746	0	68.06	12
570	906	0	63.54	12	550	835	0	62.53	3
612	852	1	60.02	12	673	905	0	67.64	8
556	890	0	43.07	2	558	844	0	54.75	2
495	834	0	77.81	12	377	511	1	60.93	2
534	869	0	77.70	1	564	814	1	61.66	2
646	981	0	57.93	1	440	725	0	57.12	3
592	927	0	57.90	1	616	951	0	70.68	1
524	859	0	76.58	1	642	976	0	91.05	2
626	961	0	69.33	1	632	966	0	57.04	2
557	892	0	58.37	1	567	901	0	74.41	2

509	834	0	63.10	11	561	885	0	55.21	12
497	822	0	63.82	11	626	951	0	62.84	11
607	818	0	55.44	10	596	731	1	47.83	3
559	813	0	71.11	7	545	669	1	88.82	11
513	842	0	77.78	7	606	700	1	45.49	12
502	837	0	64.18	1	527	851	0	72.01	12
			61.72	2	584	906	0	55.92	2
586	851	0	63.42	1	613	751	0	57.45	11
			50.23	8	546	856	0	52.25	1
644	978	0	74.38	2	545	869	0	68.11	12
			75.22	8	606	924	0	75.89	12
655	989	0	59.82	2	545	869	0	111.67	12
			57.04	8	554	876	0	84.81	2
597	931	0	64.90	2	575	789	1	52.32	1
			65.06	8	641	848	0	57.78	12
657	789	1	46.14	3	590	911	0	65.81	3
			45.26	9	664	974	1	52.28	1
587	908	0	54.75	3	437	616	1	80.48	6
			51.26	8	385	671	0	63.94	2
605	942	0	72.43	3	538	823	0	69.02	3
			68.67	8	541	780	0	65.66	1
520	852	0	65.62	4	565	804	0	55.01	1
			55.80	9	579	804	0	98.62	3
623	955	0	52.38	4	553	794	0	68.58	11
			53.12	10	434	659	0	88.71	3
647	796	0	50.66	5	460	687	0	59.33	1
			47.11	9	442	669	0	44.66	1
515	815	0	91.03	5	736	903	1	53.84	5
			93.85	9	545	844	0	67.84	1
575	900	1	78.44	5	729	1005	0	Missing	
			88.46	9	666	936	0	77.09	6
594	925	0	67.96	5	671	910	1	59.54	6
			62.68	9	669	824	0	60.25	7
649	981	0	41.94	4	721	981	0	52.33	4
			47.70	10	546	811	0	83.80	4
664	995	0	66.68	5	562	701	0	62.55	1
			69.05	10	563	863	0	59.08	12
535	630	1	73.60	5	551	850	0	69.39	1
			81.05	10	729	987	0	64.53	6
544	875	0	73.31	5	649	790	1	63.28	1
			70.45	10	663	976	0	57.82	11
601	900	0	58.19	9	676	845	0	67.76	1
			64.48	2	677	727	1	57.33	1
661	891	1	58.65	5	717	985	0	51.02	8
			61.79	11	696	882	0	49.27	7
508	839	0	98.03	5	681	890	1	50.50	7
			79.22	11	700	969	0	52.98	7
610	939	0	66.59	7	686	796	0	111.28	11
			71.63	2	682	716	0	54.47	11
584	913	0	58.15	7	672	938	0	91.76	10
			72.77	2	603	771	1	53.59	3
641	897	1	50.76	6	593	847	0	39.69	2
			45.73	1	586	884	0	56.84	2
665	995	0	54.39	6	592	826	0	53.11	2
			57.39	2	682	912	0	60.43	10
647	940	0	69.84	12	689	930	0	58.80	11

609	844	0	79.84	5	553	850	0	63.43	3
602	836	0	54.31	6				76.72	4
705	962	0	64.68	7	487	784	0	76.05	3
676	775	0	71.48	5				74.61	4
701	955	0	60.54	10	505	795	0	77.35	10
700	820	1	83.13	11				88.76	1
598	985	0	51.35	3	632	922	0	65.30	10
702	927	0	54.38	3				84.14	11
684	765	1	78.17	3	546	836	0	78.25	10
700	924	0	87.02	4	646	658	1	51.33	11
680	910	0	72.77	10	632	921	0	71.19	11
684	759	1	90.00	9	591	805	0	54.92	11
719	975	0	58.29	4	555	844	0	72.76	11
672	995	0	93.57	1				67.01	12
625	851	0	68.91	2	559	859	0	65.02	12
			63.39	3	593	893	0	82.32	12
633	943	0	37.78	2	556	856	0	77.08	12
			51.79	3	486	786	0	68.27	12
642	952	0	69.47	2	577	876	0	62.79	1
			71.14	3	604	904	0	83.50	12
563	600	0	93.51	2	594	894	0	56.30	12
			65.94	3	655	916	1	81.70	2
661	966	0	66.48	2	578	877	0	54.91	1
			68.96	3	494	793	0	79.66	1
596	906	0	56.63	2	625	924	0	69.03	1
			51.85	3	654	953	0	52.91	1
621	930	0	64.49	3	559	858	0	58.41	1
			62.28	4	504	787	0	72.38	1
479	788	0	66.92	3	628	926	0	46.72	2
			67.73	4	594	788	0	77.84	2
558	867	0	79.49	3	634	763	0	56.39	2
			72.55	4	641	890	0	74.43	3
588.	654	1	46.30	3	622	664	0	52.67	10
			44.35	4	478	768	0	68.18	10
663	972	0	58.65	3	498	781	0	68.10	5
			62.32	4				66.05	10
567	876	0	83.22	3	517	664	0	53.85	8
			74.06	4	523	820	0	51.14	8
584	893	0	59.99	3	525	651	1	48.68	8
			63.55	4	542	846	0	74.39	8
565	874	0	64.16	3	584	877	0	85.09	7
			71.77	4	693	846	0	60.95	3
487	796	0	75.16	3	517	769	0	59.97	9
			71.47	4	456	757	0	70.54	11
585	893	0	63.60	4	456	662	1	63.52	11
			67.37	5	473	774	0	49.51	11
494	802	0	61.14	4	463	764	0	43.46	11
			58.23	5	596	890	0	62.09	6
633	941	0	64.81	4	561	856	0	75.93	5
			64.91	5	578	585	0	55.40	7
532	840	0	62.94	4	565	860	0	58.63	5
			61.06	5	553	838	0	73.89	4
618	750	1	70.17	3	581	696	0	58.15	5
			76.70	5	565	852	0	70.59	1
524	821	0	72.71	3	571	803	1	66.01	10
			61.11	6	581	797	0	71.81	9

576	866	0	66.87	10				67.44	11
467	761	0	57.31	6	534	816	0	63.13	6
428	722	0	74.62	6	556	776	0	49.81	6
491	782	0	63.02	9	517	799	0	88.61	6
567	843	0	48.75	9	603	885	0	75.34	6
495	778	0	54.99	5	506	788	0	70.41	6
			67.74	11	539	821	0	76.54	6
497	780	0	76.27	5	601	878	0	103.24	11
			115.17	11	507	789	0	54.59	6
488	771	0	67.47	5	557	839	0	49.07	6
			64.14	10	568	849	0	57.77	7
574	857	0	51.91	5				63.57	2
492	770	0	82.10	10	576	857	0	52.40	7
522	805	0	66.40	5				39.75	1
641	902	0	64.88	5	602	882	0	66.36	8
493	776	0	70.87	5				65.04	2
589	871	0	59.20	6	592	872	0	47.53	8
591	874	1	55.63	6				86.07	1
535	817	0	54.88	6					

ACKNOWLEDGMENTS

I am grateful to John Kaldor of the International Agency for Research on Cancer for extended discussion, which led to the general formulation of the problem as set out in the section "A General Model." I am also indebted to Nick Day, also of IARC, for his support and encouragement of my work on this topic during a spell of study leave in 1984. I would like to thank Professor J. N. Morris and Miss Jean Marr for their permission to quote the data set analyzed in the section "An Example: Diet and Heart."

REFERENCES

Aitkin M (1985). Contribution to the discussion, in Clayton and Cuzick (1985).

Aitkin M, Anderson D, Hinde J (1981). "Statistical modelling of data on teaching styles." *Journal of the Royal Statistical Society A* 144:419–461.

Andersen EB (1973). *Conditional Inference and Models for Measuring.* Copenhagen, Mental Hygienisk Forlag.

Anderson JA (1972). "Separate sample logistic discrimination." *Biometrika* 59:19–35.

Anderson JA (1984). "Regression and ordered categorical variables." *Journal of the Royal Statistical Society B* 46:1–30.

Armstrong BG, Whittemore AS, Howe GR (1989). "Analysis of case-control data with covariate measurement error: Application to diet and colon cancer." *Statistics in Medicine* 8:1151–1158.

Baker R, Nelder J (1978). *The GLIM System, Release 3.* Oxford, Numerical Algorithms Group.

Bartholomew DJ (1980). "Factor analysis for categorical data" (with discussion). *Journal of the Royal Statistical Society B* 42:293–321.

Berkson J (1950). "Are there two regressions?" *Journal of the American Statistical Association* 39:357–365.

Berry G (1983). "The analysis of mortality by the subject-years method." *Biometrics* 39:173–184.

Breslow NE (1978). "The proportional hazards model: Applications in epidemiology." *Communications in Statistics A* 1:315–332.

Breslow NE, Day NE (1980). *Statistical Methods in Cancer Research*. Vol. 1. *The Analysis of Case-Control Studies*. Lyon, France, International Agency for Research on Cancer.

Byar DP, Gail MH (eds) (1989). "Workshop on errors-in-variables." *Statistics in Medicine* 8:1027–1160.

Chen TT (1979). "Log-linear models for categorical data with misclassification and double sampling." *Journal of the American Statistical Association* 74:481–488.

Clayton DG (1972). "The analysis of prospective studies of disease aetiology." *Communications in Statistics* 11:2129–2155.

Clayton DG (1978). "A model for association in bivariate life-tables and its application in epidemiological studies in chronic disease incidence." *Biometrika* 65:141–151.

Clayton DG (1985). "Using test-retest reliability data to improve estimates of relative risk: An application of latent class analysis." *Statistics in Medicine* 4:445–455.

Clayton DG, Cuzick J (1985). "Multivariate generalisations of the proportional hazards model" (with discussion). *Journal of the Statistical Society A* 148:82–117.

Clogg CC (1981). "New developments in latent structure analysis. In Jackson DJ, Borgatta EF (eds), *Factor Analysis and Measurement in Sociological Research*. London, Sage.

Cochran WG (1968). "Errors of measurement in statistics." *Technometrics* 10:637–666.

Cox DR (1972). "Regression models and life tables" (with discussion). *Journal of the Royal Statistical Society B* 34:187–220.

Cox DR (1975). "Partial likelihood." *Biometrika* 62:269–276.

Cuzick J (1985). "A method of analysing case-control studies with ordinal exposure variables." *Biometrics* 41:609–621.

Efron B, Morris C (1973). "Steins estimation rule and its competitors—an empirical Bayes approach." *Journal of the American Statistical Association* 68:117–130.

Ekholm A, Palmgren J (1982). "A model for binary response with misclassification." *Conference on Generalized Linear Models. GLIM 82: Proceedings of the International Conference on Generalized Linear Models*. Heidelberg, Springer, pp 128–143.

Elton RA, Duffy SW (1983). "Correcting for the effect of misclassification bias in a case-control study using data from two different questionnaires." *Biometrics* 39:659–664.

Fletcher R, Powell M (1963). "A rapidly convergent descent method for minimization." *Computer Journal* 10:392–399.

Gill RC (1985). Contribution to the discussion, in Clayton and Cuzick (1985).

Goldstein H (1979). "Some models for analysing longitudinal data on educational attainment." *Journal of the Royal Statistical Society A* 142:407–442.

Goodman LA (1974). "Exploratory latent structure analysis using both identifiable and unidentifiable models." *Biometrika* 61:215–231.

Goodman LA (1978). *Analysing Qualitative/Categorical Data*. London, Addison-Wesley.

Halperin M, Blackwelder WC, Verter JI (1971). "Estimation of the multivariate logistic risk function: A comparison of the discriminant function and maximum likelihood approaches." *Journal of Chronic Diseases* 24:125–158.

Harris RWC, Brinton LA, Cowdell RH, Skegg DCG, Smith PG, Vessey MP, Doll R (1980). "Characteristics of women with dysplasia or carcinoma in situ of the cervix uteri." *British Journal of Cancer* 42:359–369

Hougaard P (1984a). "Life table methods for heterogeneous populations:Distributions describing the heterogeneity." *Biometrika* 71:75–83.

Hougaard P (1984b) "Frailty models derived from the stable distributions." Reprint 84/7, Institute of Mathematical Statistics, University of Copenhagen, Denmark.

James W, Stein C (1961). "Estimation with quadratic loss." Proceedings of the Fourth Berkeley Symposium, Berkeley, University of California Press, vol. 1, pp 361–373.

Jöreskog KG (1973). "A general method for estimating linear structural equation system." In Goldberg AS, Duncan OD (eds), *Structural Equation Models in the Social Sciences*. New York, Seminar Press.

Jöreskog KG (1977). "Structural equation models in the social sciences: Specification, estimation and testing." In Krishaiah PR (ed), *Proceedings of the Symposium on Applications of Statistics*. Amsterdam, North Holland.

Kaldor J, Clayton DG (1985). "Latent class analysis in chronic disease epidemiology." *Statistics in Medicine* 4:327–335.

Keys A (1970). "Coronary heart disease in seven countries." American Heart Association Monograph No. 29. *Circulation* (Suppl. I) 41, 42:I-1–I211.

Keys A (1980). *Seven Countries: A multivariate Analysis of Death and Coronary Heart Disease*. Cambridge, Mass., Harvard University Press.

Laird N (1978). "Non-parametric maximum likelihood estimation of a mixing distribution." *Journal of the American Statistical Association* 73:805–811.

McClish D, Quade D (1985). "Improving estimates of prevalence by repeated testing." *Biometrics* 41:81–89.

McCullagh P (1980). "Regression models for ordinal data" (with discussion). *Journal of the Royal Statistical Society B* 42:109–142.

McCullagh P, Nelder J (1984). *Generalized Linear Models*. London, Chapman and Hall.

MacMahon S, Peto R, Cutler J, Collins R, Sorlic P, Neaton J, Abbott R, Godwin J, Dyer A, Stamler J (1990). "Blood pressure, stroke and coronary heart disease (part 1)." *Lancet* 335:765–774.

Mantel N (1973). "Synthetic retrospective studies and related topics." *Biometrics* 29:479

Maritz J (1970). *Empirical Bayes Methods*. London, Methuen.

Marr JW (1971). "Individual dietary surveys: Purposes and methods." *World Review of Nutrition and Diet* 13:105–164.

Marshall JR, Graham S (1984). "Use of dual responses to increase the validity of case-control studies." *Journal of Chronic Diseases* 37:125–136.

Michalek JE, Tripathi RC (1980). "The effects of errors in diagnosis and measurement on the estimation of the probability of an event." *Journal of the American Statistical Association* 75:713–721.

Miettinen OS (1972). "Components of the crude risk ratio." *American Journal of Epidemiology* 100:350–353.

Morris C (1983). "Parametric empirical Bayes inference: Theory and applications" (with discussion). *Journal of the American Statistical Association* 78:47–65.

Morris JN, Marr JW, Clayton DG (1977). "Diet and heart: A postscript." *British Medical Journal* 2:1301–1368.

Muthen B (1979). "A structural probit model with latent variables." *Journal of the American Statistical Association* 74:807–881.

Muthen B (1984). "A general equation model with dichotomous, ordered categorical and continuous latent variable indicators." *Psychometrika* 49:115–132.

Nelder JA, Wedderburn RWM (1972). "Generalized linear models." *Journal of the Royal Statistical Society A* 135:370–384.

Palmgren J, Ekholm A (1986). "Exponential family non-linear models for categorical data with errors of observation."

Pike MC, Hill AP, Smith PG (1980). "Bias and efficiency in logistic analysis of stratified case-control studies." *International Journal of Epidemiology* 9:89–95.

Prentice RL (1982). "Covariate measurement error and parameter-estimation in a failure-time regression model." *Biometrika* 69:331–342.

Prentice RL, Breslow NE (1978). "Retrospective studies and failure-time models." *Biometrika* 65:153–158.

Report from the Committee of Principle Investigators (1978). "A cooperative trial in primary prevention of ischaemic heart disease using clofibrate." *British Heart Journal* 60:1069–1118.

Robbins H (1956). "An empirical Bayes approach to statistics. *Proceedings of the 3rd Berkeley Symposium*. Berkeley, University of California Press, vol. 1, pp 157–163.

Rosner B, Willett WC, Spiegelman D (1989). "Correction of logistic regression relative risk estimates and confidence intervals for systematic within-person measurement error." *Statistics in Medicine* 8:1051–1071.

Smith PG, Pike MC, Hill AP, Breslow NF, Day NE (1981). "Multivariate conditional logistic analysis of stratum-matched case-control studies." *Applied Statistics* 30:190–197

Thomas DC (1981). "General relative-risk models for survival time and matched case-control analysis." *Biometrics* 37:673–686.

Truett J, Cornfield J, Kannel W (1967). "A multivariate analysis of the risk of coronary heart disease in Framingham." *Journal of Chronic Diseases* 20:511–524.

Walter SD (1984). "Commentary on 'Use of dual responses to increase validity of case-control studies'." *Journal of Chronic Diseases* 37:137–140.

Willett W (1989). "An overview of issues related to the correction of non-differential exposure measurement error in epidemiologic studies." *Statistics in Medicine* 8:1031–1040.

Wong MY (1989). "Likelihood estimation of a simple linear regression model when both variables have error." *Biometrika* 76:141–148.

13

Modeling Complex Exposure Histories in Epidemiologic Studies

JOHN KALDOR

Regression models now play a central role in the analysis of data from studies of chronic disease etiology. They are attractive conceptually because they can readily incorporate multiple continuous and discrete risk factors in the same framework. Much of the original theory and practice of regression analysis developed around linear models for uncensored, normally distributed response variables. More recently, the dichotomous or otherwise censored variables arising as outcomes in many areas of health research have inspired the development of corresponding methods based on the multiple logistic and proportional hazards models.

The routine application of regression methods involves fitting—usually by maximum likelihood or some form of least squares—models relating the outcome variable to subsets of the independent variables of interest, and then evaluating the importance of these factors by comparing how well the models describe the relationships between the outcome variable and the independent variables. When the number of independent variables is limited, it is possible to use systematic stepwise procedures to arrive at the best subset of variables (or their transformations). In this context, "best" reflects a compromise between the two competing principles of goodness of fit and economy of parameterization.

When observational studies of chronic disease etiology entail the collection of a huge number of exposure variables, a mechanical approach to model fitting is not feasible. The consequent statistical analysis frequently develops an artisanal (some might say artistic) rather than scientific flavor, as the investigator attempts to fashion a large volume of data into a coherent summary of risk in the study population. Clearly there is a need for a more systematic approach to data analysis in such situations. In this chapter we consider strategies for analyzing the effect on disease incidence of multiple exposure variables that can be considered a priori to have the same chance of being associated with the risk of disease. In the next section we describe three types of study in which variables of this kind arise, for use in illustrating the subsequent statistical methods. Although the methods are discussed in terms of longitudinal or cohort studies, most of them are equally applicable to the other main type of epidemiologic investigation, namely the case-control study. The third section consists of a brief review of the current techniques available for estimating the relationship between a single exposure variable and disease risk. In the fourth section, the extension to multiple exposure variable analysis is made via conventional statistical methods, and following this we discuss the merits of "exposure matrices" to reduce the number of exposure variables. The chapter concludes with a new proposal for a statistical analysis of multiple exposure studies based on empirical Bayes arguments, in which the prior distribution for the effect parameters is formally incorporated.

EXAMPLES

We consider epidemiologic studies in which an *exposure history* can be compiled for each individual. The exposure history in its most general form can be described by a J-dimensional vector function of time, whose components correspond to each of an ensemble of J study variables, or $[X^i(t), t_0^i \leqslant t \leqslant t_1^i]$ for the ith individual, where $X_j^i(t)$ is the jth component of the vector, associated with the jth exposure variable. Thus $X_j^i(t)$ is the value of the jth variable measured for the ith individual at time t. In some studies, X_j^i will be interpretable as the level of exposure to a specific agent, but in other cases it will denote simply the presence or absence of an exposure.

Three examples follow of studies that would yield complex exposure histories for analysis.

Occupational Studies with Multiple Job Categories

In investigations of the relationship between occupation and disease incidence or mortality, the most commonly used design is the occupational cohort study, which can be viewed as a form of longitudinal study even though the data are usually obtained historically rather than in "real" time. The cohort comprises individuals who are identified at some point in time through sources such as employment or union records and then followed up for the occurrence of health events of interest. The observed number of events is compared with the number expected based on an appropriate comparison population. For occupational groups under study for the first time, where there is no information on possible risks, broad categories of mortality would probably be the outcome variable used. Narrower endpoints, such as cancer incidence by site, would be employed if more specific hypotheses were being investigated. In any case, once an elevated risk for a particular outcome is detected in a cohort, the next step in the analysis is to investigate whether the risk can be ascribed to any particular subgroup of the cohort.

In general, however, individuals cannot be allocated uniquely to one job category, since for many their job classification will change during the course of their career. An example is provided by the employees in a South Wales nickel refinery (Doll, Morgan, & Speizer, 1970, 1976; Kaldor et al., 1986; Peto et al., 1984). No direct measurements of exposure were available, but it was possible to classify each man's employment history into a number of work areas in the refinery. There were 679 men employed during the period 1902–1930, when hazardous exposures occurred, but only 145 remained in the same area during the whole period. On average, each man worked in 2.5 areas of the refinery. An individual exposure history in an occupational study would generally consist of a series of dates marking the transitions between different employment categories. Each component of $\underline{X}^i$ then refers to a specific category, and it takes the value one when the person is employed in the category and zero otherwise. Less frequently, $\underline{X}^i$ could contain quantitative values of industrial hygiene measurements made on J specific exposures.

Studies of Long-Term Risks in Relation to Pharmaceutical Drugs

A number of classes of drugs have been the subject of epidemiologic investigation, motivated by case reports of adverse effects or by studies in laboratory animals. Often there are many different formulations aimed at producing the same effect, and it is important to be able to evaluate them separately, rather than as a group. For example, the recent debate over oral contraceptives and breast cancer has focused largely on progestagen potency and whether certain formulations are associated with a higher risk of breast cancer than others. A woman's exposure to oral contraceptives can be represented by the vector $[X^i(t)]$, where $X^i_j(t)$ is defined as the doese level of the jth type of contraceptive being taken at time t. A similar representation would be appropriate in studies of the carcinogenic effects of analgesics, or of cytotoxic drugs used in cancer therapy. In all of these examples, many individuals will have been exposed to a variety of drugs at different points in time, or even simultaneously in the case of cancer chemotherapy.

Studies of Diet and Chronic Disease

Diet is one of the most difficult and challenging areas remaining in the study of chronic disease etiology, but there is no clear consensus on the best methodology to employ, either in the measurement of diet or in the analyses of the data collected. Case-control studies, in which subjects are asked to recall their food consumption patterns at some point in the recent past, have provided some information on the relationship between disease risk and various food groups, food items, and nutrients. The results have been far from conclusive, however, and painstaking longitudinal studies, in which careful dietary measurements are taken over extended time periods, will probably be required to produce definitive results. Unfortunately, such studies are often prohibitively expensive.

Whatever design is used, studies on diet invariably produce a large volume of measurements on the frequency and quantity of various food items. Some questionnaires are sufficiently elaborate to permit the construction of a crude exposure history by dietary item although, in general, only frequency and quantity at one time point are available. In the notation just defined, the quantity of each food item consumed at time t would be represented by a component of $[X^i(t)]$.

STATISTICAL METHODS FOR ASSESSING THE EFFECT OF A SINGLE EXPOSURE VARIABLE

Since the majority of subjects in longitudinal studies do not suffer the disease under study, their observation time is censored. Most statistical methods for the analysis of censored survival data are based on the proportional hazards model, in which the effect of exposure is assumed to combine multiplicatively with a theoretical background or baseline risk of disease occurring in the absence of exposure. Although other models have been suggested, they have not yet been assimilated into current statistical practice, and they are not available on any standard commercially available computer programs. The proportional hazards model for regression in survival analysis thus plays a role similar to the normal-theory model in standard regression analysis: While no one believes it is correct in any mechanistic sense, it provides a practical and flexible tool for evaluating and interpreting relationships in the body of data being analyzed. The multiple logistic model has similar utility for dichotomous outcome variables, and in fact has also been applied extensively to the analysis of longitudinal studies such as Framingham. Although it does not incorporate length of follow-up in a natural way, the logistic model can be extended to include time parameters (see Chapter 7 in this volume).

It is not possible in the space of this chapter to give a detailed account of statistical inference using the proportional hazards model, or of its application to epidemiologic data. The reader is referred to articles by Breslow, Lubin, Marek, and Langholz (1983), Berry (1983), and Anderson et al. (1980). Here we focus on aspects of the statistical analysis that are of particular relevance when assessing the effect of exposure history on disease risk. In this section we restrict attention to a single exposure variable, $X^i(t)$. In terms of the examples given in the previous section, it could refer to a single job category, a single drug, or a single food item.

Under the proportional hazards model, it is assumed that the hazard or incidence function for the ith individual at time u after follow-up has started can be expressed as

$$\lambda_i(u) = r\{[X^i(v), v \leqslant u]\} \cdot \lambda_0(u) \tag{1}$$

where $\lambda_0(u)$ is the hazard function in the absence of exposure and r is the relative risk function, which relates the exposure history to time u to the relative risk at time u. In utilizing relationships of the kind expressed by (1), it is necessary to consider the choice of time scale, how to deal with the nuisance parameter $\lambda_0(t)$, and the specific form of the relative risk function r. We discuss each of these issues in turn.

Choice of Time Scale

At least three time scales are of importance in longitudinal studies of disease:

1. The *age* of study subjects is strongly related to risk for many diseases, particularly chronic diseases such as cancer and cardiovascular disease. Any statistical evaluation of the effects of exposure must therefore take into account age, whether by matching in the design or adjustment in the analysis.
2. Where observation occurs over an extended period, factors related to *calendar time* can modify the risk of disease. Diagnostic changes, and the introduction of preventive measures, influence incidence; therapeutic advances have the possibility of reducing mortality.
3. The third time scale to be considered is the *time on study*, or the time since follow-up began. Although this scale has little biologic relevance, it is the one on which the study is conducted at an individual and is routinely used in clinical trials.

Other time scales that have been utilized in cancer epidemiology are the time since first exposure to the factor under study, the duration of exposure, and the time since exposure ceased.

The dependence of λ_i and λ_0 on K time scales is readily expressed by defining $s_k(u)$ as the time attained on the kth scale at follow-up time u, and then specifying that $\lambda_i(u) = \lambda_i[s_k(u), k = 1, 2, \ldots, K]$ and $\lambda_0(u) = \lambda_0[s_k(u), k = 1, 2, \ldots, K]$. Thus if $K = 2$ and age and calendar time are the scales used, $s_1(u)$ would be the subject's age at follow-up time u, and $s_2(u)$ would be the calendar time.

Several criteria are relevant in the choice of time scale for analyzing epidemiologic data. First, if valid external baseline rates are available (see the next section) it is appropriate to use the time scales on which they are based (generally age and calendar time). Second, the principle of parsimony would support a scale on which the proportionality assumption could be satisfied using as simple a parameterization of r as possible, preferably with a minimal dependance on u (see equation [1]). The degree of proportionality can be examined by graphic methods for any single scale of interest (Clayton & Kaldor, 1986a), and the effect of temporal variables on λ_i can be formally tested if they are included as categorical covariates influencing r in equation (1) (see the section "The Relative Risk Function r").

The Baseline Hazard λ_0

For some outcomes, such as cause-specific mortality and site-specific cancer incidence, population rates are available on a regional or countrywide basis, generally annually by five-year age groups. In classic cohort study methods based on the standardized mortality ratio (SMR), epidemiologists have implicitly used these rates as if they were appropriate for unexposed individuals. More recently, Poisson regression methods have been developed in which the relative risk function r is modeled as a function of exposure variables, and the unexposed baseline λ_0 is assumed to be known from population rates.

There are a number of potential problems in assuming that general population rates can be used as if they were known rates in unexposed individuals. Serious difficulties can arise if the study cohort and general population differ with regard to important risk factors for the disease under study. For example, studies of lung cancer in occupational groups are often criticized on the grounds that smoking habits in the study cohort may differ from those in the general population. Thomas (1986) has suggested methods for adjusting population rates when data on such important risk factors are available. General population rates are of little use in studies where membership in the cohort is not the principal factor of interest. Indeed, in many cohort studies of diet the goal in sampling the study population is to choose a group that represents the general population as far as possible. Finally, for rare diseases, even reference rates may be based on relatively few events, and the SMR and Poisson regression methods do not take the resulting uncertainty into account.

When there is doubt about the validity of population rates, or if they are unavailable or inappropriate, it is necessary to resort to methods in which the baseline λ_0 is estimated. Two approaches are available. Under the first, λ_0 is assumed to have some specific parametric form, and the unknown parameters are estimated simultaneously with those of the relative risk function r. The parameterization can be either a continuous one, such as the Weibull distribution to account for age effects, or a step function, defined to be constant over, for example, five-year age and calendar time groups. In the latter case, the number of parameters to be estimated can become excessive (e.g., with ten 5-year age groups and five 5-year calendar periods, fifty parameters are required), and it may be necessary to assume that the effects of different time scales are multiplicative with each other.

The second option is to employ the methods of partial or conditional likelihood, under which the unknown function λ_0 is effectively removed from the estimation problem and the resulting likelihood function contains only the parameters of the relative risk function. Although this method is computationally more burdensome than parametric estimation, the computational load can be reduced by sampling a subset of the healthy subjects to carry out a "synthetic" case-control analysis within the study cohort (Breslow et al., 1983; Mantel, 1973; Thomas, 1977).

Whichever course is taken with regard to λ_0, there remains the fundamental question of the validity of the multiplicative nature of the model relating λ_0 to λ_i. A few recent papers have been devoted to methods of checking these assumptions (Breslow & Langholz, 1986, Clayton & Kaldor, 1986b; Moreau, O'Quigley & Mesbah, 1985).

The Relative Risk Function r

The function r is generally assumed to depend on a small number of parameters that represent the relationship between an exposure X and the risk of disease. Of the number of different parametric forms that have been utilized, some have a clear biological basis, while others are pragmatic choices motivated by simplicity and statistical identifiability. The simplest form for r is the "ever-never" relative risk function, defined by

$$r(u) = \begin{pmatrix} \alpha & \text{if the individual has ever been exposed up to time } u \\ 1 & \text{otherwise} \end{pmatrix} \qquad (2)$$

resulting in a hazard of $\lambda_0(u)$ for unexposed individuals and of $\alpha\lambda_0(u)$ after exposure has occurred. A model of this kind is implicit when a single SMR is calculated for a study cohort as a whole, regardless of the duration, type, and level of exposure experienced by individuals in the cohort, and the SMR is in fact the maximum likelihood estimate of α (Breslow, 1977).

At the next level of analysis, duration of exposure is taken into account, most crudely by a log-linear model

$$r(u) = \exp[\beta C_1(u)] \qquad (3)$$

or a linear model

$$r(u) = 1 + \beta C_1(u) \qquad (4)$$

where

$$C_1(u) = \int_0^u X(v)dv$$

the cumulative exposure up to time u. The adoption of a parametric form for the relationship between $C_1(u)$ and $r(u)$ can be avoided by defining the step function

$$r(u) = \beta_s \qquad a_{s-1}^1 < C_1(u) \leqslant a_s^1 \qquad (5)$$

where $a_0^1 = 0$ and $s = 1, 2, \ldots, S$.

Under models (3) and (4), only the single parameter β is to be estimated and the hypothesis that exposure has no effect on risk is equivalent to $\beta = 0$. Under model (5) the number of parameters is equal to the number of categories chosen to divide up the scale of $C_1(u)$, and the null hypothesis is that $\beta_s = 1$ for all categories i.

In addition to duration, the relative risk may be influenced by a number of other temporal variables, including the age and calendar time at which exposure occurred, the time elapsed since it occurred (sometimes referred to as *latency*), and the age and calendar time at risk. Their effect on risk can be investigated by including additional terms in the models (3), (4), or (5). For example, to incorporate the time since exposure began, define $C_2(u) = u - t_0$, where t_0 is the time at which exposure first occurred. The effect of C_2 on risk can then be estimated using the model

$$r(u) = \exp[\beta_1 C_1(u) + \beta_2 C_2(u)]$$

and (4) can be extended similarly. The model (5) requires the categorization of $C_2(u)$, resulting in

$$r(u) = \beta_s \gamma_t \qquad a^1_{s-1} < C_1(u) \leqslant a^1_s$$
$$a^2_{t-1} < C_2(u) \leqslant a^2_t$$

It is also possible to construct composite indices of several temporal variables, such as the total duration of exposure occurring at least ten years ago, which take into account aspects of both duration and latency. These variables can be used in the same way as C_1 and C_2 in regression equations.

Thomas (1983) has criticized the use of C_2 on the grounds that the time since first exposure does not account for the intensity of subsequent exposure in its effect on risk, and has suggested the use of a weighted integral of dose over time. Similar modifications can be made to the age at exposure, to account for changing exposure levels. Unfortunately, in many situations the level of exposure is unknown and must be assumed to be constant. In this case, the dose-weighted integral becomes the difference between the midpoint of the exposure interval and the age at risk.

In the methods just described, there is no attempt to construct a mechanistic model of the effect of exposure on disease risk. Temporal variables that are thought to have an influence on risk are entered into the model as if they were independent variables in a regression. However, a number of these variables are closely related, and collinearity problems are likely to arise in many data sets. For example, in an occupational cohort, the duration of exposure will be identical to the time since exposure began, for individuals who are currently employed. In most situations, only two or three temporal variables can feasibly be entered into a regression model if collinearity is to be avoided.

An alternative to the regression model is to formulate the effect of exposure in terms of a mathematical model of the disease process. This kind of approach has mainly been confined to cancer, for which various forms of the "multistage" model have been proposed over the past thirty years (Armitage & Doll, 1961; Moolgavkar & Venzon, 1979). Although none has been validated on a wide variety of experimental and epidemiologic data, they do allow temporal and dose effects to be incorporated in a way that is biologically interpretable. Nevertheless, they have some practical drawbacks. First, they cannot be readily fitted with routinely available software. Their second difficulty is that the range of possibilities they offer is too broad. It is often possible to fit the same set of data with a wide range of mechanistic models, although the same argument applies to purely descriptive models and, in fact, useful comparisons can be made within classes of models, even if the overall model cannot be validated. Another difficulty with mechanistic models is that they are nonstandard from a statistical point of view, and the properties of inferential procedures based on the models have not been well scrutinized. Thomas (1983) has used two forms of the multistage model to estimate the dose and temporal effects of cigarette smoking and asbestos exposure on lung cancer risk in a cohort of Canadian miners and millers, and Brown and Chu (1982) have applied it to a study of lung cancer among workers exposed to arsenic.

STATISTICAL PROBLEMS IN EVALUATING THE EFFECT OF MULTIPLE EXPOSURE VARIABLES

When multiple exposures are measured, the statistical methods must take into account a number of problems in addition to the issues discussed in the previous section. Principal among them are confounding and multiple inference.

Confounding

Since epidemiology is generally an observational rather than an experimental discipline, it is not possible to assign randomly the level of covariables when studying the relationship between a specific exposure and disease risk. Accordingly, a large part of the statistical methodology has been developed with the aim of controlling or adjusting for the confounding that occurs when a covariable is related to both disease risk and the exposure variable under study.

The most straightforward means of controlling for confounding is to stratify the subjects according to values of the confounding variable or variables. The effect of exposure can then be examined within each stratum of the confounding variable. This approach is fully satisfactory if the number of potentially confounding variables is small, and if their values can be sensibly grouped into a small number of categories. Each variable of interest can be examined in this way in turn. However, in the studies referred to in the "Examples" section, a large number of risk variables are under simultaneous investigation. The required stratification would result in very few individuals per stratum on average, even if each variable was dichotomous (Breslow & Day, 1980). There are some ad hoc procedures that can be employed to minimize the consequent loss of information. For example, in analyzing the data on the South Wales nickel workers, Peto and colleagues (1983) first carried out an analysis in which the effect of each job category on risk was examined separately. Then all men who had ever worked in the category showing the strongest effect were excluded, and the analysis was repeated on the remaining men. This process was repeated until no further categories appeared with a significantly elevated risk.

The alternative to stratified analyses is the simultaneous estimation of the effect of all study variables, whether they are the exposure variables of interest or confounding variables. Under the relative risk model (1), this is accomplished by regression methods. It is generally assumed that the effects of different risk factors on the relative risk function r combine multiplicatively, although interaction terms can of course be included in the model. The simplest multiplicative model is the natural extension of (2), in which

$$r(u) = \prod_{j=1}^{J} \alpha_i^{\delta_j(u)}$$

$$\text{where } \delta_j(u) = \begin{cases} 1 & \text{if the individual has been exposed} \\ & \text{to the } j\text{th variable before time } u \\ 0 & \text{otherwise} \end{cases}$$

The models (2) and (3) for the effect of duration can be similarly extended, with a single parameter β_j expressing the relationship between the jth exposure and relative risk. Table 13-1 shows the results of fitting model (2) to the data on lung and nasal sinus cancer among nickel refinery workers in South Wales (Kaldor et al., 1986). The computer program PECAN (Storer, Wacholder, & Breslow, 1985) was used to fit the model, after choosing matched controls for the cancer cases. In these situations, the incorporation of temporal effects other than duration must generally be left to a later stage in the analysis, when all but a few important risk factors have been excluded from consideration by application of stepwise regression procedures.

Thomas (1983) has suggested a more general family of relative risk functions, which include the possibility of additive effects among variables. The multiplicative model has also been generalized by Breslow (1986), using a power transformation, and by Clayton and Kaldor (1985), who introduced an extra parameter for interindividual heterogeneity in response.

Regression methods achieve the simultaneous adjustment of multiple risk factors for each other provided the factors exert their effect in the manner specified by the model. If they do not, the adjustment can either create spurious relationships or overly attenuate true ones. Thus there is a price to pay in our ability to verify model validity when multiple regression analysis is applied to large data sets. The price may be acceptable, provided regression methods are viewed as, at best, crude if convenient tools for detecting relationships. Detailed investigations of the nature of the relationships can follow once they have been identified.

Table 13-1. Regression coefficients (and standard errors) for duration in each job category, considering all categories simultaneously

Category	Lung cancer		Nasal sinus cancer		Lung and nasal sinus cancer combined	
Calcining I						
(general and furnace)	0.17[a]	(0.052)	0.063	(0.075)	0.14[a]	(0.042)
Calcining II (crushing)	0.27[a]	(0.11)	0.081	(0.18)	0.21[a]	(0.092)
Copper sulphate	0.094[a]	(0.041)	0.070	(0.051)	0.087	(0.032)
Reduction	0.077[a]	(0.043)	−0.030	(0.061)	0.039	(0.034)
Nickel sulphate	0.094	(0.059)	0.076	(0.070)	0.088[a]	(0.046)
Furnaces	0.16[a]	(0.058)	0.16[a]	(0.071)	0.16[a]	(0.046)
Concentrates	0.12[a]	(0.067)	−0.054	(0.13)	0.067	(0.060)
Gas, steam, and power						
production	0.024	(0.047)	−0.47	(0.19)	−0.047	(0.043)
General engineering	0.043	(0.048)	−0.021	(0.065)	0.021	(0.038)
General trades	−0.057	(0.049)	−0.10	(0.075)	−0.033	(0.040)

[a]Ratio of the parameter to its standard error exceeds 1.645, indicatiang significance at the 0.05 level (one-sided test).

Multiple Inference

The other important issue when many factors are under study is what is known as the *problem of multiple inference*. Under the classic theory of statistical inference, which still dominates most biomedical areas of application, attention is focused on a "null hypothesis," which is supposed to reflect a conservative subset of the parameter space being considered. The credibility of any relationship estimated to be outside this subset is evaluated not by its magnitude but by its likelihood of occurring if the true value of the parameter is in the region of conservatism. When this probability (or p value) is small (or significant), the observed relationship is considered to be evidence against the null hypothesis. Clearly the simultaneous calculation of many such p values could result in some being small by chance, even when all parameters are in the null hypothesis subset. Statisticians operating in the classic, or frequentist, tradition have long been concerned about this "type I" error, and have produced a number of corresponding classic solutions to the problem. These generally involve strengthening the criterion for significance so that the overall probability of at least one estimated relationship being significant when in fact all are null is below some desired level. Thomas et al. (1985), who reviewed the problem of multiple inference in epidemiology, pointed out that this approach can lead to unnecessarily stringent significance criteria in studies where many exposures are under investigation, and when taken to its logical conclusion would oblige the adoption of criteria that allow p values from multiple studies to be considered simultaneously. In addition it takes no account of the magnitude of the estimated effects, so that a very precisely estimated weak effect may be judged more important than a stronger effect that happens to have been estimated less accurately.

EXPOSURE MATRICES TO REDUCE THE DIMENSIONALITY OF THE PROBLEM

In most studies, multiple exposure variables are recognized to be surrogates for a much small number of etiologically important variables, whose relationship to the measured variables may or may not be known. For example, job categories are utilized as exposure variables in many occupational studies simply because exposure measures to known or suspected toxicants are unavailable. Similarly, in studies of diet the risk or protection associated with the consumption of a particular food item is usually considered to be attributable to specific components, rather than the item per se. Thus one solution to the problem of evaluating multiple exposures is to reduce them to a small number of variables that reflect specific hypotheses under investigation. In occupational studies, job exposure matrices have been used to convert a job title, either qualitatively or quantitatively, into the specific agents that are present in the working environment (Medical Research Council, 1983). Siemiatycki et al. (1982) reconstructed the employment history of individual workers and thereby obtained exposure estimates for a variety of potential carcinogens. Food tables serve a similar function in dietary studies: A long list of individual food items can be reduced to a smaller number of nutrients of interest, such as specific vitamins (Willett et al., 1985). In studies of drug exposures, the dose of a specific active ingredient can serve as the exposure variable, replacing a variety of formulations or brand names for which data were originally collected. The crudest means of variable reduction is adding over variables that a priori seen to be related, such as items in the same food group.

Once a conversion has been made to a derived set of exposure variables, the statistical analysis proceeds in much the same way as it would have with the original variables, except that the problem of multiple exposures is considerably alleviated. There are, nonetheless, some unsatisfactory aspects to this strategy.

First, the exposure information obtained in epidemiologic studies is generally rather crude, and to use it as a basis for quantifying exposure to individual substances may be unjustified. For example, in occupational studies even reliable industrial hygiene measurements made at some point in time may not be representative of the long-term exposure profile. In dietary studies the information obtained from one food frequency questionnaire does not necessarily provide a picture of lifetime consumption.

Another problem is that it may not be possible to come up with a generally agreed exposure matrix for a given set of measured variables. In the South Wales nickel refinery (Doll et al., 1970; Kaldor et al., 1986; Peto et al., 1984), there has been considerable uncertainty about the nickel compounds to which workers in each job were exposed in the refinery. It is unlikely that a definitive answer will ever be obtained, since the refining processes used during the period when exposure was high have since been changed. The use of "progestogen potency" by Pike et al. (1983) as a means of quantifying exposure to oral contraceptives was heavily criticized on the grounds that its experimental basis was inadequate (Swyer, 1983). Dietary studies encounter similar controversy. For example, there are at least three different ways of measuring dietary fibre, which can produce substantially different results when applied to individual food items (Bingham, 1986). While the exposure variables actually measured in a study may be crude, they do have the advantage that they can be interpreted unambiguously and do not depend on a conversion table.

The final argument against the use of exposure matrices applies to studies of an exploratory nature, in which we are searching for etiologic factors rather than attempting to verify the hazard associated with a specific agent. The exposure matrix imposes on the investigator a fixed set of risk variables, most of which have been identified on the basis of prior information, thus limiting the potential for discovering new relationships.

EMPIRICAL BAYES METHODS FOR THE ANALYSIS
OF MULTIPLE EXPOSURES

In the preceding sections, the problems associated with analyzing the effect of many exposure variables have been presented, and the conventional solutions outlined. Clearly none are fully satisfactory, and the problem is unlikely to diminish as epidemiologists utilize increasingly meticulous questionnaires and interviewing techniques to gather exposure data. There is a need for a more flexible approach, which can take into account the possibility of confounding but permits simultaneous evaluation of many relationships. This latter consideration leads naturally into the *Bayesian* statistical philosophy, according to which unknown parameters, such as the effect measures in epidemiology, are only defined probabilistically. Instead of being used to estimate the "true" value of a parameter, the data collected in a study are used to refine the *prior* probability distribution of a parameter into its *posterior* distribution. Hypothesis tests are replaced by statements about the probability that the parameter lies in a specified region, and a point estimate is provided by the mean of the posterior distribution. The question of multiple inference does not arise, since the control of type I error is not a concern.

The practical difficulty in Bayesian methods has always been the necessarily subjective specification of a prior distribution. Scientists are generally uncomfortable with the idea that one's "prior belief" of where a parameter lies can formally influence the resulting parameter estimate, even though such a process takes place implicitly when data are evaluated. However, when many parameters of the same kind are being estimated, the possibility arises of ascribing to them the same prior distribution. In Bayesian terminology, such parameters would be said to have *exchangeable prior distributions*. The essence of the *empirical Bayes method* is to estimate the common prior distribution from the data. It is criticized by "pure Bayesian" statisticians on the grounds that the unknown parameters of the prior distribution should also be viewed probabilistically and be assigned their own prior distribution. Nevertheless, it is appealing to those who prefer to work with classic statistical concepts, since it does not require the specification of any subjective prior distributions and yet circumvents many of the difficulties of multiple inference.

Thomas et al. (1985) have applied empirical Bayes estimation in evaluating multiple relative risks estimated in an epidemiologic study, but the approach taken was oversimplified in that it did not take account of the covariance between estimates. Hui and Berger (1983) used empirical Bayes techniques to estimate individual rates of change in longitudinal studies, and such techniques have also been used by Tsutakawa, Shoop, and Marienfeld (1985) and Clayton and Kaldor (1986b) in the estimation of disease rates by geographic region. The common feature in all of these applications is a multiplicity of parameters, about which we have roughly the same amount of prior information. Clayton and Kaldor (1986b) discussed the situation where prior information involves some degree of correlation between parameters, but in most cases it has been supposed that the two are independent.

Other epidemiologic applications of methods that have an empirical Bayes flavor have been in modeling heterogeneity in response (Clayton & Kaldor, 1985) and measurement error (Clayton, Chapter 12 in this volume).

In the following we briefly outline the empirical Bayes arguments for a standard normal-theory regression model, under which the empirical Bayes estimates can be obtained straightforwardly. In subsequent work, it will be necessary to make the extension to the dichotomous and censored outcome variables that occur in epidemiologic studies.

Suppose that for the ith individual there are k independent variables measured, $(X_{i1}, \ldots, X_{ik})$, which are a priori believed to have the same relationship to the dependent variable y_i, and that the standard regression model applies so that y_i has a normal distribution conditional on $(X_{i1}, \ldots, X_{ik})$, with mean $\alpha + \Sigma \beta_j x_{ij}$ and variance σ^2. The prior knowledge about β is reflected in the further assumption that the parameters β_j constitute a random sample of size k from a normal distribution with mean u_β and variance γ^2. Then, following Lindley and Smith (1972), it is possible to derive the distribution of the parameter β conditional on the observations γ, and it is the mean of this distribution that provides the empirical Bayes estimates of β. Expressed in matrix form, we have

$$E(\beta|y) = \left(\frac{1}{\sigma^2}X^T X + \frac{1}{\gamma^2}I_k\right)^{-1} \left(\frac{1}{\sigma^2}X^T(y - \alpha 1_k) + \frac{1}{\gamma^2}u_\beta 1_k\right) \qquad (6)$$

where X is the $(n \times k)$ matrix whose ith row is the vector $(X_{i1}, \ldots, X_{ik})$, I_k is the $(k \times k)$ identity matrix, and 1_k is a $(k \times 1)$ column vector of 1's. Supposing for the moment that σ^2, γ^2, u_β, and α are known, this estimate is in fact a weighted average of the usual least-squares regression estimates $\hat{\beta}$ of the β, and the mean of the prior distribution u_β. This can be seen more clearly by considering the simplified situation where the regression variables are orthogonal, so that $X^T X$ is diagonal. Then we have

$$E(\beta_j|y) = \frac{\hat{\beta}_j + (\sigma^2/\gamma^2 \Sigma_i x_{ij}^2)u_\beta}{1 + (\sigma^2/\gamma^2 \Sigma_i x_{ij}^2)}$$

The estimate is weighted toward u_β when the prior variance γ^2 is low, or when $\sigma^2/(\Sigma_i x_{ij}^2)$, the usual estimation error associated with $\hat{\beta}_j$, is high. In other words, imprecisely estimated regression coefficients are "shrunk" substantially toward the overall mean of the coefficients, while precisely estimated ones resemble the usual least-squares estimate. If the prior variance is high compared with the estimation error of all the coefficients, all of the empirical Bayes estimates will be nearly the same as the least-squares estimates.

In practice σ^2, γ^2, u_β, and α are unknown. They can be estimated by maximum likelihood from the marginal distribution of y, which after integrating out the parameters β, is normal, with mean $(\alpha 1_n + u_\beta \times 1_n)$ and variance $\sigma^2 I_n + \gamma^2 \times X^T$. Substitution of the estimates back into (6) yields the empirical Bayes estimates. The likelihood could be maximized using the EM algorithm (Dempster et al., 1977), in which the parameters β are treated as missing data. The algorithm proceeds iteratively, successively updating the empirical Bayes estimates of the slope coefficients β and the parameters of the marginal distribution of the observations (y_i) at each step. The posterior covariance matrix of β could also be derived and estimated in the same way, again substituting the maximum likelihood estimates of the parameters $\sigma^2, \gamma^2, u_\beta$, and α where appropriate. If n, the number of observations, and k, the number of slope coefficients, are large, these estimates are likely to be rather precise, and the posterior variance estimate for the ith coefficient can be used to construct confidence intervals about the empirical Bayes estimate. Modifications would be required if k is small to moderate, but the resulting intervals can still be shown to be on average shorter than the usual linear model intervals (Morris, 1983). Confidence intervals for u_β and γ^2 can also be constructed and used to test the hypotheses that the slope coefficients β are centered around zero ($u_\beta = 0$) or that they are equal ($\gamma^2 = 0$). Thomas et al. (1985) used a prior distribution—a mixture of a Gaussian density and a mass at zero—to represent the prior belief that many associations are null. For each association under study they computed the posterior probability that it came from the mass at zero.

This basic model can be extended to include multiple groups of risk variables. For example, in a study of dietary variables it might be assumed that the coefficient for all meat items came from one prior distribution, that those for all green vegetables came from a second, and so on. Then the empirical Bayes estimate of the coefficients of each groups would be drawn toward each other, to an extent determined by the precision with which individual coefficients were estimated, and the amount of variance estimated for each food group. The coefficient estimates obtained under a model of this kind would have taken account of the a priori belief that items in the same food group should have a similar effect on the outcome variables. However, they retain the possibility of differing, unlike the estimates that would result from transforming the items in a food group to specific quantitative values on the basis of a food table. Related hierarchical mixing distributions have been used by Manton, Woodbury, and Stallard (1982) in the estimation of geographic clustering.

The challenge remains to extend these ideas and methods to regression for nonnormal outcomes, in particular the proportional hazards model. Work is continuing in this direction, and should ultimately provide a powerful tool for the analysis of multiple exposure variables in epidemiologic studies.

CONCLUSION

We have tried to outline the difficulties that arise in the analysis of multiple exposure variables in epidemiologic studies. Sophisticated methods exist for assessing the relationship between a single exposure variable and the risk of disease. The extension to multiple exposures necessitates the adoption of a regression model, but the problem of multiple inference limits the application of standard methods. The empirical Bayes approach is proposed as an alternative; it takes account of prior beliefs about parameter groupings.

REFERENCES

Anderson S, Auguier A, Hauck WW, Oakes D, Vandaele W, Weisberg HI (1980). *Statistical Methods for Comparative Studies.* New York, Wiley.
Armitage P, Doll R (1961). "Stochastic models of Carcinogenesis." In Neyman J (ed),

Proceedings of the Fourth Berkeley Symposium on Mathematical Statistics and Probability, Vol. 4. Berkeley, University of California Press, pp 19–38.

Berry G (1983). "The analysis of mortality by the subject-years method." *Biometrics* 39:173–184.

Bingham S (1986). "Epidemiology of dietary fiber and colorectal cancer; current status of the hypothesis." In Bahouny GV, Kritchevsky D (eds), *Dietary Fiber: Basic and Clinical Aspects.* New York, Plenum pp 523–543.

Breslow NE (1977). "Some statistical models useful in the study of occupational mortality." In Whittemore AS (ed), *Environmental Health: Quantitative Methods.* Philadelphia, Society for Industrial and Applied Mathematics, pp 88–103.

Breslow NE, Day NE (1980). Statistical Methods in Cancer Research. Vol. I: *The Analysis of Case-Control Studies.* Lyon, France, International Agency for Research on Cancer.

Breslow NE, Langholz B (1986). "Nonparametric estimation of relative mortality functions." *Journal of Chronic Diseases* 40, Suppl 2:89S–99S.

Breslow NE, Lubin JH, Marek P, Langholz B (1983). "Multiplicative models and cohort analysis." *Journal of the American Statistical Association* 78:1–12.

Brown CC, Chu KC (1982). "Approaches to epidemiologic analysis of prospective and retrospective studies: Example of lung cancer and exposure to arsenic." In Prentice RL, Whittemore AS (eds), *Environmental Epidemiology: Risk Assessment.* Philadelphia, Society for Industrial and Applied Mathematics, pp 94–106.

Clayton DC, Kaldor JM (1985). "Heterogeneity models as an alternative to proportional hazards in cohort study data." *Bulletin of the International Statistical Institute* 32:1–16.

Clayton DG, Kaldor JM (1986a). "Diagnostic plots for departures from proportional hazards in cohort study data." *Journal of Chronic Diseases* 40, Suppl 2:125S–132S.

Clayton DG, Kaldor JM (1986b). "Empirical Bayes estimates of age-standardized relative risks for use in disease mapping." *Biometrics* 43:671–681.

Doll R, Morgan JG, Speizer FE (1970). "Cancers of the lung and nose in nickel workers." *British Journal of Cancer* 24:623–632.

Hui SL, Berger JO (1983). "Empirical Bayes estimation of rates in longitudinal studies." *Journal of the American Statistical Association* 78:753–760.

Kaldor J, Peto J, Easton D, Doll R, Hermon C, Morgan L (1986). "Models for respiratory cancer in nickel workers." *Journal of the National Cancer Institute.*

Lindley DV, Smith AFM (1972). "Bayes estimates for the linear Model" (with discussion). *Journal of the Royal Statistical Society B* 34:1–41.

Mantel N (1973). "Synthetic retrospective studies and related topics." *Biometrics* 29:479–486.

Manton KG, Woodbury MA, Stallard E (1981). "A variance component approach to categorical data models with heterogeneous cell populations: Analysis of spatial gradients in lung cancer mortality rates in North Carolina counties." *Biometrics* 37:259–269.

Medical Research Council Environmental Epidemiology Unit (1983). *Job Exposure Matrices. Proceedings of a Conference held in April 1982 at the University of Southampton.* Scientific Report, no. 2. Southampton, England, Medical Research Council.

Moolgavkar SH, Venzon DJ (1979). "Two-event models for carcinogenesis: Incidence curves for childhood and adult tumors." *Mathematical Biosciences* 47:55–xx.

Moreau T, O'Quigley J, Mesbah M (1985). "A global goodness-of-fit statistic for the proportional hazards model." *Applied Statistics* 34:212–218.

Morris CN (1983). "Parametric empirical Bayes inference: Theory and applications."

Journal of the American Statistical Association 78:47–65.

Peto J, Cuckle H, Doll R, Hermon C, Morgan LG (1984). Respiratory cancer mortality of Welsh nickel refinery workers." In Sunderman PFW (ed), Jr, *Nickel in the Human Environment*. Lyon, France, International Agencya for Research on Cancer, pp 37–46.

Pike MC, Henderson BE, Krailo MD, Duke A, Roy S (1983). "Breast cancer in young women and use of oral contraceptives: Possible modifying effect of formulation and age at use." *Lancet* 2:926–929.

Siemiatycki J, Gerin M, Richardson L, et al. (1982). "Preliminary report of an exposure-based, case-control monitoring system for discovering occupational carcinogens." *Teratogenesis, Carcinogenesis, Mutagenesis* 2:169–177.

Storer BE, Wacholder S, Breslow NE (1983). "Maximum likelihood fitting of general risk models to stratified data." *Applied Statistics* 32:172–181.

Swyer GIM (1983). "Oral contraceptives and cancer" (letter to the editor). *Lancet* 2:1019.

Thomas DC (1977). "Addendum to FDK Liddell and DC Thomas, "Methods of cohort analysis: Appraisal by application to asbestos mining." *Journal of the Royal Statistical Society A* 140:469–491.

Thomas DC (1983). "Statistical methods for analyzing effects of temporal patterns of exposure on cancer risks." *Scandinavian Journal of Work, Environment and Health* 9:353–366.

Thomas DC (1986). "Use of auxiliary information in fitting nonproportional hazards models." In Moolgavkar SH, Prentice R (eds), *Modern Statistical Methods in Chronic Disease Epidemiology*. Philadelphia, Society for Industrial and Applied Mathematics, pp 197–210.

Thomas DC, Siemiatycki J, Dewar R, Robins J, Goldberg M, Armstrong BG (1985). "The problem of multiple inference in studies designed to generate hypotheses." *American Journal of Epidemiology* 122:1080–1095.

Tsutakawa RK, Shoop GL, Marienfeld CJ (1985). "Empirical Bayes estimation of cancer mortality rates." *Statistics in Medicine* 4:201–212.

Willett WC, Sampson ML, Stampfer MJ, Rosner B, Bain C, Witschi J, Hennekens CH, Speizer FE (1985). "Reproducibility and validity of a semiquantitative food frequency questionnaire." *American Journal of Epidemiology* 122:51–65.

IV
Future Directions

14

Use of Biologic Models to Analyze Epidemiologic Data
Application: Stochastic Models of Carcinogenesis, Gene–Environment Interactions, and Breast and Lung Cancer

DUNCAN THOMAS

A large portion of epidemiologic research concerns the determinants of a dichotomous disease variable, such as disease incidence or mortality. The most commonly used longitudinal designs for studying these outcomes are the case-control study and the cohort study. In these designs, at most a single transition from a healthy to a diseased state is observed, and the objective of the analysis is to relate the rate of these transitions to the subjects' histories of exposure to various causal, confounding, and modifying factors. (Methods for modeling an entire history of changes in a categorical outcome variable are discussed in Chapters 8 and 9 in this volume.)

In recent years, the logistic and proportional hazards models have been widely used in the analysis of case-control and cohort studies. These techniques are thoroughly described by Breslow (Chapter 7) and Kaldor (Chapter 13) in this volume; they are reviewed briefly in the second section in this chapter to establish the notation for the extensions to be developed later. In the terminology of this introduction, such techniques are "weak models", in the sense that they provide a description of the data and allow hypotheses to be tested about the influence of explanatory variables but do not exploit any biologic theories about the underlying disease mechanisms. Such theories can either be used to develop a set of predictions that can be compared with observed patterns of disease incidence, or be formulated in statistical terms as "strong models" and fitted directly to epidemiologic data on individuals. This chapter is concerned with the latter approach.

The second section introduces the concept of a "general relative risk model," which provides the basic machinery for applying maximum likelihood methods for case-control and cohort studies to more complex biologic models. Further subtleties involved in fitting nonstandard models are discussed. The techniques of fitting biologic models are illustrated by a discussion of theories of the carcinogenic process.

The third section provides a general review of a few stochastic models of carcinogenesis—their rationales, mathematical formulations, and predictions—and illustrates their application to a number of epidemiologic data sets. In the fourth section, a few other types of biologic processes related to cancer are explored: some preliminary work on modeling the metabolic pathways that relate exposure histories to tissue dose, and the use of the multivariate extensions of the proportional hazards model discussed by Kaldor (Chapter 13 in this volume) to modeling gene–environment interactions, using data on breast cancer in twins.

In the fifth section, the question of whether this kind of analysis can distinguish between alternative biologic theories is addressed. We have developed a Monte Carlo simulation program to generate data in the form of typical epidemiologic studies, where the underlying model is known. These data are then analyzed using both the simulated and alternative models in order to assess the ability of the methods to distinguish between different submodels within a particular class of models (e.g., early- vs. late-stage action in the multistage model), to distinguish between fundamentally different models, and to arrive at qualitatively correct conclusions when the assumed model is incorrect.

Biologic models have important implications for risk assessment. In addition to the widely discussed uncertainties about the form of the dose-response relationship (e.g., Crump, 1979), there are major uncertainties about the evolution of risk over time beyond the observed period of observation of exposed populations. The use of models that include explicit consideration of such time-related modifying factors as age at exposure, duration and intensity of exposure, time since exposure, and age at event should allow more precise projections of lifetime risk or at least better quantify the reasonable range of this component of uncertainty. The use of models for risk assessment is not addressed specifically here; the interested reader is referred to Thomas (1983, 1985, 1988).

BASIC APPROACHES TO FITTING RISK MODELS TO BINARY OUTCOME DATA

Review of Basic Logistic and Proportional Hazards Models

Suppose we have $i = 1, \ldots, N$ subjects under study, of whom $i = 1, \ldots, D$ have developed the disease under study and $i = D + 1, \ldots, D + S$ are free of disease. Let d_i be an indicator variable for disease status (1 = case; 0 = noncase), s_i the age at which observation began, and t_i the age at which the subject was diagnosed (if a case) or last seen disease free. (In analysis of clinical trial data, time since diagnosis or start of treatment is often taken as the time scale, but in modeling disease incidence, age is generally the strongest determinant and hence the natural choice of time scale.) Extensions of the approaches described below are available to allow the disease rates to depend on calendar time as well as age, either by stratifying on year of birth or by incorporating external rates (Breslow, Lubin, Marek, & Langholz, 1983.) Finally, let $z_i(t)$ denote a vector of (possibly time-dependent) exposure variables that are thought to influence the disease rate at time t. In fitting biologic models, the major challenge is the appropriate choice of such time-dependent covariates, which must generally be developed from the histories of exposures $x_i(.) = \{x_i(u), u \leqslant t\}$ by some process of integration.

In an unmatched case-control study or a cohort study in which all subjects are followed for the same length of time, the usual model is the logistic

$$P(d_i = 1 \mid z_i) = \frac{1}{1 + \exp(-\alpha - \beta' z_i)}$$

where the unknown regression parameters α and β are estimated using the unconditional likelihood function (Breslow & Day, 1980)

$$L = \prod_{i=1}^{D} P(d_i = 1 \mid z_i) \prod_{i=D+1}^{N} P(d_i = 0 \mid z_i)$$

The logistic model is not appropriate when the length of observation varies between individuals; even when it is constant there may be some gain in efficiency if the exact times of diagnosis are used. The most commonly used model for survival time is the proportional hazards model

$$\lambda(t, z) = \lambda_0(t) \exp[\beta'/z(t)] \tag{1}$$

where λ is the hazard function, the instantaneous probability density of the event given that it has not occurred prior to t. This can be fitted either using the full survival likelihood

$$L = \prod_{i=1}^{N} \lambda[t_i, z_i(t_i)]^{d_i} S[s_i, t_i, z_i(.)]$$

where $S(s, t, z) = \exp\{-\int_s^t \lambda[u, z(u)] \, du\}$ is the probability of surviving from age s to age t, or using Cox's (1972) "partial" likelihood

$$L = \prod_{i=1}^{D} \frac{\lambda[t_i, z_i(t_i)]}{\sum_{k \in R_i} \lambda[t_i, z_k(t_i)]} \tag{2}$$

where R_i is the set of subjects at risk at time t_i. This same likelihood can be used for matched case-control studies, with the modification that R_i now refers to the set containing case i and its matched controls.

General Relative Risk Models

The formulation of the proportional hazards model in (1) assumes not only that covariates act multiplicatively on the background rates $\lambda_0(t)$, but also that the dependence of relative rates on covariates is exponential and that multiple covariates combine multiplicatively. This model has a number of convenient mathematical properties but may be too restrictive for fitting the types of models we wish to consider. We therefore express the proportional hazards model more generally in terms of some "general relative risk model" $r(\beta, z)$ as

$$\lambda(t, z) = \lambda_0(t) r[\beta, z(t)] \tag{3}$$

where r can be any nonnegative parametric function with continuous first derivatives with respect to β. This model can then be substituted in the full or partial likelihoods just described. Applications of this model to comparing simple exponential and linear or multiplicative and additive models have been described in Thomas (1981).

Incorporation of Absolute Rates

Models that can be expressed in relative risk form (equation [3]), can be fitted using partial likelihood methods without knowledge of the form of $\lambda_0(t)$. There may be a gain in efficiency by exploiting such knowledge, but the gain appears to be small and may be outweighed by the bias that would result if such knowledge were incorrect (Breslow et al., 1983).

In contrast, models that are not expressible in relative risk form cannot be fitted at all without knowledge of the form of $\lambda_0(t)$. This knowledge can come either from parametric assumptions or from observed rates in some reference population. The multistage model discussed in the third section (Armitage and Doll's) provides an example of a parametric assumption: here $\lambda_0(t)$ is given by αt^{k-1}, where α and k are estimated from the data. Reference population rates $\lambda^*(t)$ might be used as a direct estimate of $\lambda_0(t)$ if $\underline{z} = 0$ for the reference population and the reference rates are thought to reflect the rates the study population would have experienced if it had been unexposed (i.e., no healthy worker effect or differences in unmeasured confounding variables).

Once $\lambda_0(t)$ has been specified, virtually any model can be expressed in relative risk form and partial likelihood methods applied. For example, first suppose the $\lambda_0(t) = \lambda^*(t)$, a set of external rates. Then the additive model $\lambda(t, \underline{z}) = \lambda_0(t) + \underline{\beta}'/\underline{z}$ can be written in this form by letting $r(\underline{\beta}, \underline{z}) = 1 + \underline{\beta}/\underline{z}^*(t)$ where $\underline{z}^*(t) = \underline{z}/\lambda_0(t)$. Now suppose instead that the reference population has the same distribution of exposure as the study cohort, so that $\lambda^*(t) = \lambda_0(t) + \underline{b}'\underline{\bar{z}}(t)$, where $\underline{\bar{z}}(t)$ is the mean exposure of the reference population at age t. Then solving for $\lambda_0(t)$, one obtains the same expression for r, with $\underline{z}^*(t) = [\underline{z} - \underline{z}(t)]/\lambda^*(t)$.

Although in principle any model can be fitted using the partial likelihood approach if the baseline rates are modeled parametrically, the parameters of the baseline rates may not be estimable very precisely. For example, in the multistage model, k cannot be estimated using the partial likelihood approach because the dependence of relative rates on k is very weak, while the strong dependence of λ_0 on k cancels out in the partial likelihood (2). Methods for supplementing the partial likelihood approach by using external rates in a cohort study or cohort rates in a nested case-control study to obtain a more efficient estimate of the parameters of the baseline rates are described in Thomas (1986).

USE OF STOCHASTIC MODELS OF CARCINOGENESIS TO ANALYZE EPIDEMIOLOGIC DATA

There is an extensive literature on mathematical theories of the carcinogenic process. For comprehensive reviews see Armitage and Doll (1961) and Whittemore and Keller (1978). Most of this literature describes the mathematical formulation of various models and develops some of their theoretical predictions concerning the shape of the age incidence curve and its modification by age at start of exposure, time since stopping exposure, and other factors. Several authors (e.g., Day & Brown, 1980; Peto, 1977; Pike, Henderson, & Casagrande, 1981; Whittemore, 1977) have examined the rates of cancer in various exposed groups in relation to these factors and tried to infer whether the carcinogen acted at an early or late stage in the process. But because age, duration, and time since exposure are closely interrelated, it is difficult to interpret such comparisons (Thomas, 1988, 1990). A more powerful approach is to fit the models directly to epidemiologic data on individuals, so that these interrelations can be controlled. In this section several different models are described and their applications to various data sets are illustrated.

Simple Initiation-Latency Model

One of the most important features of cancer is that it never develops immediately after exposure but always after a "latent" period that can be several decades long and is always quite variable. The different ways in which the term *latency* has been used has led to considerable confusion in the literature; for a discussion of the problems of definition, see Peto (1985), Thomas (1983, 1988), and Armenian (1987). In this chapter, it will be defined as a distribution of intervals from each increment of exposure to an increase in risk attributable to that exposure increment.

This leads to perhaps the simplest model of carcinogenesis, which postulates that cancer results from a two-stage process of initiation and development. Each increment of exposure is assumed to cause cells to be "initiated" at a rate $v(x)$ proportional to the tissue dose $x(t)$ at that time. Each initiated cell then remains "latent" for an interval d having some probability density function $f(d)$ independent of age at initiation or number of other initiated cells; this process, determined by subsequent transformations and growth of the clone, is simply treated as a "black box." The incidence rate of cancer is then determined by the time to appearance of the first malignant clone. Armitage and Doll (1961) showed that this is simply given by

$$\lambda[t, x(.)] = \int_0^t v[x(u)] f(t - u) du$$

To allow for background incidence in the absence of exposure to the carcinogens under study, the initiation rate can be taken to be a linear function of dose $v(x) = \beta_0 + \beta'x$. The distribution of latent periods has been reviewed by Armenian and Lilienfeld (1974), who concluded that for the vast majority of cancers, it could be adequately described by a log-normal distribution, with parameters median μ and dispersion e^σ. One would then wish to estimate the parameters β, μ, and σ simultaneously. A widely discussed hypothesis proposes that higher doses may be associated with shorter latent periods (e.g., Druckery, 1967; Guess & Hoel, 1977). To test this hypothesis, one could fit a regression model for the median latency μ_i for subject i, say $\mu_i = \exp(\gamma - \eta'\underline{X}_i)$, where $\underline{X}_i$ is the total dose for individual i, estimating the parameters γ and $\underline{\eta}$ together with $\underline{\beta}$ and σ.

The model has been applied to a nested case-control study of lung cancer in a cohort of Quebec asbestos workers (Thomas, 1983). The cohort consisted of about 11,000 men born between 1881 and 1920 who had worked in the Quebec asbestos mines or mills for at least one month (Liddell, McDonald, & Thomas, 1977; McDonald et al., 1980). Each of the 245 lung cancer deaths occurring before 1975 was matched with three controls drawn from those who were born in the same year, worked in the same mining area, and outlived the case. For each case and control, estimates of annual asbestos exposure were obtained from employer's payroll records, combined with historical dust measurements or estimates. Information on smoking was obtained by questionnaire and consisted of the age at starting and stopping cigarette smoking and the average number of cigarettes per day.

The simplest version of the model, with $\eta = 0$ (i.e., no modification of latent periods by dose), showed a strong dependence of initiation rates on both smoking and asbestos, with an expected latent period of $\hat{\mu} = e^{\hat{y}} = 11$ years. Paradoxically, asbestos and smoking appeared to have opposite effects on the latent period distribution, a phenomenon that could be explained by longer latent periods for asbestos-initiated cells ($\hat{\mu}_A = 16$ years) compared with smoking-initiated cells ($\hat{\mu}_S = 7$ years). This difference is plausible because the dose variable used was the current exposure level, but it is known that asbestos is retained in the lung for long periods (see the fourth section). Allowing for different baseline latencies γ for asbestos and smoking, both appeared to be significantly associated with shorter latent period distributions (i.e., $\eta_A > 0$ and $\eta_B > 0$).

A similar approach was taken by Lundin, Archer, and Wagoner (1979) in their analysis of lung cancer in the Colorado plateau uranium miners. A series of "effective exposure variables" were computed as time-dependent accumulations of past exposures, weighted by a log-normal distribution of intervals with various choices of the median and dispersion. These were then used in standard person-years methods of analysis and the best fit was found for a median of five years and a dispersion factor of 2. Our use of likelihood methods with general relative risk models allows these parameters to be estimated directly rather than by trial and error.

A quite different approach, known as the "serially additive expected dose model," has been suggested by Smith, Waxweiler, and Tyroler (1980) and refined by Lubin (1983). In this method, the average annual exposures of cases and their risk sets are compared as a function of time prior to diagnosis of the case. The attractive feature of this approach is that it provides a "nonparametric" estimate of the latent period distribution $f(d)$.

One problem with this simple model is that it predicts that the age-incidence curve in the general population should begin to taper off at ages corresponding to the median latent period. The fact that the incidence of cancer continues to rise into old age would imply that the median latent period is over 100 years, which conflicts with observations in heavily exposed populations. This would not be a problem if latency is indeed shorter at higher doses, though there is little good evidence to support this hypothesis (Guess & Hoel, 1977). Another possibility, which follows naturally from the multistage model discussed in the following, is that the latency distribution depends on age as well as time since exposure.

Armitage and Doll's Multistage Model

Perhaps the most widely discussed mathematical theory of carcinogenesis is the multistage model of Armitage and Doll (1961), which postulates that cancer arises from a single cell undergoing a series of k distinct, heritable mutations in a particular sequence. Each of the transition rates might depend on the tissue dose of carcinogens but is otherwise not an explicit function of time. Denoting these rates from stage j to $j + 1$ for subject i by $v_{ij}(t)$, the incidence rate of cancer is given by integrating the product of the transition probabilities over all possible times $t_{i1} < \cdots < t_{ik}$ each transition might have occurred, that is,

$$\lambda_i(t) = v_{ik}(t) \int_0^t \int_0^{t_{k-1}} \cdots \int_0^{t_2} v_{i1}(t_1) v_{i2}(t_2) \cdots v_{i,k-1}(t_{k-1}) dt_1 \ldots dt_{k-1} \qquad (4)$$

Now suppose that a single carcinogen acts linearly on a single transition rate j, that is, that $v_{ij}(t) = v_{0j}[1 + \beta_j x_i(t)]$. Whittemore (1977) has shown that the incidence rate, relative to a nonexposed subject, is simply

$$r[t, x(.)] = 1 + \beta_j z_{ijk}(t) \qquad (5a)$$

where

$$z_{ijk}(t) = \int_0^t x(u) f_{jk}(t, u) du \qquad (5b)$$

and

$$f_{jk}(t, u) = \frac{u^{j-1}(t - u)^{k-j-1}}{t^{k-1}} \qquad (5c)$$

Equation (5c) describes a family of latency distributions ranging from continuously increasing for first-stage effects to continuously decreasing for penultimate-stage effects, with various skewed distributions for intermediate-stage effects (Thomas, 1982).

This model is easily fitted to case-control data simply by evaluating the indices $z_{ijk}(t)$ at the age at death of the case for a variety of choices of j and k and then fitting the linear relative risk model to these indices. For the Quebec data described earlier, both asbestos and smoking appeared to act at relatively late stages, but the conditional likelihood was nearly flat with respect to k (Thomas, 1983). As noted earlier, one would need to use absolute rates to estimate k with any precision. On the basis of general population rates, k was fixed at 6 for all further analyses.

For two carcinogens x_1 and x_2 acting at different stages j_1 and j_2 with relative slopes β_1 and β_2, respectively (or a single carcinogen acting at two stages), the relative incidence rate is

$$r[t, x_1(.), x_2(.)] = 1 + \beta_1 z_{i1}(t) + \beta_2 z_{i2}(t) + \beta_1 \beta_2 z_{i3}(t) \tag{6}$$

where z_{i1} and z_{i2} are given by equation (5b) and

$$z_{i3}(t) = \int_0^t \int_u^t \frac{x_{i1}(u) x_{i2}(v) u^{j_1-1} (v-u)^{j_2-j_1-1} (t-v)^{k-j_2-1}}{t^{k-1}} \, dv \, du$$

For the Quebec data, the best fit was obtained with asbestos acting at the fourth and smoking at the fifth stage. Because the product term z_{i3} vanishes when the two carcinogens act at the same stage and is approximately equal to the product of z_{i1} and z_{i2} otherwise, this suggests that the joint effect is more nearly multiplicative than additive in form. However, the timing of the two exposures can modify this interaction: if the later stage carcinogen is applied entirely before the earlier stage one, z_{i3} is zero and the joint effect is simply additive; on the other hand, if the later stage carcinogen is applied at a suitable interval after the first, the joint effect can be many times more than multiplicative (Thomas, 1982).

Brown and Chu (1983) have described similar analyses for a cohort of smelter workers in relation to arsenic. As in Lundin's approach, time-dependent variables z_{i1k} and $z_{i,k-1,k}$ for first and penultimate stage effects, respectively, were computed using equation (5b); these variables were used for categorical comparisons in standard person-years and case-control methods. Again, the penultimate stage effects appeared to better describe the data.

They later applied similar methods to a case-control study of smoking and lung cancer (Brown & Chu, 1987). Relative risks were estimated for categorical levels of intensity, age at start, age at stop, and duration of smoking in continuing smokers relative to nonsmokers and in exsmokers relative to continuing smokers. These relative risks were then fitted to equation (6) using a nonlinear least-squares procedure. Brown and Chu concluded that the long lag from start of smoking to increase in risk and the rapid decline in relative rates after cessation of smoking could only be explained if smoking acted at both an early and a late stage of the process.

Biologic Time Scales

If the transition rates in the multistage model are constant over time, then equation (4) is simply proportional to t^{k-1}. This well describes the population incidence rates for most epithelial tumors, with k about 5 to 7. An interesting exception, however, is breast cancer, which shows a much larger slope on a log-log scale before age 45 than after. Pike, Henderson, and Casagrande (1981) have reviewed the epidemiologic evidence concerning the influence of age and other modifying factors on incidence rates. They suggested that if instead of taking chronologic age t as the time scale one used "breast tissue age" $\tau(t)$, defined as the cumulative rate of cell division, then many of the features of breast cancer epidemiology could be explained in terms of multistage models. They further suggested that the cell division rate $v(t)$ was zero until menarche and was constant from then until first full-term pregnancy, when there was a sudden burst of proliferation followed by a lower rate until menopause and an even lower rate thereafter. These rates were later estimated from population rates together with aggregate data on relative risk and age distributions for the three events (Pike et al., 1983a).

We have since fitted the same basic model to individual data from Pike et al.'s (1983b) case-control study of breast cancer in young women, allowing us to incorporate a number of other factors including benign breast disease, use of oral contraceptives, and family history (Krailo, Thomas, & Pike, 1987). Essentially, we modeled the cell division rate $v_i(t)$ as a log-linear function of various time-dependent covariates $z_i(t)$ and fitted the relative risk model $r_i(t) = \tau_i(t)^{k-1}$ where $\tau_i(t)$, "breast tissue age," is given by $\int_0^t v_i(u)du$.

Moolgavkar and Knudson's Two-Stage Model

Although the multistage model can explain many features of cancer epidemiology, it has difficulty explaining childhood cancers and the genetics of cancer. Also, the existence of as many as six distinct stages has never been demonstrated experimentally (although there is good support for the hypothesis that the process consists of several discrete events at a cellular level, rather than a continuous process). These considerations led Moolgavkar and Knudson (1981) to propose a two-stage model, involving mutations of normal to intermediate and intermediate to malignant cells, with proliferation and death of normal and intermediate cells. Letting $N(t)$ be the number of normal cells at time t, $v_1(t)$ and $v_2(t)$ be the rate of first and second mutations, and $\phi(t)$ be the net growth (division minus death) rate of intermediate cells, they showed that the incidence rate of cancer was given by

$$\lambda(t) = v_2(t) \int_0^t N(u)v_1(u)\exp\left[\int_u^t \phi(v)dv\right]du \qquad (7a)$$

In fitting this model to the breast cancer data, we expressed $N(u)v_1(u)$, $\phi(v)$, and $v_2(t)$ as log-linear functions of the same time-dependent covariates as for the multistage model and identified the terms to which each covariate seemed to have the strongest effect by a stepwise selection procedure (Krailo, Thomas, & Pike, 1987).

In an attempt to explain cancers that followed an autosomal dominant pattern of inheritance, Moolgavkar and Knudson postulated that subjects who inherited the gene would begin life with all cells in the intermediate stage, so that their cancer incidence would be simply

$$\lambda(t) = v_2(t)N(0)\exp\left[\int_0^t \phi(v)dv\right] \qquad (7b)$$

Thus an individual's rate would be a sum of (7b) and (7a), weighted by the probabilities of having the gene or not. In fitting this variant of the model, we chose to model these probabilities as a logistic function of the number of affected family members, weighted by their degrees of relatedness. We were unable to distinguish whether the strong familial aggregation in these data was a reflection of a major gene effect (as described in this model) or of a general influence on transition rates (e.g., as mediated through an effect on hormone levels). This issue is addressed further in the next section.

OTHER ASPECTS OF MODELING THE CARCINOGENIC PROCESS

Metabolic Processes

In the discussion of the asbestos example above, the difference in latency between asbestos and smoking effects was hypothesized to be the result of differences in the rates at which the two carcinogens were eliminated from the lung. A simple approach to this issue would be to model the retained dose $z(t)$ as a one-compartment exponential washout process with parameter ζ, that is,

$$z(t) = \int_0^t x(u) \exp[-(t - u)\zeta] \, du$$

More complex models for respiratory particles have been discussed by Smith (1987). This model has been combined with the two-stage initiation-latency model described in the third section and fitted to the Quebec asbestos data. The best fit was obtained with a washout parameter corresponding to a half-life of about twenty years, but the data are also compatible with any value from about two years to infinity. (Berry et al., 1979, found similar results in an analysis of dose-response relations for asbestosis.)

The problem with this model is that the estimate of this washout parameter is strongly correlated with the estimate of the median latent period. Adequate testing of a metabolic model therefore requires that other correlated parameters relating to the carcinogenic process be estimable separately. A promising approach appears to be to fit a common model of carcinogenesis to data on two carcinogens that would be metabolized differently but might have similar carcinogenic actions. In the Quebec data, for example, one might force asbestos and smoking to have similar median latent periods in the two-stage model but different retention parameters. Another example would be a comparison of bone sarcoma in two series of subjects exposed to radium, dial painters exposed primarily to ^{226}Ra and German injection patients exposed to ^{224}Ra. Results of these analyses will be reported elsewhere.

Models for Gene–Environment Interactions

Geneticists have developed a wide variety of models for describing the familial aggregation of traits. Although some of these models attempt to separate the effects of genes and environment in general terms, seldom do they include explicit environmental covariates. Also, for binary diseases the classic methods of genetics generally ignore the censored nature of the outcome. Both aspects are central to studies of breast cancer in twins in which we are currently involved (Thomas, Langholz, Mack, and Floderus, 1990). The recent multivariate extensions of the proportional hazards model discussed by Kaldor (Chapter 13 in this volume) are directly relevant to both of these issues.

In particular, we have been working with an approach developed by Self and Prentice (1985). Suppose $i = 1, \ldots, I$ families are under observation, each consisting of $j = 1, \ldots, n_i$ members. As in the previous sections, let t_{ij} represent their ages at onset of the disease or censoring, d_{ij} indicate their disease status, and $\underline{z}_{ij}$ be a vector of environmental covariates (possibly time dependent). To allow for the correlated rates of family members, Self and Prentice proposed extending the proportional hazards model by the addition of a "latent" variable (in the terminology of Bentler, Dwyer, and Clayton in their respective chapters in this volume), ε, which they called "frailty" and geneticists call "liability":

$$\lambda(t, \underline{z}_{ij}, \varepsilon_i) = \lambda_0(t) \exp(\underline{\beta}'\underline{z}_{ij} + \varepsilon_i) \tag{8}$$

The frailties ε_i were then postulated to have a log-gamma distribution with between-family variance σ^2. Self and Prentice then showed that the marginal (observable) incidence rates have the form

$$\lambda(t, \underline{z}_{ij}) = \lambda_0(t) \exp(\underline{\beta}'\underline{z}_{ij}) \frac{1 + \sigma^2 N_i(t)}{1 + \sigma^2 E_i(t)} \tag{9}$$

where $N_i(t)$ is the number of cases in the family by time t and $E_i(t)$ is the expected number based on the baseline rates $\lambda_0(t)$ and the times and covariate values of the family members at risk. This model is then used in place of the usual proportional hazards model to construct a "partial" likelihood as a product of contributions L_{ij} from all subjects that became cases, in the form

$$L_{ij} = \frac{\lambda(t_{ij}, \underline{z}_{ij})}{\Sigma_{k \varepsilon R(t_{ij})} \lambda(t_{ij}, \underline{z}_k)}$$

where $R(t)$ is the set of all subjects at risk at time t (irrespective of their family membership) and $\lambda(t, \underline{z})$ is given by equation (9). In the foregoing presentation it is assumed that all family members share the same genetic risk ε_i, but extensions of the techniques to allow for more comples patterns of correlation in frailty are currently being explored (Mack, Langholz, and Thomas, 1990).

The basic model just described can be extended to allow for gene–environment interactions by adding various products of the measured covariates z with the unmeasured frailties ε in model (8). The approach is essentially the same as that described by Martin, Eaves, and Heath (1987), who partitioned the measured covariates into components relating to genotype (e.g., measurements of specific genetic markers, such as alleles at the Ha-Ras locus that has recently been associated with cancer (Krontiris, Dimartino, Colb, & Parkinson, 1985)) and those related to environment, and the frailty into two components relating to residual genotype (with correlations depending on the degree of relationship) and residual environment (identical within families). They show that in principle the main effects of measured genotype, measured environment, residual genotype, and residual genotype and most of their two-way interactions are estimable, although very large sample sizes are required for many of the interactions.

CAN EPIDEMIOLOGIC DATA DISTINGUISH BIOLOGIC MODELS?

In any analysis, whether fitting simple descriptive models or more elaborate mechanistic models, one should always be concerned about the validity of the conclusions, particularly when there is doubt about the validity of the assumptions. In the present context, one might well have several types of concerns:

1. Is it possible by fitting different models to infer the correct mechanism (e.g., multistage versus two-stage models)?
2. Even if one cannot distinguish fundamentally different models, can one make valid inferences about the parameters within a particular model (e.g., early- vs. late-stage action within the multistage model)?
3. If the assumed model is incorrect, can one nevertheless arrive at qualitatively meaningful conclusions (e.g., about latent periods and their modification by dose in the two-stage model, if the multistage model is correct)?

Because of the complexity of these models, there does not seem to be much prospect of an analytic answer to these questions, so we are therefore approaching them by simulation (Thomas, 1987). Our basic approach can be summarized as follows. First, we generate simulated data from hypothetical nested case-control studies for which the underlying mechanism would be known. Presently this is done by generating cohorts with randomly selected exposure histories, calculating the age-specific cancer incidence rates under the multistage model (equations [5] and [6]), generating cases as a Poisson process, and then sampling age-stratified controls from the age-specific exposure distribution of survivors. The resulting exposure histories are then corrupted by various patterns of systematic and random error. These data are then analyzed using the standard and model-fitting approaches described above.

Preliminary results (Thomas, 1987) indicate that comparison of fitted multistage models can correctly identify the stage of action for an occupational exposure (even with substantial time-related measurement errors) but not for smoking. This may be because the exposure histories for occupation were simulated to be much more detailed and heterogeneous over time than for smoking, as is often the case. For occupation, there was a substantial loss of information when a simple summary index such as total exposure was used in the analysis instead of the correct multistage model indices, whereas for smoking, most of the indices produced fairly similar results. We have not yet addressed the issue of robustness when the model is incorrect, but if these results are supported in further simulations, it would at least offer hope that valid comparisons could be made within a particular class of models.

DISCUSSION

One may question whether biologists would consider the models described here as "biologic models" and whether they should not be better described as "statistical models" taken to a level of unobservable phenomena—cellular changes in the case of the models of carcinogenicity, or frailty in the models of genetic effects. Beyond the question of nomenclature, the deeper question of whether there is a scientific purpose in models that specify random processes *below the level of observation* may be posed. With regard to the carcinogenesis models, they imply a belief that changes at the cellular level should be describable by fairly simple models. On the other hand, in cardiovascular epidemiology, it appears likely that the underlying disease process is a very complex one and modeling it at a lower level brings no gain in simplicity. With regard to the genetic models, the same model can be derived either "statistically" starting from a single-parameter model for association in bivariate survival data, or somewhat more "biologically" by postulating the unobservable frailty variable corresponding to shared genotype. Ultimately, we must choose between general models chosen for their tractability, which may require many parameters to adequately describe the data, or mechanistic models, which offer simpler descriptions at some underlying level but rely on unobservable characteristics.

There is a prevalent view that because several models may give similar fits to a set of data it is potentially misleading to try to interpret a fitted model (see, e.g., Vandenbroucke, 1987). Certainly in the asbestos example, the best fitting two-stage and multistage models gave very similar likelihoods, as did the multistage and Moolgavkar models in the breast cancer example. The different numbers of free parameters and the fact that the comparisons are not nested preclude formal comparison of their fits, but it is certainly true that each provided adequate descriptions of the data. This, of course, does not establish the truth of either model; at most one can hope to reject an ill-fitting model. Rather than trying to discriminate between models of fundamentally different form, the point of the exercise is to make comparisons within a general class of models, for example, to compare early- with late-stage hypotheses in the multistage model, or to test hypotheses about the effect of exposure on latency in the two-stage model or on growth rates in the Moolgavkar model. Thus the models are distinguishable not in terms of their fits to data but in the usefulness of the inferences they allow.

Whether or not valid inferences about mechanisms can be drawn from biologic models, such models do have clear utility for risk assessment. Because few populations have been followed to extinction, an important question is how excess risk due to exposure will continue to evolve in the future. Interim answers to this question must come from exposure-time-response models fitted to the presently available data. Such models can be simple descriptions of the data ("weak models," in the terminology of Chapter 1 in this volume), such as relative risk models with age or time-since-exposure interactions as needed. But intellectually more satisfying models are based on some biologic theory of the underlying disease process ("strong models"). Only further follow-up will tell whether such biologically based models will also provide better predictions of future trends in disease rates.

REFERENCES

Armenian HK (1987). "Incubation periods of cancer: Old and new." *Journal of Chronic Disease* 40, Suppl. 2:9–15.

Armenian, HK, Lilienfeld A (1974). "The distribution of incubation periods of neoplastic diseases." *American Journal of Epidemiology* 99:92–100.

Armitage P, Doll R (1961). "Stochastic models of carcinogenesis." in Neyman J (ed), *Proceedings of the 4th Berkeley Symposium on Mathematical Statistics and Probability*. Berkeley, University of California Press, pp 19–38.

Berry G, Gilson JC, Holmes S, et al. (1979). "Asbestosis: A study of dose-response relationships in an asbestos textile factory." *British Journal of Industrial Medicine* 36:98–112.

Breslow NE, Day NE (1980). *Statistical Methods in Cancer Research. I. The Analysis of Case-Control Studies*. Lyon, France, International Agency for Research on Cancer.

Breslow NE, Lubin JH, Marek P, Langholz B (1983). "Multiplicative models and cohort analysis." *Journal of the American Statistical Association* 78:1–12.

Brown CC, Chu KC (1983). "Implications of the multistage theory of carcinogenesis applied to occupational arsenic exposure." *Journal of the National Cancer Institute* 70:455–463.

Brown CC, Chu KC (1987). "Use of multistage models to infer stage affected by carcinogenic exposure: Example of lung cancer and cigarette smoking." *Journal of Chronic Diseases* 40, Suppl. 2:171–179.

Cox DR (1972). "Regression models and life tables" (with discussion). *Journal of the Royal Statistical Society B* 34:187–220.

Crump KS (1979). "Dose response problems in carcinogenesis." *Biometrics* 35:157–167.

Day NE, Brown CC (1980). "Multistage models and primary prevention of cancer." *Journal of the National Cancer Institute* 64:977–989.

Druckery H (1967). "Quantitative aspects of chemical carcinogenesis." In Truhaut R (ed), *Potential Carcinogenic Hazards from Drugs*. UICC Monograph, no. 7. New York, Springer-Verlag, pp 60–78.

Guess HA, Hoel DG (1977). "The effect of dose on cancer latency period." *Journal of Environmental Pathology and Toxicology* 1:279–286.

Krailo M, Thomas DC, Pike MC (1987). "Fitting models of carcinogenesis to case-control data on breast cancer." *Journal of Chronic Diseases* 40, Suppl. 2:181–189.

Krontiris TG, Dimartino NA, Colb M, Parkinson DR (1985). "Unique allelic restriction fragments of the human Ha-ras locus in leukocyte and tumour DNAs of cancer patients." *Nature* 313:369–373.

Lidell FDK, McDonald JC, Thomas DC (1977). "Methods of cohort analysis: Appraisal by application to asbestos mining" (with discussion). *Journal of the Royal Statistical Society A* 140:469–491.

Lubin JH (1983). "A reformulation of the serially additive expected dose method for occupational cohort data." *American Journal of Epidemiology* 118:592–598.

Lundin FE, Archer VE, Wagoner JK (1979). "An exposure-time-response model for lung cancer mortality in uranium miners: Effects of radiation exposure, age, and cigarette smoking." In Breslow NE, Whittemore AS (eds), *Energy and Health* Philadelphia, Society for Industrial and Applied Mathematics, pp 243–264.

McDonald JC, Liddel FDK, Gibbs GW, et al. (1980). "Dust exposure and mortality in chrysotile mining, 1910–75." *British Journal of Industrial Medicine* 37:11–24.

Mack W, Langholz B, Thomas DC (1990). "Survival models for familial aggregation of cancer." *Environmental Health Perspectives* 81:27–36.

Martin NG, Eaves LJ, Heath AC (1987). "Prospects for detecting genotype X environment interactions in twins with breast cancer." *Acta Geneticae Medicae Et Gemellologiae* 36:5–20.

Miettinen O (1982). "Design options in epidemiologic research: An update." *Scandinavian Journal of Work and Environmental Health* 8, suppl 1:7–14.

Moolgavkar SH, Knudson AG JR (1981). "Mutation and cancer: A model for human carcinogenesis." *Journal of the National Cancer Institute* 66:1037–1052.

Peto J (1977). "Epidemiology, multistage models, and short-term mutagenicity tests." In Hiatt HH, Watson JD Winster JA (eds), *Origins of Human Cancer*. New York, Cold Spring Harbor Publications, pp 1402–1428.

Peto J (1985). "Some problems in dose-response estimation in cancer epidemiology." In Voug VB, Butler GB, Hoel DG, Peakall DB (eds), *Methods for Estimating Risk of Chemical Injury: Human and Non-Human Biota and Ecosystems*. New York, Wiley, pp 361–380.

Pike MC, Henderson BE, Casagrande JT (1981). "The epidemiology of breast cancer as it relates to menarche, pregnancy, and menopause." In *Banbury Report 8: Hormones and Breast Cancer*. New York, Cold Spring Harbor Laboratory, pp 3–18.

Pike MC, Henderson BE, Krailo MD, et al. (1983b). "Breast cancer in young women and use of oral contraceptives: Possible modifying effect of formulation and age at use." *Lancet* 2:926–930.

Pike MC, Krailo MD, Henderson BE, et al. (1983a). "'Hormonal' risk factors, 'breast tissue age' and the age-incidence of breast cancer." *Nature* 303:767–770.

Self SG, Prentice RL (1985). "Incorporating random effects into multivariate relative risks regression models." In Moolgavkar SH, Prentice RL (eds), *Modern Statistical Methods in Chronic Disease epidemiology*. New York, Wiley, pp 167–177.

Smith AH, Waxweiler RJ, Tyroler HA (1980). "Epidemiologic investigation of occupational carcinogenesis using a serially additive expected dose model." *American Journal of Epidemiology* 112:787–797.

Smith TJ (1987). "Development and application of a model for estimating alveolar and interstitial dust levels." *Annals of Occupational Hygiene* 29:495–516.

Thomas DC (1981). "General relative-risk models for survival time and matched case-control analysis." *Biometrics* 37:673–686.

Thomas DC (1982). "Temporal effects and interactions in cancer: Implications of carcinogenic models." In Prentice R, Whittemore AS (eds), *Environmental Epidemiology: Risk Assessment*. Philadelphia, Society for Industrial and Applied Mathematics, pp 107–122.

Thomas DC (1983). "Statistical methods for analyzing effects of temporal patterns of exposure on cancer risks." *Scandinavian Journal of Work and Environmental Health* 9:353–366.

Thomas DC (1986). "Use of auxiliary information in fitting nonproportional hazards models." In Moolgavkar SH, Prentice RL (eds), *Modern Statistical Methods in Chronic Disease Epidemiology*. New York, Wiley, pp 197–210.

Thomas DC (1987). "Use of computer simulation to explore analytical issues in tested case-control studies of cancer involving extended exposures: Methods and preliminary findings." *Journal of Chronic Diseases* 40, Suppl. 2:201–208.

Thomas DC (1988). "Exposure-time-response relations in cancer epidemiology." *Annual Review of Public Health* 9:451–482.

Thomas DC (1990). "A model for dose rate and duration of exposure effects in radiation carcinogenesis." *Environmental Health Perspectives* 87:163–172.

Thomas DC, Langholz B, Mack W, Floderus B (1990). "Bivariate survival models for analysis of genetic and environmental effects on twins." *Genetic Epidemiology* 7:121–135.

Thomas DC, McNeill KG, Dougherty C (1985). "Estimates of lifetime lung cancer risks resulting from Rn progeny exposure." *Health Physics* 49:825–846.

Vandenbroucke JP (1987). "Should we abandon statistical modeling altogether?" *American Journal of Epidemiology* 126:10–13.

Whittemore AS (1977). "The age distribution of human cancers for carcinogenic exposures of varying intensity." *American Journal of Epidemiology* 106:418–432.

Whittemore AS, Keller JB (1978). "Quantitative theories of carcinogenesis." *SIAM Review* 20:1–30.

15

Toward a General Model for Longitudinal Change in Categorical and Continuous Variables Observed with Error

GERHARD ARMINGER AND ULRICH KÜSTERS

MEASUREMENT ERRORS AND MEASUREMENT MODELS

Research in epidemiology as well as in psychology, sociology, and econometrics often faces the problem that variables of interest either can be measured only with error or can be measured only indirectly by using a set of indicator variables. Typical examples for variables measured with error are blood pressure or body weight, as discussed by Dwyer (1991) in this volume. Variables that may be observed only indirectly are social support and drug abuse, as used by Bentler and Newcomb (1991) in this volume. In both cases, the latent variables "true blood pressure" and "drug abuse" are assumed to be metric variables that are to be predicted from explanatory variables in a regression model. As long as the latent variables as well as the observed variables that are used as indicators are metric, the relation among observed indicators, latent variables, and explanatory variables is often described in joint mean- and covariance structure models as discussed by a number of authors (Bentler, 1986; Jöreskog & Sörbom 1984). While authors like Browne (1984) devised robust estimation strategies for mean- and covariance structure models without assuming multivariate normality of the indicators of the endogenous variables, their models retain the assumption that the observed indicators are metric variables. These robust estimation procedures have been implemented in EQS (see Chapter 6). The assumption of metric variables is unrealistic because more often than not dichotomous or ordinal variables such as test items or Likert scales are used to describe attitudes or habits of individuals. However, dichotomous or ordinal variables are characterized by the fact that the distances between categories are unknown. Hence, statistical measures such as means, variances, coefficients of skewness, and curtosis cannot be computed meaningfully from the raw scores. Therefore, we focus on the construction of joint regression and measurement models that allow explicitly the inclusion of indicators with any kind of measurement level. Such construction principles may yield more realistic models for epidemiological research than the treatment of raw scores in dichotomous or ordinal data like metric variables. The type of model that we believe to be more realistic has the structure shown in Figure 15-1. This model is characterized by the following properties:

1. The latent variables of interest denoted by η_1 and η_2 are metric and are called *latent traits*. They are dependent on each other and on exogenous variables $\underline{x}$. The variables in $\underline{x}$ are either metric or dummy variables for

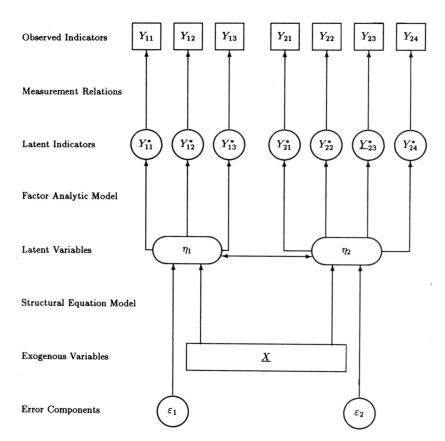

Figure 15–1. Combined regression and measurement models in latent variables with metric and non-metric indicators.

Y_{11} metric indicator connected with metric Y_{11}^* through the identity relation.
Y_{12} censored metric indicator connected with metric Y_{12}^* through a tobit threshold model.
Y_{13} ordered categorical indicator connected with metric Y_{13}^* through an ordered probit threshold model.
Y_{21} ordered categorical indicator connected with metric Y_{21}^* through an ordered logit model.
Y_{22} metric indicator (a count variable) connected with metric Y_{22}^* through a loglinear model.
Y_{23} unordered categorical indicator connected with metric vector $\mathbf{Y}_{23}^*$ through a multinomial logit model.
Y_{24} metric indicator connected with metric Y_{24}^* through the identity relation.

categorical variables. This dependence will usually be described by a structural equation model.

2. The latent traits η_1 and η_2 are connected to indicator sets $\{Y_{11}^*, Y_{12}^*, Y_{13}^*\}$ and $\{Y_{21}^*, Y_{22}^*, \mathbf{Y}_{23}^*, Y_{24}^*\}$ via a factor analytic model with a simple structure. If all the observed indicators $\{Y_{11}, Y_{12}, Y_{13}\}$, $\{Y_{21}, Y_{22}, Y_{23}, Y_{24}\}$ are metric, the starred variables are identical with the observed variables and a classic mean-covariance structure model of the LISREL or EQS type is defined. It should be noted that the latent indicator $\underline{Y}_{23}^*$ corresponding to an unordered categorical observed indicator is a vector-valued variable. All of the latent indicators are assumed to be metric variables.

3. Each latent indicator is connected to one and only one observed indicator through a measurement relation. If the observed indicator is metric the measurement relation is the identity relation. For the pair (Y_{12}, Y_{12}^*) we have assumed a Tobit threshold relation, for (Y_{13}, Y_{13}^*) an ordered Probit threshold relation.

The last two models are special cases of threshold models based on normal distribution theory (Maddala 1983). Models for such indicators are termed MCO(*metric, censored metric, ordered probit*) models. Since they allow estimation strategies based on normal theory, classic mean-variance and covariance structure models may be constructed and estimated.

The latent indicators $\{Y_{21}^*, Y_{22}^*, \underline{Y}_{23}^*, Y_{24}^*\}$ of the second latent variable η_2 are connected to their corresponding observed indicators $\{Y_{21}, Y_{22}, Y_{23}, Y_{24}\}$ via an ordered logit, a log-linear, a multinomial logit, and an identity relation model, respectively. All of these measurement relations are examples of models not based on normal theory. Hence, as shown below, different and computationally much more cumbersome estimation strategies than in the MCO case have to be employed.

MODELS FOR NORMAL-THEORY MEASUREMENT RELATIONS

Model Construction

The class of models discussed in this section generalizes the approach of Muthén (1984) to include censored metric variables in addition to dichotomous and ordinal variables. Let $\boldsymbol{\eta} \sim (n \times 1)$ be a vector of endogenous latent traits and $\mathbf{x} \sim (p \times 1)$ a vector of exogenous variables related to each other in the structural equation model

$$\mathbf{B}\boldsymbol{\eta} = \boldsymbol{\Gamma}\mathbf{x} + \tilde{\boldsymbol{\varepsilon}} \tag{1}$$

with $\tilde{\boldsymbol{\varepsilon}} \sim N_n(\mathbf{O}, \tilde{\boldsymbol{\Omega}})$, $E(\mathbf{x}\tilde{\boldsymbol{\varepsilon}}^T) = \mathbf{O}$, $\mathbf{B}$ regular, and $\tilde{\boldsymbol{\Omega}}$ positive definite (cf. Schmidt, 1976). The reduced form of the system is given by

$$\boldsymbol{\eta} = \boldsymbol{\Pi}\mathbf{x} + \boldsymbol{\varepsilon} \tag{2}$$

with $\boldsymbol{\Pi} = \mathbf{B}^{-1}\boldsymbol{\Gamma}$ and $\boldsymbol{\varepsilon} = \mathbf{B}^{-1}\tilde{\boldsymbol{\varepsilon}} \sim N_n(\mathbf{O}, \boldsymbol{\Omega})$ with $\boldsymbol{\Omega} = \mathbf{B}^{-1}\tilde{\boldsymbol{\Omega}}\mathbf{B}^{-1T}$. We assume that each equation i, $i = 1, \ldots, n$ is identified by a normalization restriction $(B_{ii} = 1)$ and at least $n - 1$ exclusion restrictions on the coefficients

$\mathbf{B}_{i.} = (B_{i1}, \ldots, B_{in})$ and $\mathbf{\Gamma}_{i.} = (\Gamma_{i1}, \ldots, \Gamma_{ip})$. The relationship between the latent variables $\mathbf{\eta}$ and their latent indicators $\mathbf{Y}^* \sim m \times 1 (m \geqslant n)$ is not restricted to simple structure factor analytic models such as depicted in Figure 15-1, but may be of the general type

$$\mathbf{Y}^* = \mathbf{\Lambda}\mathbf{\eta} + \mathbf{\delta} \tag{3}$$

with $\mathbf{\delta} \sim N_m(\mathbf{O}, \mathbf{\Omega}_0)$ and $E(\mathbf{\eta}\mathbf{\delta}^T) = \mathbf{O}$. The matrix $\mathbf{\Lambda} \sim m \times n$ denotes the usual factor loading parameters. Similar to the identification restrictions in the simultaneous equation system, uniqueness conditions in $\mathbf{\Lambda}$ and $\mathbf{\Omega}_0$ must hold (cf. Dunn, 1973). The mean and covariance structure of $\mathbf{Y}^*$ is given by

$$E(\mathbf{Y}^*) = \mathbf{\Lambda}\mathbf{B}^{-1}\mathbf{\Gamma}\mathbf{x} \equiv \mathbf{\Delta}(\mathbf{\theta})\mathbf{x} \tag{4}$$

$$V(\mathbf{Y}^*) = \mathbf{\Lambda}\mathbf{B}^{-1}\tilde{\mathbf{\Omega}}\mathbf{B}^{-1}\mathbf{\Lambda}^T + \mathbf{\Omega}_0 \equiv \mathbf{\Sigma}(\mathbf{\theta}) \tag{5}$$

$\mathbf{\Delta}(\mathbf{\theta})\mathbf{x}$ is the conditional mean structure and $\mathbf{\Sigma}(\mathbf{\theta})$ the covariance structure of $\mathbf{Y}^*$ such that $\mathbf{Y}^* \sim N_m(\mathbf{\Delta}(\mathbf{\theta})\mathbf{x}, \mathbf{\Sigma}(\mathbf{\theta}))$.

The distinct parameters $\mathbf{B}$, $\mathbf{\Gamma}$, $\tilde{\mathbf{\Omega}}$, and $\mathbf{\Omega}_0$, which are allowed to vary freely, are collected in a vector $\mathbf{\theta}$ of parameters to be estimated. $\mathbf{\Delta}(\mathbf{\theta})$ and $\mathbf{\Sigma}(\mathbf{\theta})$ are reduced-form coefficients as functions of $\mathbf{\theta}$.

It should be noted that the mean-variance and covariance structure in $\mathbf{Y}^*$ may be extended to incorporate hierarchical systems with exogenous variables on each hierarchy level (Küsters, 1987; Küsters & Arminger, 1986). It is also possible to write in $\mathbf{Y}^*$ all of the models for panel data found in Jöreskog and Sörbom (1977) or in Arminger (1986a).

The measurement relations between latent indicators $Y_j^*, j = 1, \ldots, m$ and observed indicators $Y_j, j = 1, \ldots, m$ are given by one of the following relations.

1. Y_j is metric. The measurement relation is the identity mapping

$$Y_j = r(Y_j^*) = Y_j^* \tag{6}$$

The density of Y_j is given by

$$P(Y_j = y_j|\mathbf{x}) = \phi(Y_j|\Delta_{j.}\mathbf{x}, \Sigma_{jj}) \tag{7}$$

where $\phi(\cdot|\cdot, \cdot)$ is the univariate normal density with mean $\Delta_{j.}\mathbf{x}$ and variance Σ_{jj}.

2. Y_j is metric, but is censored at a known lower bound τ_j. The measurement relation is the Tobit relation (Amemiya, 1984):

$$Y_j = r(Y_j^*) = \begin{cases} Y_j^* & \text{if } Y_j^* > \tau_j \\ \tau_j & \text{otherwise} \end{cases} \tag{8}$$

The density of Y_j is given by

$$P(Y_j = y_j|\mathbf{x}) = \begin{cases} \phi(Y_j|\Delta_{j.}\mathbf{x}, \Sigma_{jj}) & \text{if } Y_j^* > \tau_j \\ \displaystyle\int_{-\infty}^{\tau_j} \phi(y_j^*|\Delta_{j.}\mathbf{x}, \Sigma_{jj})dy_j & \text{if } Y_j^* \leqslant \tau_j \end{cases} \tag{9}$$

The Tobit relation above can be reversed and may be extended to deal with a lower and an upper bound (Rosett & Nelson, 1975) in the same relation.

3. Y_j is ordinal with c_j categories. The measurement relation is an ordered Probit threshold model (McKelvey & Zavoina, 1975).

$$Y_j = r(Y_j^*) = k \Leftrightarrow \tau_{j,k-1} < Y_j^* \leqslant \tau_{j,k} \qquad k = 1, \dots, c_j \tag{10}$$

with $-\infty = \tau_{j,0} < \tau_{j,1} < \cdots < \tau_{j,cj} = +\infty$.

The threshold parameters $\tau_{j,k}$ describe the distance between ordered categories and must be estimated. To be able to identify the regression constant in Δ_j and the scale of the regression coefficients, the threshold $\tau_{j,1}$ is set to 0 and the variance Σ_{jj} is set to 1 (Nelson, 1976). However, this restriction is not meaningful if panel data are collected. With panel data it is important to check whether the variance of Y_j^* changes in time. Otherwise questions of asymptotic stability (cf. Arminger, 1986a) and reliability of the measurement in the factor analytic part of the model cannot be discussed. In the panel case we assume the threshold parameters $\tau_{j,k}^{(t)}$ where t denotes the number of the panel wave to be constant and $\Sigma_{jj}^{(t)}$ equals 1 only for the first panel wave $t = 1$. $\Sigma_{jj}^{(t)}$ is allowed to vary freely in the succeeding panel waves.

Increasing values of $\Sigma_{jj}^{(t)}$ for $t > 1$ indicate a relative loss of reliability. Decreasing values of $\Sigma_{jj}^{(t)}$ for $t > 1$ indicate a relative gain of reliability in the factor analytic measurement model. However, the restrictions on the threshold values and the possibility of variation in the variances of the specific factors will be brought into effect during the discussion of the estimation procedure, rather than in the model formulation presented here.

Returning to the general case, the univariate density of Y_j is given by

$$P(Y_j = k|\mathbf{x}) = \int_{\tau_{j,k-1}}^{\tau_{j,k}} (y_j^*|\Delta_j.\mathbf{x}, \Sigma_{jj})dy_j^* \tag{11}$$

with the restrictions $\tau_{j,1} = 0$ and $\Sigma_{jj} = 1$.

The multivariate density of the vector of all observed indicators $\mathbf{Y}$ jointly is given by

$$P(\mathbf{Y}|\mathbf{x}) = \int_{r_1^-(Y_1)} \cdots \int_{r_m^-(Y_m)} \phi(\mathbf{y}^*|\Delta\mathbf{x}, \Sigma)d\mathbf{y}^*. \tag{12}$$

The integration interval $r_j(Y_j)$ of variable Y_j is defined by the inverse measurement relation $r_j^-(Y_j) = [y_j^*:r(y_j^*) = Y_j]$. If Y_j is metric, then $r_j^-(Y_j) = Y_j^*$. If the integration interval consists of one point only, the integral sign disappears. Otherwise the threshold values occur in the integrals. The univariate densities given above (equations (7), (9), (11)) are the marginal densities of equation (12).

A more general approach to model construction is given by the fact that the density of $\mathbf{Y}$ may be rewritten as a mixture density by using the following decomposition substituting the structural parameters of equations (1) and (3) in the reduced-form parameters Δ and Σ.

$$\begin{aligned}
P(\mathbf{Y}|\mathbf{x}) &= \int_{r_1^-(Y_1)} \cdots \int_{r_m^-(Y_m)} \phi(\mathbf{y}^*|\Delta\mathbf{x}, \Sigma)d\mathbf{y}^* \\
&= \int_{r_1^-(Y_1)} \cdots \int_{r_m^-(Y_m)} \left[\int_{\mathbb{R}^n} \phi(\mathbf{y}^*|\Lambda\boldsymbol{\eta}, \Omega_0)\phi(\boldsymbol{\eta}|\mathbf{B}^{-1}\Gamma\mathbf{x}, \mathbf{B}^{-1}\tilde{\Omega}\mathbf{B}^{-1T})d\boldsymbol{\eta} \right] d\mathbf{y}^* \\
&= \int_{\mathbb{R}^n} P(\mathbf{Y}|\boldsymbol{\eta})\phi(\boldsymbol{\eta}|\mathbf{B}^{-1}\Gamma\mathbf{x}, \mathbf{B}^{-1}\Omega\mathbf{B}^{-1T})d\boldsymbol{\eta} \tag{13}
\end{aligned}$$

where $\phi(\boldsymbol{\eta}|\cdot,\cdot)$ is the mixing density and

$$P(\mathbf{Y}|\boldsymbol{\eta}) = \int_{r_1^-(Y_1)} \cdots \int_{r_m^-(Y_m)} \phi(\mathbf{y}^*|\boldsymbol{\Lambda}\boldsymbol{\eta}, \boldsymbol{\Omega}_0)dy^* \tag{14}$$

is the conditional density of $\mathbf{Y}$ given $\boldsymbol{\eta}$. If the assumption of local (conditional) independence of $(Y_j|\eta)$ holds true, $\boldsymbol{\Omega}_0$ is a diagonal matrix.

If we additionally assume that each indicator Y_j loads on one latent variable η_i only, we may write $P(\mathbf{Y}|\boldsymbol{\eta})$ in the product form

$$P(\mathbf{Y}|\boldsymbol{\eta}) = \prod_{i=1}^{n} \prod_{j=1}^{m_i} P(Y_j|\eta_i) \tag{15}$$

where m_i is the number of indicators Y_j loading on the latent variable η_i.

Model Estimation

We assume a sample of independent identically distributed drawings $(\mathbf{y}, \mathbf{x})_t$, $t = 1, \ldots, T$ where the distribution of $\mathbf{x}$ is not specified but is not degenerate except for a regression constant, that is, $V(\mathbf{X})$ is positive definite. The parameters to be estimated are collected in a vector $\tilde{\boldsymbol{\theta}}$ which consists of $\boldsymbol{\theta}$ and the threshold values $\tau_{j,k}, k \geqslant 2, \ldots, c_{j-1}$ of the ordinal variables in the data if cross-sectional data are considered. If panel data are analyzed, the threshold values $\tau_{j,k}, k \geqslant 2, \ldots, c_{j-1}$ of the first panel wave and the variances Σ_{jj} for the ordinal variables from the second wave on will be added as free parameters to $\boldsymbol{\theta}$. For both cases the likelihood for an individual is given by

$$L_t(\tilde{\boldsymbol{\theta}}) = \int_{r_1^-(y_1)} \cdots \int_{r_m^-(y_m)} \phi(\mathbf{y}^*|\boldsymbol{\Delta}\mathbf{x}_t, \Sigma)dy^* \tag{16}$$

The log likelihood $l(\tilde{\boldsymbol{\theta}}) = \Sigma_{t=1}^{T} \ln L_t(\tilde{\boldsymbol{\theta}})$ of the sample contains multivariate normal integrals and is obviously too cumbersome to compute by numerical integration at the present time. Hence the outline of a four-stage estimation procedure generalizing Muthèns's (1984) method is presented.

The first stage consists of the estimation of the reduced-form regression coefficients $\boldsymbol{\Delta}_j$. and of Σ_{jj} by maximizing the univariate marginal log likelihood for each observed indicator Y_j.

$$l(\boldsymbol{\Delta}_j, \Sigma_{jj}) = \sum_{t=1}^{T} l_t(\boldsymbol{\Delta}_j, \Sigma_{jj}) \tag{17}$$

with

$$l_t(\boldsymbol{\Delta}_j, \Sigma_{jj}) = \int_{r_j^-(y_t)} \phi(y_j^*|\boldsymbol{\Delta}_j.\mathbf{x}_t, \Sigma_{jj})dy_j^* \tag{18}$$

Depending on the measurement level of the indicator y_j, either a multiple regression of y_j on $\mathbf{x}$ is computed or a ML estimate for a Tobit model (Amemiya, 1984), respectively, for an ordinal Probit model is calculated.

In the second stage the correlation coefficient ρ_{jh} between two latent indicators Y_j^* and Y_h^* is estimated conditional on the results $\hat{\tau}_j, \hat{\tau}_h, \hat{\Delta}_{j\cdot}, \hat{\Delta}_{h\cdot}, \hat{\Sigma}_{jj}$, and $\hat{\Sigma}_{hh}$ from the first stage by using bivariate conditional ML methods.

$$l(\rho_{jh}|\hat{\tau}_j, \hat{\tau}_h, \hat{\Delta}_{j\cdot}, \hat{\Delta}_{h\cdot}, \hat{\Sigma}_{jj}, \hat{\Sigma}_{hh}) = \sum_{t=1}^{T} \ln P(y_{j,t}, y_{h,t}|x_t) \tag{19}$$

with

$$P(y_{j,t}, y_{h,t}|x_t) = \int_{r^-(y_{j,t})} \int_{r^-(y_{h,t})} \phi(y_j^*, y_h^*|\hat{\Delta}_{j\cdot}x_t, \hat{\Delta}_{h\cdot}x_t, \hat{\Sigma}_{jj}, \hat{\Sigma}_{hh}, \rho_{jh}) dy_h^* dy_j^* \tag{20}$$

The correlation coefficient $\hat{\rho}_{jh}$ is a generalization of the polychoric (Olsson, 1979) and polyserial (Olsson, Drasgow, & Dorans 1982) correlation coefficient incorporating censored metric variables and a mean structure conditional on x. Hence $\hat{\rho}_{jh}$ is called the polytobiserial correlation coefficient. The coefficients $\hat{\rho}_{jh}$ are collected in the correlation matrix $\hat{R}$. In the third stage the covariance matrix $\hat{\Sigma}$ is computed by setting $D^2 = \text{diag } \{\Sigma_{jj}\}$ and taking the correlation matrix $\hat{R}$ from the second stage:

$$\hat{\Sigma} = \hat{D}\hat{R}\hat{D} \tag{21}$$

The thresholds $\hat{\tau}$, regression coefficients $\hat{\Delta}$, and covariances $\hat{\Sigma}_{jh}$ $j \leqslant h$, $h = 1, \ldots, m$ are collected in a vector $\hat{\gamma}$. The asymptotic covariance matrix W of $\hat{\gamma}$ is then estimated by using a double Taylor expansion of the conditional log likelihood function of the second stage in analogy to Amemiya (1978a) to derive the asymptotic covariance matrix of the parameters in Δ and $\hat{R}$ and by applying the multivariate δ method (Rao, 1973) to the transformation in equation (21). The necessary derivations and computational formulae, which are rather cumbersome, are found in detail in Küsters (1987).

In the final stage the parameter vector $\hat{\gamma}$ is considered as a function of the structural parameters $\tilde{\theta}$. A weighted least-squares approach is used to estimate $\tilde{\theta}$ by minimizing the function

$$Q(\tilde{\theta}) = (\hat{\gamma} - \gamma(\tilde{\theta}))^T \hat{W}^{-1} (\hat{\gamma} - \gamma(\tilde{\theta})) \tag{22}$$

To find the first derivatives of $Q(\tilde{\theta})$ the matrix differentiation rules of McDonald and Swaminathan (1973) are used. In this stage the special restrictions necessary for analyzing panel data are brought into effect. The parameters $\tau_{j,k}, k \geqslant 2$ are restricted to be equal across panel waves, while parameters Σ_{jj} are allowed to differ from 1 from the second wave on. As a small example consider an ordered categorical variable Y with four categories, which has been measured in two panel waves. The estimated threshold values are $\hat{\tau}_2^{(1)}, \hat{\tau}_3^{(1)}$ for the first and $\hat{\tau}_2^{(2)}, \hat{\tau}_3^{(2)}$ for the second panel wave. The estimated reduced-form coefficients are $\hat{\Delta}^{(1)}$ and $\hat{\Delta}^{(2)}$. The reduced-form variances $\Sigma_{11}(\tilde{\theta})$ and $\Sigma_{22}(\tilde{\theta})$ have been set to 1. If we assume now that the thresholds are equal across panel waves but that the structural form variance in the second wave, denoted by σ_2^2, is allowed to vary, the estimated parameters $\hat{\tau}_2^{(1)}, \hat{\tau}_3^{(1)}, \hat{\Delta}^{(1)}, \hat{\tau}_2^{(2)}, \hat{\tau}_3^{(2)}, \hat{\Delta}^{(2)}$, and $\hat{\rho}_{12}$ (correlation between waves) collected in γ may be written as a function of the structural parameters τ_2, τ_3, $\Delta^{(1)}$, σ_2, $\Delta^{(2)}$, and ρ_{12} collected in $\tilde{\theta}$.

$$\hat{\tau}_2^{(1)} = \tau_2 \qquad \hat{\tau}_3^{(1)} = \tau_3 \qquad \hat{\Delta}^{(1)} = \Delta^{(1)} \tag{23}$$

$$\hat{\tau}_2^{(2)} = \frac{\tau_2}{\sigma_2} \qquad \hat{\tau}_3^{(2)} = \frac{\tau_3}{\sigma_2} \qquad \hat{\Delta}^{(2)} = \frac{\Delta^{(2)}}{\sigma_2}$$

$$\hat{\rho}_{12} = \rho_{12} \tag{24}$$

Note that the estimated regression coefficients $\hat{\Delta}^{(2)}$ are also transformed by σ_2.

Under covariance structure models, which are more general than LISREL type models, for example general hierarchical systems, $Q(\tilde{\theta})$ must sometimes be estimated with restrictions on $\tilde{\theta}$. In this case routines for optimization under restrictions such as Lagrange multiplier or penalty function methods must be employed (Luenberger, 1984).

The four stage estimation just described has recently been implemented in the computer programs LISCOMP by Muthén (1988) and MECOSA by Schepers (1991).

MODELS FOR GENERAL MEASUREMENT RELATIONS

Model Construction

The class of models discussed in this section comprises the models outlined above as well as non-normal-theory measurement relations and models formulated by psychometricians and statisticians such as Bock (1972), Bock and Aitkin (1981) and Bartholomew (1980, 1983, 1984). The structural model for the latent variables η is the same as given previously, that is, $(\eta|x)$ follows the multivariate normal density

$$\phi(\eta | B^{-1}\Gamma x, B^{-1}\tilde{\Omega}B^{-1T}) \tag{25}$$

with the reduced-form density $\phi(\eta|\Pi x, \Omega)$. The marginal density for each latent variable η_i is given by a univariate normal density

$$\phi(\eta_i | \Pi_i . x, \Omega_{ii}) \tag{26}$$

The factor analytic model may be formulated in principle as general as the model for Y^* in the previous section. We consider now the joint density of all observed indicators $(Y|x)$ conditional on x as a mixture distribution:

$$P(Y|x) = \int_{\mathbb{R}^n} P(Y|\eta)\phi(\eta | \Pi x, \Omega)d\eta \tag{27}$$

In general, parameters in mixture density cannot be estimated because the evaluation of the multivariate integral is not feasible with today's numerical methods. Hence we simplify $P(Y|\eta)$ by employing concepts of local independence and simple factor structures. We consider first the case of cross-sectional data, and next the formulation of a model for two-wave panel data.

In the case of a cross-sectional sample, the notion of local independence of the observed indicators means that the dependence structure between the observed indicators is a function only of the dependence structure between the latent variables. Hence we use the following product form for the conditional density $P(\mathbf{Y}|\boldsymbol{\eta})$:

$$P(\mathbf{Y}|\boldsymbol{\eta}) = \prod_{k=1}^{m} P(Y_k|\boldsymbol{\eta}) \tag{28}$$

$P(Y_k|\boldsymbol{\eta})$ is the conditional density of the kth observed indicator, $k = 1, \ldots, m$ given the vector of latent variables $\boldsymbol{\eta}$. If we additionally assume a simple structure in the sense that the variation in an observed indicator $(Y_k|\boldsymbol{\eta})$ conditional on $\boldsymbol{\eta}$ can be attributed to one factor $\eta_i, i = 1, \ldots, n$ only, the following equation holds true:

$$P(Y_k|\boldsymbol{\eta}) = P(Y_k|\eta_i) \tag{29}$$

if Y_k loads on variable η_i.

If we partition the set of m observed indicators in n subsets indexed by the latent variable η_i with elements $Y_{j,i}, j = 1, \ldots, J_i$ for each subset, the product form of equation (28) may be written as

$$P(\mathbf{Y}|\boldsymbol{\eta}) = \prod_{i=1}^{n} \prod_{j=1}^{J_i} P(Y_{j,i}|\eta_i) \tag{30}$$

Substitution of the last equation into the general mixture $P(\mathbf{Y}|\mathbf{x})$ and integrating over all latent variables except for the ith variable η_i yields the marginal density for the ith indicator set $(\mathbf{Y}_i|\mathbf{x})$

$$P(\mathbf{Y}_i|\mathbf{x}) = \int_{\mathbb{R}} \prod_{j=1}^{J_i} P(Y_{j,i}|\eta_i)\phi(\eta_i|\boldsymbol{\Pi}_i \cdot \mathbf{x}, \Omega_{ii})d\eta_i \tag{31}$$

Note that the integration now involves a univariate integral only, which may be computed by standard numerical integration procedures.

The simplification employed in the last paragraph cannot be applied meaningfully if panel data are analyzed. Assume a one-dimensional latent variable η and a corresponding indicator set $\mathbf{Y}$ that is observed in two panel waves. The variables are denoted by η and $\mathbf{Y}$ in the first and by $\tilde{\eta}$ and $\tilde{\mathbf{Y}}$ in the second wave. The structural equation system is formulated for $(\eta, \tilde{\eta})^T$. In the most general case the conditional density $P(\mathbf{Y}, \tilde{\mathbf{Y}}|\eta, \tilde{\eta})$ implies dependence of $\mathbf{Y}$ and $\tilde{\mathbf{Y}}$ on η and $\tilde{\eta}$ as well as on each other. Typical for panel models is the assumption that each indicator $\tilde{Y}_j$ in the second panel wave is stochastically dependent on the corresponding indicator Y_j in the first wave, but each pair $(Y_j, \tilde{Y}_j|\eta, \tilde{\eta})$ is stochastically independent of the remaining pairs $(Y_h, \tilde{Y}_h|\eta, \tilde{\eta})$ with $h \neq j$. Hence the joint conditional density of $(\mathbf{Y}, \tilde{\mathbf{Y}}|\eta, \tilde{\eta})$ can be written as a product of *bivariate* conditional densities

$$P(\mathbf{Y}, \tilde{\mathbf{Y}}|\eta, \tilde{\eta}) = \prod_{j=1}^{m} P(Y_j, \tilde{Y}_j|\eta, \tilde{\eta}) \tag{32}$$

This equation is similar to the introduction of an autoregressive term in the error structure of the measurement part of a LISREL model for a one-dimensional latent variable η. The corresponding LISREL formulation is

$$\mathbf{Y} = \mathbf{\Lambda}\eta + \boldsymbol{\varepsilon} \quad \text{for the first wave} \tag{33}$$

$$\tilde{\mathbf{Y}} = \mathbf{\Lambda}\tilde{\eta} + \tilde{\boldsymbol{\varepsilon}} \quad \text{for the second wave} \tag{34}$$

with

$$E(\boldsymbol{\varepsilon}^T, \tilde{\boldsymbol{\varepsilon}}^T)^T = \mathbf{0} \qquad E(\varepsilon_j^2) = \Omega_{jj} \qquad E(\tilde{\varepsilon}_j^2) = \Omega_{j+m,j+m}$$

$$E(\varepsilon_j\tilde{\varepsilon}_j) = \Omega_{j,j+m} \qquad E(\varepsilon_j\varepsilon_h) = 0 \quad \text{for } j \neq h$$

$$E(\tilde{\varepsilon}_j\tilde{\varepsilon}_h) = 0 \quad \text{for } j \neq h \quad E(\varepsilon_j\tilde{\varepsilon}_h) = 0 \quad \text{for } j \neq h$$

Note that the conditional density of equation (32) involves the specification of the serial dependence structure of Y_j and $\tilde{Y}_j$, which is simple in the usually considered case of two metric variables as shown in the LISREL formulation above. Specification becomes much more complicated, however, if conditional densities not based on normal theory are used. Also note that the mixture density $P(\mathbf{Y}, \tilde{\mathbf{Y}}|\mathbf{x}, \tilde{\mathbf{x}})$ conditional on the exogenous variables $\mathbf{x}$ and $\tilde{\mathbf{x}}$ from panel wave one and two must be computed as a two-dimensional integral:

$$P(\mathbf{Y}, \tilde{\mathbf{Y}}|\mathbf{x}, \tilde{\mathbf{x}}) = \int_{\mathbb{R}^2} \prod_{j=1}^{m} P(Y_j, \tilde{Y}_j|\eta, \tilde{\eta})\phi(\eta|\mathbf{B}^{-1}\mathbf{\Gamma}\mathbf{z}, \mathbf{B}^{-1}\tilde{\mathbf{\Omega}}\mathbf{B}^{-1T})d\boldsymbol{\eta} \tag{35}$$

with $\boldsymbol{\eta} = (\eta, \tilde{\eta})^T$ and $\mathbf{z} = (\mathbf{x}^T, \tilde{\mathbf{x}}^T)^T$.

Returning to the case of cross-sectional data with a simple factor loading structure, we now have to specify the conditional density $P(Y_{j,i}|\eta_i)$ describing the dependence of an indicator $Y_{j,i}$ on the latent variable η_i. For notational convenience, we drop the index i for the moment. Let Y_j^* be again the latent indicator for the observed variable Y_j. The measurement relations $Y_j = r(Y_j^*)$ proposed here are only examples. More general measurement relations and conditional densities may be conceived.

1. Y_j is metric. The measurement relation is again the identity mapping

$$Y_j = r(Y_j^*) = Y_j^* \tag{36}$$

Again, a normal conditional density is assumed.

$$P(Y_j = y_j|\eta) = \phi(y_j|\alpha_j + \lambda_j\eta, \sigma_{jj}^*) \tag{37}$$

The variance σ_{jj}^* corresponds to the variance of the specific factor in Y_j as in classic factor analysis. λ_j is the factor loading of Y_j on the latent trait η and α_j corresponds to a mean value or regression constant.

2. Y_j is metric, but is censored at a known lower bound τ_j. The measurement relation is the Tobit relation as above:

$$Y_j = r(Y_j^*) = \begin{cases} Y_j^* & \text{if } Y_j^* > \tau_j \\ \tau_j & \text{otherwise} \end{cases} \tag{38}$$

$$P(Y_j = y_j|\eta) = \begin{cases} \phi(y_j|\alpha_j + \lambda_j\eta, \sigma_{jj}^*) & \text{if } Y_j^* > \tau_j \\ \int_{-\infty}^{\tau_j} \phi(y_j^*|\alpha_j + \lambda_j\eta, \sigma_{jj}^*)dy_j^* & \text{if } Y_j^* \leqslant \tau_j \end{cases} \tag{39}$$

Again, σ_{jj}^* corresponds to the variance of the specific factor in Y_j^*.

3. Y_j is ordinal with c_j categories. The measurement relation is a threshold model

$$Y_j = r(Y_j^*) = k \Leftrightarrow \tau_{j,k-1} < Y_j^* \leqslant \tau_{j,k} \qquad k = 1, \ldots, c_j \qquad (40)$$

with $-\infty = \tau_{j,0} < \tau_{j,1} < \cdots < \tau_{j,cj} = +\infty$.

If we assume that the distribution of Y_j^* is a univariate normal with the identification restriction of variance $\sigma_{jj}^* = 1$, the conditional density follows an ordered Probit model with

$$P(Y_j = k|\eta) = \int_{\tau_{j,k-1}}^{\tau_{j,k}} \phi(y_j^*|\alpha_j + \lambda_j\eta, 1)dy_j^* \qquad (41)$$

$$= \Phi(\tau_{j,k} - (\alpha_j + \lambda_j\eta)) - \Phi(\tau_{j,k-1} - (\alpha_j + \lambda_j\eta)).$$

where $\Phi(\cdot)$ denotes the cumulative normal distribution function.

Until now we have considered only conditional densities based on univariate normal distribution theory. A much more general formulation is necessary if we consider observed indicators such as counts or unordered categorical variables.

1. Y_j is a count variable. The commonly used distribution function for modeling counts is the Posson distribution with expected value μ_j. Assume a loglinear model $\ln \mu_j = \alpha_j + \lambda_j\eta$. Then the conditional density is given by

$$P(Y_j = k|\eta) = \mu_j^k e^{-\mu_j}/k! \qquad (42)$$

2. Y_j is an unordered categorical variable with c_j categories. For each category k we assume the existence of an indicator variable $Y_{j,k}^*$ that describes the utility of choosing category k (McFadden, 1974). Category k is actually chosen if $Y_{j,k}^* > Y_{j,h}^*$ for all alternatives $h \neq k$. Hence the measurement relation is defined by the random utility maximization principle

$$Y_j = k \quad \text{if} \quad Y_{j,k}^* > Y_{j,h}^* \quad \text{for } h = 1, \ldots, c_j \qquad h \neq k \qquad (43)$$

The utilities $Y_{j,k}^*$ consist of a systematic and a random component

$$Y_{j,k}^* = \mu_{j,k} + \zeta_{j,k} \qquad k = 1, \ldots, c_j \qquad (44)$$

$$\mu_{j,k} = \alpha_{j,k} + \lambda_{j,k}\eta \qquad (45)$$

It is assumed that the random components $\zeta_{j,k}$ are independently extreme-value distributed with distribution function

$$F(\zeta_{j,k}) = \exp(-\exp(-\zeta_{j,k}))$$

Hence Y_j follows a conditional multinomial logit probability function (McFadden, 1974)

$$P(Y_j = k|\eta) = \frac{\exp(\alpha_{j,k} + \lambda_{j,k}\eta)}{\sum_{h=1}^{c_j} \exp(\alpha_{j,h} + \lambda_{j,h}\eta)} \qquad (46)$$

The first category $Y_{j,1}$ serves as reference category. Therefore $\alpha_{j,1}$ and $\lambda_{j,1}$ are set to 0 for identification. An additional identification restriction is necessary if an unordered categorical variable has been chosen as the first indicator for η, that is, $\alpha_{1,2} = 0$.

Special cases of the multinomial logit in equation (46) comprise models for ordered categorical indicators that are not based on ordered probits. Examples are ordered logits with the restrictions $0 = \alpha_{j,1} < \alpha_{j,2} \cdots < \alpha_{j,k-1} < \infty$ and $\lambda_{j,k} = \lambda_j$ for all $k \geqslant 2$, or Anderson's (1984) stereotype logit model with $0 = \alpha_{j,1} < \alpha_{j,2} \cdots < \alpha_{j,k-1} < \infty$ and $\lambda_{j,1} = 0 < \lambda_{j,2} < \cdots < \lambda_{j,k} < \infty$. Another special case is the Rasch model for dichotomous outcomes (Fischer, 1973) with $\lambda_{j,1} = 0$ and $\lambda_{j,2} = 1$ where $\alpha_{j,2}$ denotes the item score of item Y_j and η denotes the ability of a person to solve item Y_j.

The conditional densities for count variables and unordered categorical variables in equations (42) and (46) are special members of generalized linear models with canonical or noncanonical link functions (McCullagh & Nelder, 1983). Hence the whole class of generalized linear models can be used to construct conditional densities, thereby yielding many more models than discussed here.

Model Estimation

Here we focus on models for cross-sectional data with simple factor loading structures. Hence local independence of the observed indicators and univariate normality of the missing density are assumed. Again, a sample of independent identically distributed drawings $(\mathbf{Y}, \mathbf{x})_t$, $t = 1, \ldots, T$ is considered. The distribution of $\mathbf{x}$ is not specified but is not degenerate. The joint likelihood for each observation t is given by

$$L_t(\tilde{\theta}) = \int_{\mathbb{R}^n} P(\mathbf{Y}|\eta)\phi(\eta|\mathbf{B}^{-1}\Gamma\mathbf{x}, \mathbf{B}^{-1}\tilde{\Omega}\mathbf{B}^{-1T})d\eta \qquad (47)$$

The parameters of the structural equation system, of the measurement model, and of the measurement relations are all collected in $\tilde{\theta}$. To use full information maximum likelihood methods, the multivariate normal integral of equation (47) must be evaluated. This evaluation is practically impossible with today's numerical methods and computational tools. Hence a limited marginal maximum likelihood method is employed for estimation. A detailed description of the estimation method is found in Arminger and Küsters (1988); we give only a short outline. In the first step, the marginal likelihood for each latent variable η_i with indicator set $\mathbf{Y}_i$ is considered (cf. equation [31])

$$L_t^M(\theta_i) = \int_{\mathbb{R}} \prod_{j=1}^{J_i} P(Y_{i,j}|\eta_i)\phi(\eta_i|\Pi_{i.}, \mathbf{x}, \Omega_{ii})d\eta_i \qquad (48)$$

The reduced-form parameters pertaining to η_i only are collected in the vector θ_i. The marginal likelihood equations are either solved directly or by application of the EM algorithm. The direct solution also yields an estimate of the asymptotic covariance matrix of θ_i. The vector θ_i does not contain estimates of the structural parameters $\mathbf{B}$, $\boldsymbol{\Gamma}$, and $\tilde{\boldsymbol{\Omega}}$, but only the reduced form parameters $\boldsymbol{\Pi}_{i\cdot}$ and Ω_{ii}, $i = 1, \ldots, n$.

In the second step, Amemiyas principle (Amemiya, 1978b, 1979) is applied to estimate the structural parameters $\mathbf{B}_{i\cdot}$ and $\boldsymbol{\Gamma}_{i\cdot}$ separately for each equation i from the estimates $\hat{\boldsymbol{\Pi}}_{i\cdot}$ of the reduced-form parameters using ordinary or weighted least squares. Also the asymptotic covariance matrix of $\hat{\mathbf{B}}_{i\cdot}$ and $\hat{\boldsymbol{\Gamma}}_{i\cdot}$ is computed.

In a third optional step the correlations ρ_{ij} between latent variables η_i and η_j are estimated conditional on the results of the first step using the marginal likelihood of two latent variables η_i and η_j. This procedure involves numerical integration of a bivariate integral and its derivative with respect to ρ_{ij}. This estimation procedure generalizes the computation of the polychoric and polyserial correlation coefficients (Olsson, 1979; Olsson, Drasgow, & Dorains, 1982) to the general concept of latent trait correlation. From the latent trait correlation ρ_{ij}, the reduced-form covariances Ω_{ij} and the structural form covariances $\tilde{\Omega}_{ij}$ between η_i and η_j may be computed.

In a fourth optional step the latent trait scores $\hat{\eta}_{i,t}$, $t = 1, \ldots, T$ for each individual are calculated by computing a posteriori expected value. This procedure follows Bartholomew (1981).

At present, there is no computer program available that handles latent trait models with indicators of any measurement level. A first version of a program for the estimation procedure outlined above is currently being developed.

SUMMARY AND OUTLOOK

We have outlined the construction of a general model that deals with latent traits. These latent traits may depend on exogenous variables as well as on each other in the form of a structural equation system. The indicators for the latent traits need not be metric; they may be measured on a metric, censored metric, ordinal, or nominal scale.

The estimation procedures differ with respect to the measurement level of the indicators contained in the model. If only metric, censored metric, or ordered categorical variables with a normal-theory threshold model are used as indicators, a generalization of Muthén's (1984) estimation procedure may be used. This procedure allows the inclusion of autoregressive terms for the analysis of panel data in a straightforward way. If, however, the set of observed indicators also includes count data or unordered categorical data, the estimation procedure becomes computationally much more cumbersome because numerical integration is needed. The formulation and estimation of autoregressive models for panel data becomes also much more difficult and in fact has not yet been considered thoroughly.

Finally, we have pointed out that the models discussed here may be generalized to include latent variables η_i, which are not metric but rather unordered categorical. A special case of such a model is Lazarsfelds latent class analysis (Goodman, 1974; Lazarsfeld, 1950). However, the flexibility of the simultaneous equation structure of latent trait models is lost if the latent variables consist of latent classes (cf. Arminger, 1986b).

REFERENCES

Amemiya T (1978a). "On a two-step estimation of a multivariate logit model." *Journal of Econometrics* 8:13–21.

Amemiya T (1978b). "The estimation of a simultaneous equation generalized probit model." *Econometrica* 46:1193–1205.

Amemiya T (1979). "The estimation of a simultaneous equation tobit model." *International Economic Review* 20:169–181.

Amemiya T (1984). "Tobit models: A survey." *Journal of Econometrics* 24:3–61.

Anderson JA (1984). "Regression and ordered categorical variables" (with discussion). *Journal of the Royal Statistical Society B* 46:1–30.

Arminger G (1986a). "Linear stochastic differential equation models for panel data with unobserved variables." In Tuma N (ed), *Sociological Methodology*. San Francisco, pp 187–212.

Arminger G (1986b). "Latente Variablen Modelle auf der Basis von Mischverteilungen." In Beckmann M, Gaede K, Ritter K, Schneeweiß H (eds), *Methods of Operations Research 53, Part I*. Meisenheim, pp 483–506.

Arminger G, Küsters U (1988). "Latent trait models with indicators of mixed measurement level." In Langeheine R, Rost J (eds), *Latent Trait and Latent Class Models*. New York.

Bartholomew DJ (1980). "Factor analysis for categorical data." *Journal of the Royal Statistical Society B* 42:293–321.

Bartholomew DJ (1981). "Posterior analysis of the factor model." *British Journal of Mathematical and Statistical Psychology* 34:93–99.

Bartholomew DJ (1983). "Latent variable models for ordered categorical data." *Journal of Econometrics* 22:229–243.

Bartholomew DJ (1984). "The foundations of factor analysis." *Biometrika* 71:221–232.

Bentler P (1986). "Structural modeling and psychometrika: An historical perspective on growth and achievements." *Psychometrika* 51:35–51.

Bock RD (1972). "Estimating item parameters and latent ability when responses are scored in two or more nominal categories." *Psychometrika* 37:29–51.

Bock RD, Aitkin M (1981). "Marginal maximum likelihood estimation of item parameters: Application of an EM algorithm." *Psychometrika* 46:443–459.

Browne MW (1984). "Asymptotically distribution-free methods for the analysis of covariance structures." *British Journal of Mathematical and Statistical Psychology* 37:62–83.

Dunn JE (1973). "A note on a sufficient condition for uniqueness of a restricted factor matrix." *Psychometrika* 38:141–143.

Fischer G (1973). *Einführung in die Theorie psychologischer Tests–Grundlagen und Anwendungen*. Bern.

Goodman LA (1974). "Exploratory latent structure analysis using both identifiable and unidentifiable models." *Biometrika* 61:215–231.

Jöreskog KG, Sörbom D (1977). "Statistical models and methods for analysis of longitudinal data." In Aigner DJ, Goldberger AS (eds), *Latent Variables in Socioeconomic Models*. Amsterdam, pp 285–324.

Jöreskog KG, Sörbom D (1984). *LISREL VI–Analysis of Linear Structural Relationships by Maximum Likelihood, Instrumental Variables and Least Squares Methods*. Mooresville, Ind.

Küsters U (1987). *Hierarchische Mittelwert- und Kovarianzstrukturmodelle mit nichtmetrischen endogenen Variablen*. Heidelberg.

Küsters U, Arminger G (1986). "Hierarchische Mittelwert- und Kovarianzstruktur-modelle mit nichtmetrischen endogenen Variablen." In Streitferdt L, Hauptmann H, Marusev AW, Ohse D, Pape U (eds), *Operations Research Proceedings 1985*. Berlin, pp 347–357.

Lazarsfeld PF (1950). "The logical and mathematical foundation of latent structure analysis." In Stouffer SA, et al. (eds), *Studies in Social Pychology in World War II. Vol. IV, Measurement and Prediction*. Princeton, pp 363–412.

Luenberger DG (1984). *Linear and Nonlinear Programming*. Reading, Mass.

McCullagh P, Nelder JA (1983). *Generalized Linear Models*. London.

McDonald RP, Swaminathan H (1973). "A simple matrix calculus with applications to multivariate analysis." *General Systems* 18:37–54.

McFadden D (1974). "Conditional logit analysis of qualitative choice behavior." In Zarembka P (ed), *Frontiers in Econometrics*. New York, pp 105–142.

McKelvey RD, Zavoina W (1975). "A statistical model for the analysis of ordinal level dependent variables." *Journal of Mathematical Sociology* 4:103–120.

Maddala GS (1983). *Limited-dependent and Qualitative Variables in Econometrics*. Cambridge, Mass.

Muthén B (1984). "A general structural equation model with dichotomous, ordered categorical, and continous latent variable indicators." *Psychometrika*. 49:115–132.

Muthén B (1988). *LISCOMP – Analysis of Linear Structural Equations with a Comprehensive Measurement Model*. Mooresville, Ind.

Nelson FD (1976). "On a general computer algorithm for the analysis of models with limited dependent variables." *Annals of Economic and Social Measurement* 5:493–509.

Olsson U (1979). "Maximum likelihood estimation of the polychoric correlation coefficient." *Psychometrika* 44:443–460.

Olsson U, Drasgow F, Dorans NJ (1982). "The polyserial correlation coefficient." *Psychometrika* 47:337–347.

Rao DR (1973). *Linear Statistical Inference and its Applications*. New York.

Rosett RN, Nelson FD (1975). "Estimation of the two-limit probit regression model." *Econometrica* 43:141–146.

Schepers A (1991). "Numerische Verfahren und Implementation der Schätzung von Mittelwert—und Kovarianz struktur modellen mit nicht metrischen variablem." Ph.D diss., Wuppertal.

Schmidt P (1976). *Econometrics*. New York.

Index